Behavior: A Guide for Practitioners

Editors

GARY M. LANDSBERG
VALARIE V. TYNES

VETERINARY CLINICS OF NORTH AMERICA: SMALL ANIMAL PRACTICE

www.vetsmall.theclinics.com

May 2014 • Volume 44 • Number 3

ELSEVIER

1600 John F. Kennedy Boulevard • Suite 1800 • Philadelphia, Pennsylvania, 19103-2899
http://www.vetsmall.theclinics.com

VETERINARY CLINICS OF NORTH AMERICA: SMALL ANIMAL PRACTICE Volume 44, Number 3
May 2014 ISSN 0195-5616, ISBN-13: 978-0-323-29729-5

Editor: Patrick Manley
Developmental Editor: Susan Showalter

Veterinary Clinics of North America: Small Animal Practice (ISSN 0195-5616) is published bimonthly by Elsevier Inc., 360
Park Avenue South, New York, NY 10010-1710. Months of issue are January, March, May, July, September, and
November. Business and Editorial Offices: 1600 John F. Kennedy Blvd., Ste. 1800, Philadelphia, PA 19103-2899.
Customer Service Office: 3251 Riverport Lane, Maryland Heights, MO 63043. Periodicals postage paid at New York,
NY and additional mailing offices. Subscription prices are $310.00 per year (domestic individuals), $500.00 per year
(domestic institutions), $150.00 per year (domestic students/residents), $410.00 per year (Canadian individuals),
$621.00 per year (Canadian institutions), $455.00 per year (international individuals), $621.00 per year (international
institutions), and $220.00 per year (international and Canadian students/residents). To receive student/resident rate,
orders must be accompanied by name of affiliated institution, date of term, and the *signature* of program/residency
coordinator on institution letterhead. Orders will be billed at individual rate until proof of status is received. Foreign air
speed delivery is included in all *Clinics* subscription prices. All prices are subject to change without notice. **POSTMAS-
TER:** Send address changes to *Veterinary Clinics of North America: Small Animal Practice*, Elsevier Health Sciences
Division, Subscription Customer Service, 3251 Riverport Lane, Maryland Heights, MO 63043. Customer Service
(orders, claims, online, change of address): Elsevier Periodicals Customer Service, Elsevier Health Sciences Division
Subscription Customer Service 3251 Riverport Lane Maryland Heights, MO 63043. Tel: 1-800-654-2452 (U.S. and
Canada); 314-447-8871 (outside U.S. and Canada). Fax: 314-447-8029. E-mail: journalscustomerservice-
usa@elsevier.com (for print support); journalsonlinesupport-usa@elsevier.com (for online support).

Reprints. For copies of 100 or more of articles in this publication, please contact the Commercial Reprints Department,
Elsevier Inc., 360 Park Avenue South, New York, NY 10010-1710. Tel.: 212-633-3874; Fax: 212-633-3820; E-mail:
reprints@elsevier.com.

Veterinary Clinics of North America: Small Animal Practice is also published in Japanese by Inter Zoo Publishing
Co., Ltd., Aoyama Crystal-Bldg 5F, 3-5-12 Kitaaoyama, Minato-ku, Tokyo 107-0061, Japan.

Veterinary Clinics of North America: Small Animal Practice is covered in *Current Contents/Agriculture, Biology and Environmental Sciences, Science Citation Index, ASCA, MEDLINE/PubMed (Index Medicus), Excerpta Medica, and BIOSIS.*

Contributors

EDITORS

GARY M. LANDSBERG, BSc, DVM, MRCVS
Diplomate, American College of Veterinary Behaviorists; Diplomate, European College of Animal Welfare and Behavioural Medicine; Veterinary Behaviourist, North Toronto Veterinary Behaviour Specialty Clinic, Thornhill, Ontario, Canada

VALARIE V. TYNES, DVM
Diplomate, American College of Veterinary Behaviorists; Premier Veterinary Behavior Consulting, Sweetwater, Texas

AUTHORS

MELISSA BAIN, DVM, MS
Diplomate, American College of Veterinary Behaviorists; Associate Professor, Clinical Animal Behavior Service, University of California School of Veterinary Medicine, Davis, California

DESIREE BROACH, DVM
JBSA-Lackland, San Antonio, Texas

DEBORAH BRYANT, DVM
Sartell, Minnesota

DIANE FRANK, DVM
Diplomate, American College of Veterinary Behaviorists; Department of Clinical Sciences, Centre Hospitalier Universitaire Vétérinaire, Saint-Hyacinthe, Quebec, Canada

SARAH HEATH, BVSc, CCAB, MRCVS
Diplomate, European College of Animal Welfare and Behavioural Medicine (Behavioural Medicine); Behavioural Referrals Veterinary Practice, Upton, Chester, United Kingdom

MEGHAN E. HERRON, DVM
Diplomate, American College of Veterinary Behaviorists; Department of Veterinary Clinical Sciences, The Ohio State University College of Veterinary Medicine, Columbus, Ohio

DEBRA F. HORWITZ, DVM
Diplomate, American College of Veterinary Behaviorists; Owner, Veterinary Behavior Consultations, St Louis; Adjunct Professor, Department of Veterinary Medicine and Surgery, University of Missouri, College of Veterinary Medicine, Missouri

CHRISTOS KARAGIANNIS, DVM, MSc, MRCVS
Animal Behaviour, Cognition and Welfare Group, School of Life Sciences, University of Lincoln, Lincoln, United Kingdom

GARY M. LANDSBERG, BSc, DVM, MRCVS
Diplomate, American College of Veterinary Behaviorists; Diplomate, European College of Animal Welfare and Behavioural Medicine; Veterinary Behaviourist, North Toronto Veterinary Behaviour Specialty Clinic, Thornhill, Ontario, Canada

RACHEL MALAMED, DVM
Diplomate, American College of Veterinary Behaviorists; Dr. Rachel Malamed Behavior Consulting, Los Angeles, California

DEBBIE MARTIN, RVT, CPDT-KA, KPA CTP, VTS (Behavior)
Animal Behavior Technician, Veterinary Behavior Consultations, LLC, Spicewood, Texas; Owner, TEAM Education in Animal Behavior, LLC, Spicewood, Texas; Karen Pryor Academy Dog Trainer Professional Faculty, Karen Pryor Academy, Waltham, Massachusetts

KENNETH M. MARTIN, DVM
Diplomate, American College of Veterinary Behaviorists; Owner, Veterinary Behavior Consultations, LLC and TEAM Education in Animal Behavior, LLC, Spicewood, Texas

DANIEL MILLS, BVSc, PhD, CBiol, FSBiol, FHEA, CCAB, MRCVS
Diplomate, European College of Animal Welfare and Behavioural Medicine (Behavioural Medicine Subsection); European & RCVS Recognised Specialist in Veterinary Behavioural Medicine, Animal Behaviour, Cognition and Welfare Group, School of Life Sciences, University of Lincoln, Lincoln, United Kingdom

KAREN L. OVERALL, MA, VMD, PhD, CAAB
Diplomate, American College of Veterinary Behaviorists; Glen Mills, Pennsylvania

CHRISTOPHER L. PACHEL, DVM
Diplomate, American College of Veterinary Behaviorists; Owner, Animal Behavior Clinic, Portland, Oregon

CAROLINE PERRIN, BVSc, MACVSc
(Veterinary Behaviour), Veterinary Behaviourist, Sydney Animal Behaviour Service, Seaforth, New South Wales, Australia

AMY L. PIKE, DVM
Resident, Veterinary Behavior Consultations, St Louis, Missouri

KERSTI SEKSEL, BVSc (Hons), MRCVS, MA (Hons), FACVSc
Diplomate, American College of Veterinary Behaviorists; Diplomate, European College of Animal Welfare and Behavioural Medicine, Registered Veterinary Specialist in Behavioural Medicine; Registered Veterinary Specialist in Behavioural Medicine, Adjunct Senior Lecturer, Charles Sturt University, Sydney Animal Behaviour Service, Seaforth, New South Wales, Australia

JULIE K. SHAW, RVT, KPA CTP, VTS (Behavior)
Owner, TEAM Education in Animal Behavior, LLC, Spicewood, Texas; Karen Pryor Academy Dog Trainer Professional Faculty, Karen Pryor Academy, Waltham, Massachusetts

TRACI SHREYER, MA
Veterinary Medical Center, The Ohio State University College of Veterinary Medicine, Columbus, Ohio

LESLIE SINN, DVM, CPDT-KA
Professor, Northern Virginia Community College, Veterinary Technology Program, Sterling; Behavior resident, American College of Veterinary Behavior, Behavior Solutions, Hamilton, Virginia

ELIZABETH STELOW, DVM
Resident, Clinical Animal Behavior Service, University of California School of Veterinary Medicine, Davis, California

KAREN LYNN C. SUEDA, DVM
Diplomate, American College of Veterinary Behaviorists; Behavior Service, Veterinary Behaviorist, VCA West Los Angeles Animal Hospital, Los Angeles, California

KATRIINA TIIRA, PhD
Canine Genomics Research Group, Research Program's Unit, Molecular Neurology, Department of Veterinary Biosciences, The Folkhälsan Institute of Genetics, University of Helsinki, Helsinki, Finland

VALARIE V. TYNES, DVM
Diplomate, American College of Veterinary Behaviorists; Premier Veterinary Behavior Consulting, Sweetwater, Texas

CLARE WILSON, MA, VetMB, CCAB, MRCVS
Post Graduate Diplomate, Companion Animal Behaviour Counselling; Behaviour Veterinary Practice, Bramley House, Church Lawford, United Kingdom

HELEN ZULCH, BVSc (Hons), MRCVS
Diplomate, European College of Animal Welfare and Behavioural Medicine (Behavioural Medicine Subsection); European Specialist in Veterinary Behavioural Medicine, Animal Behaviour, Cognition and Welfare Group, School of Life Sciences, University of Lincoln, Lincoln, United Kingdom

Contents

> Behavioral concerns are the principal cause of a weakened human-animal bond and pet relinquishment. Triaging behavioral concerns and providing early intervention may be the difference between a patient remaining in its current home or relinquishment. Prevention and intervention behavior services using a team approach may also improve pet retention through client education and appropriate assistance. Identifying and integrating qualified animal behavior professionals to assist with the hospital's behavior team ensures appropriate support is provided to the client and patient.

> Behavior problems are often given as a reason for pet relinquishment to shelters. When presented with any behavior problem, veterinarians should perform a thorough physical examination (including neurologic and orthopedic examination) and a minimum database, including a complete blood cell count, chemistry panel, and total T4 and free T4 by equilibrium dialysis if the T4 value is low to rule out any medical contributions. Veterinarians should be a source of information regarding management, safety, and basic behavior modification for common behavior problems. Additionally, various control devices offer pet owners the ability to better manage their pets in difficult situations.

> As general veterinary practitioners, we have a duty of care that applies not only to the physical health needs of our patients but also to their mental well-being. Advising clients about how to enrich their home and kennel environments is an important part of fulfilling that duty of care and will also enrich the relationship between the veterinary practitioner and client. This article discusses how to optimize welfare for dogs and cats in the home and kenneled environments through appropriate environmental enrichment and understanding of species-typical behavioral requirements.

> Low-stress handling is important for the safety of the veterinary staff and for the welfare of the patient. The commitment to ensuring the emotional well-being of the patient should be equal to that shown toward the physical

well-being of the animals under a veterinarian's care. Before handling animals it is essential to assess the environment and the patient's response to it. Taking the time to create a behavior handling plan makes future visits easier and bonds clients to the practice. Understanding how and when to use handling tools is key to making patient visits safer, more humane, and more efficient.

Phenotyping behavior is difficult, partly because behavior is almost always influenced by environment. Using objective terms/criteria to evaluate behaviors is best; the more objective the assessment, the more likely underlying genetic patterns will be identified. Behavioral pathologies, and highly desirable behavioral characteristics/traits, are likely complex, meaning that multiple genes are probably involved, and therefore simple genetic tests are less possible. Breeds can be improved using traditional quantitative genetic methods; unfortunately, this also creates the possibility of inadvertently selecting for covarying undesirable behaviors. Patterns of behaviors within families and breed lines are still the best guidelines for genetic counseling in dogs.

Disease is always associated with changes in behavior such as disappearance of normal behaviors or appearance of new behaviors. These changes are often considered as abnormal behavior, indicating illness and/or pain. The aim of this article is to illustrate some examples of cases that might present as behavioral disorders but are in fact medical conditions. Subtle behavioral signs of disease are also discussed.

Stressors impact on all areas of a pet's life, potentially to the detriment of their well-being. In addition, should this lead to behavior change, it is likely to cause strain in the owner-pet relationship with an increased risk of relinquishment. Understanding why events may be perceived as stressful to a given individual is essential in remedying their effect. Clinicians need to be skilled in recognizing and categorizing potential stressors as well as auditing the background stress in the animal's environment as only once this has been accomplished can specific measures be implemented to reduce the effects of the stress load.

Abnormal repetitive behaviors (ARBs) represent a diverse group of behaviors whose underlying mechanism is poorly understood. Their neurobiology likely involves several different neurotransmitter systems. These behaviors have been referred to as compulsive disorders, obsessive compulsive disorders and stereotypies. Underlying medical conditions and pain can often cause changes in behavior that are mistaken for ARBs. A complete medical work-up is always indicated prior to reaching a presumptive diagnosis. The frequency of ARBs can be reduced but not always eliminated with the use of selective serotonin reuptake inhibitors (SSRIs) or tricyclic antidepressants (TCAs) in conjunction with behavior modification and environmental enrichment.

Intercat aggression is a common problem within multicat households. Diagnosis and treatment requires an understanding of the social structure of free-living cats and of how those interactions are impacted by confinement and household management practices. There are multiple causes of aggression between cats within a home, and treatment plans should be customized to account for the diagnosis and behavior pattern identified. Some cases of intercat aggression can be treated successfully without requiring full separation of the involved cats. In cases where separation is required, treatment includes steps for successful reintroduction and reintegration. Several situational and maintenance medication options can be used to improve the response to treatment.

Feline aggression toward people is a common and potentially dangerous problem. Proper diagnosis of the underlying cause of the aggression is key in effective treatment. A complete history, including information on the people in the home, other pets, and specific incidents, is necessary to make this diagnosis. A comprehensive treatment plan typically includes management, enhancement of the cat's living environment, techniques for replacing the aggressive behavior with more appropriate behaviors, and, potentially, medication. The treatment plan must reflect the abilities and commitment of the owner.

This article reviews the various causes of human-directed aggression in dogs and provides a step-by-step plan guiding the general practitioner through history taking, behavior observations, diagnosis, consultation, treatment, and follow-up care. Charts summarizing how to obtain behavioral information, the client's management options, treatment recommendations, diagnosis and treatment of human-directed aggression, and the clinician's role in preventing human-directed aggression are included. A graphic illustration of canine body language is also provided.

For many medications, the pharmacokinetics and pharmacodynamics in pets have not been established and even where studies have been done, there is widespread species and individual variation. Practitioners should start with the lower end of the dose range and titrate up to maximum doses where there is insufficient therapeutic effect and no adverse effects or contraindications. Complete blood count, serum chemistry profile, and urinalysis should be performed before initiating the use of any medication, especially with off-label medications. Pharmacologic intervention for the treatment of behavior problems should be considered just one aspect of a comprehensive behavioral management and treatment protocol.

VETERINARY CLINICS OF NORTH AMERICA: SMALL ANIMAL PRACTICE

THE CLINICS ARE NOW AVAILABLE ONLINE!
Access your subscription at:
www.theclinics.com

VETERINARY CLINICS OF
NORTH AMERICA: SMALL
ANIMAL PRACTICE

FORTHCOMING ISSUES

July 2014
Clinical Nutrition
Dottie P. Laflamme, Editor

September 2014
Advances in Oncology
Annette N. Smith, Editor

November 2014
Advances in Veterinary Neurology
Natasha J. Olby and Nicholas D. Jeffery, Editors

RECENT ISSUES

March 2014
Pediatrics
Autumn Davidson, Editor

January 2014
Canine and Feline Respiratory Medicine
Lynelle R. Johnson, Editor

November 2013
Clinical Pathology and Diagnostic Testing
Mary Jo Burkhard and
Maxey L. Wellman, Editors

RELATED INTEREST

Veterinary Clinics of North America: Small Animal Practice
March 2014 (Vol. 42, Issue 2)
Exotic Animal Training and Learning
Barbara Heidenreich, Editor

THE CLINICS ARE NOW AVAILABLE ONLINE!

Access your subscription at:
www.theclinics.com

Preface
Behavior: A Guide for Practitioners

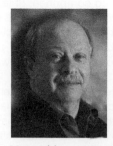 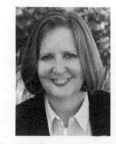

Gary M. Landsberg, BSc, DVM,   Valarie V. Tynes, DVM, DACVB
MRCVS, DACVB, DECAWBM
Editors

There have been several issues of *Veterinary Clinics of North America: Small Animal Practice* dedicated to the subject of companion animal behavior. Since the last issue, the College of Veterinary Behaviorists (dacvb.org) has grown steadily, considerable research has been published in the field, and attendance at continuing education meetings pertaining to behavior continues to be "standing room only."

Many veterinary schools still do not teach behavioral medicine, and many veterinarians have the misconception that dealing with their clients' behavior complaints is too time-consuming. Yet attention to a pet's behavior should be an integral part of every veterinary curriculum and a focus of every veterinary visit. As the reader will see, behavior problems are not simply a result of a doting, permissive owner but rather a complex result of genetics, early developmental experiences and learning, and the effects of stress and physical health. Veterinarians must have a sound understanding of normal species behavior, learning principles, and how to manage and modify undesirable behavior. Behavior screening must be an essential element of every veterinary visit since a change in behavior might be the first or only sign of underlying medical problem, or a mental health disorder. In addition, the complex role that stress plays in the development of many health and behavioral issues is only just now beginning to be recognized. In this issue, we have invited a diverse group of veterinary behaviorists, behavioral technicians, and behavior residents to provide a guide for practitioners to better understand the interplay of genetics, stress, and health in the development of behavior problems and how some of the most common canine and feline behavior problems can be managed.

The first article in this issue helps the clinician understand how adding behavioral counseling to a practice can be a sound financial decision as well as one that saves lives. The authors provide guidelines on behavioral triage, including how practitioners can incorporate a full range of behavioral services into the veterinary practice,

Vet Clin Small Anim 44 (2014) xiii–xv
http://dx.doi.org/10.1016/j.cvsm.2014.02.001
0195-5616/14/$ – see front matter © 2014 Elsevier Inc. All rights reserved.

integrating staff into a team approach to behavior counseling, and guidelines for referring problem behaviors. The following article presents the science behind learning in a simple and straightforward manner, providing the practitioner with the information needed to help their clients effectively modify their pet's behavior, tools for safe and effective management, and case examples of common problems. The next article explains why and how to implement environmental enrichment for pets in the home and in the kennel. While enrichment is a mandated component of laboratory animals and others kept in captivity, enriching the lives of our pets is all too often overlooked. By considering what is biologically relevant for dogs and cats living in our homes, this article provides guidance for offering behavioral choices and encouraging the species-typical behaviors that are critical to our pets' mental well-being.

"Pet-Friendly Veterinary Practice" explains why and how attention to the experience that animals have while in our practices can drastically reduce the number of clients who avoid bringing their pets to the veterinary clinic, reduce the fear and stress associated with veterinary visits for the pet and owner, and help to insure safe and positive experiences for all. This article provides a detailed guide for practitioners for the prevention and management of fear of the veterinary clinic.

The genetics behind behavior has long been a mystery but in this rapidly advancing field of medical science and technology, the veil is slowly being lifted in our understanding of how genotype contributes to behavior. While the subject is complex, no single gene directs a particular behavior; epigenetics, gene-gene interactions, and gene-environment interactions are all at play. Next article reviews the current state research and provides a basic primer for answering our clients' questions about the heritability of canine behavioral traits.

The contribution of medical conditions to problem behaviors can be easily overlooked, especially if finances limit the level of diagnostics available to a pet owner. When no obvious medical condition is found, the practitioner might all too quickly consider the problem "behavioral." Next article takes a systematic approach to how different medical conditions might contribute to behavioral signs, and how they are complexly intertwined.

Because of the integral role it plays in mental, physical, and social health, and how it impacts on human-pet relationships, the editors felt that an entire article on the role of stress was pertinent for this issue. Next article reviews the importance of being observant to the visual cues of stress that animals demonstrate, as well as the role that stress may play in the development of specific medical conditions. In addition, this article provides guidelines for stress auditing, stress management, and stress prevention.

The next four articles address some of the most common and serious behavior problems referred to veterinary behaviorists. Abnormal repetitive behaviors are behaviors that are also likely to have their basis in stress. In other cases, they are due to underlying and overlooked medical conditions causing pain, discomfort, or altered sensations. In the last 20 years much research on these types of behaviors in humans, laboratory animals, and captive wild animals has contributed to improved understanding. Rather than a single disorder, this article reviews what is likely to be a heterogeneous group of behaviors that have serious implications in pet health and welfare. This is followed by three articles on aggression: canine aggression to people, feline intraspecific aggression, and feline aggression to people. The articles provide extensive guidance for practitioners for understanding canine and feline communication and signaling, diagnosis, prevention, risk assessment and prognosis, management, and treatment.

The final article is included as an "appendix summary" of drug doses used in veterinary behavior, many of which are mentioned throughout the text. However, the reader is warned to fully explore the indications, contraindications, and potential side effects; screen for any underlying medical problems; weigh the evidence, benefits, and risks; and insure informed consent before dispensing any medication.

As editors, we wish to thank each of the authors for the time, effort, and commitment in advancing the field of veterinary clinical behavior. In continuing education, in research and in their extensive body of publications. In fact, we congratulate our colleagues in veterinary behavior on a great new resource co-authored entirely by American College of Veterinary Behaviour diplomates, entitled Decoding your Dog, from Houghton Mifflin Harcourt. As described by the title, in this book they decipher the latest studies, explain common dog behaviors and describe how to prevent or change unwanted behaviors. We hope that the articles in this issue provide, as the title suggests, a useful and practical Guide for Practitioners to advance their knowledge and improve their skills in the growing field of veterinary behavioral medicine.

Gary M. Landsberg, BSc, DVM, MRCVS, DACVB, DECAWBM
North Toronto Veterinary Behaviour Specialty Clinic
99 Henderson Avenue
Thornhill, ON L3T 2K9, Canada

Valarie V. Tynes, DVM, DACVB
Premier Veterinary Behavior Consulting
PO Box 1413
Sweetwater, TX 79556, USA

E-mail addresses:
behaviourvet@rogers.com (G.M. Landsberg)
pigvet@hughes.net (V.V. Tynes)

Small Animal Behavioral Triage:
A Guide for Practitioners

Kenneth M. Martin, DVM[a,b,*],
Debbie Martin, RVT, CPDT-KA, KPA CTP, VTS (Behavior)[a,b,c],
Julie K. Shaw, RVT, KPA CTP, VTS (Behavior)[b,c]

KEYWORDS

- Human-animal bond • Behavior wellness • Behavior triage • Behavior professionals

KEY POINTS

- Developing, maintaining, and enhancing the human-animal bond through prevention and intervention behavior services may help to prevent relinquishment of pets and consequent client/patient attrition.
- Because early intervention generally improves the case outcome, early detection through routine behavioral screening is imperative.
- Being able to triage safety and prognostic factors when faced with a behavioral crisis can minimize risk to veterinary staff and safeguard the pet and the public.
- It is vital to know how to evaluate a behavior professional's qualifications, because when referring clients to behavioral professionals, the methodology and philosophy used will directly reflect on you and your hospital.
- A team approach to addressing animal behavior provides a comprehensive approach that is better able to meet the needs of the client and patient.

INTRODUCTION
The Human-Animal Bond

The human-animal bond is the dynamic and mutually beneficial relationship between people and animals. This relationship includes attitudes, emotions, and the profound physical and psychological interactions between people, animals, and the environment.[1-3] In the United States many pets are viewed as members of the family, and

Conflict of Interest: Book and online course published through Sunshine Books/Karen Pryor Academy (K.M. Martin). Book and online course published through Sunshine Books/Karen Pryor Academy. Independent contractor for Karen Pryor Academy for teaching their dog trainer professional program (D. Martin). Independent contractor for Karen Pryor Academy for teaching their dog trainer professional program. Editor and writer for Vetstreet.com (J.K. Shaw).
[a] Veterinary Behavior Consultations, LLC, 580 Alta Vista Road, Spicewood, TX 78669, USA;
[b] TEAM Education in Animal Behavior, LLC, 580 Alta Vista Road, Spicewood, TX, 78669, USA;
[c] Karen Pryor Academy, 49 River Street, Suite 3, Waltham, MA, 02453, USA
* Corresponding author.
E-mail address: vbcdvm@yahoo.com

are obtained with the intent of being a human companion rather than having a utilitarian purpose.

Pet Relinquishment

Although data vary widely on specific numbers, millions of dogs and cats are relinquished to shelters annually. Species and/or breed-specific genetic predispositions, though normal, are not always adaptable to the urban domestic environment and may lead to the development of undesirable behaviors. Similarly, negative experiences or the lack of positive experiences during sensitive periods of development can also contribute to the development of undesirable behaviors. A weakening of the human-animal bond occurs when owners perceive their pets' behavior as undesirable (**Fig. 1**).

Problem behaviors can also negatively affect the animal's welfare. Behavior problems are cited as the primary reason for relinquishment of dogs (40%) and the second most common cause for cat relinquishment (28%).[4] Findings associated with relinquishment to shelters included the following[4,5]:

- Inappropriate elimination was the most common behavioral reason cited for relinquishment in dogs and cats.
- Aggression (toward people and/or other animals) was the second most common behavioral reason for relinquishment in cats and dogs.
- Other behavioral reasons for relinquishment were destructiveness, disobedience, being too active, escaping (dogs), not being friendly (cats), and demanding too much attention (cats).

The general practitioner can play a pivotal role in helping to decrease relinquishment resulting from behavioral problems. Recognizing the common issues that contribute to

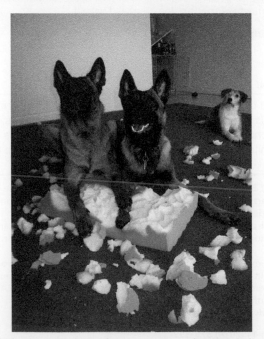

Fig. 1. Destructive behavior, although often a normal exploratory behavior of young dogs, can be damaging to the human-animal bond.

the demise of the human-animal bond and relinquishment allows the practitioner to implement a preventive behavioral plan of care for his or her clients. Through education, preventive behavioral advice, and early identification of potential behavioral concerns, the veterinary staff can maintain and enhance the human-animal bond, thus decreasing the rates of relinquishment and euthanasia.

TRIAGING BEHAVIORAL CONCERNS

Behavior problems rarely occur overnight; behavior is influenced by learning, and problems often develop over time. However, acute changes in behavior, especially in an animal that is middle aged or older, are suggestive of medical disease. A physical examination and medical workup to rule out contributing medical factors are an essential component of baseline screening for each behavior case.

Predictors of future behavior problems often include fear, anxiety, and/or aggression in the young or adolescent dog or cat.[6-9] A gradual escalation of a behavior problem, such as initially avoiding and then later growling at visitors in the home, can become a crisis when an incident occurs, such as when the dog bites a house guest. When faced with a behavioral crisis, it is important to be able to triage the situation and provide immediate relief/safety until further assistance can be provided (**Fig. 2**).

Signs of urgent behavior problems:
- There is significant damage to the human-animal bond; the owner is at his or her "wits' end" or is afraid of the pet. Regardless of the severity of the behavior, the owners' inability to tolerate the pet's behavior indicates that the pet may be close to being relinquished if immediate assistance is not provided.
- There is a risk of injury to the pet, other animals, or people. This scenario would include a dog suffering from severe separation anxiety who escapes the home by breaking out of a kennel and jumping through windows, or a cat that is unpredictably aggressive toward the owner and causing physical injury.

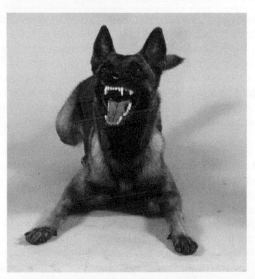

Fig. 2. A behavioral crisis may be brought on by an escalation in aggressive displays by the pet.

- The owner is unable to identify and/or avoid triggers for the behavior. The pet may be in a constant heightened state of arousal or vigilance, affecting the pet's welfare; a dog that paces aimlessly or a cat that hides under the bed for most of the day. Another example would be a dog or cat that is attacking the other resident pet in the home without an identifiable or preventable trigger.

Providing Immediate Assistance

The client may contact the veterinarian on the phone or mention the behavior concerns, in passing, at the conclusion of an appointment. It is difficult to obtain an adequate behavioral history and address behavioral concerns within the confines of a 15- to 20-minute appointment. It is important to let the client know that their concerns are valid and that help is available. It is necessary to schedule an appropriate amount of time to address the client's behavioral concerns or offer a referral to an appropriate behavior professional.

Suggestions for immediate assistance include:
- Show empathy; let pet owners know there is help and that they are not alone. Empathizing can provide instant relief for the client.
- Advise the pet owner to avoid triggers of the behavior if possible, not only for the safety of all involved but also to avoid the practicing of the undesirable behavior. For the dog that is reactive to stimuli on walks, walks should be avoided. For the cat that is showing aggression to another cat in the household, managing the cats separately in the home may be necessary.
- Cease all forms of punishment, including verbal or physical corrections; punishment can often exacerbate behavior problems and does not address the underlying motivation for the pet's behavior.[10,11]
- In some cases temporarily boarding the pet, if it is safe to do so, will provide the pet owner with a necessary reprieve until further assistance can be provided.

Medical Problems with Underlying Behavioral Issues

Patients may present with medical conditions that are influenced by an underlying behavioral issue. Although not intended to be all-inclusive, **Table 1** lists examples of medical conditions that potentially have underlying behavioral causes. Medical conditions can cause behavioral changes, and behavioral conditions can cause medical changes. Taking a complete and holistic approach to patient care includes ruling out and treating all factors, medical and behavioral. All behavior conditions have medical rule-outs (see the article by Frank elsewhere in this issue). The veterinarian's role is paramount to the successful treatment of concerns that involve medical and/or behavioral conditions.

Case Example (name and breed of dog has been changed for confidentiality): Tulip, a 6-year-old, female spayed terrier mix, presented for a fear of thunderstorms and occasional urine and stool accidents in the house when left home alone. Her medical history indicated several episodes of hemorrhagic gastroenteritis (HGE) requiring frequent hospitalization and symptomatic treatment during the summer months. Once behavior medications and behavior modification were implemented to address her underlying thunderstorm anxiety and separation anxiety, Tulip ceased to have any further episodes of HGE. It is documented that chronic stress can result in gastrointestinal disorders.[12] Through successful treatment of Tulip's behavioral conditions and alleviation of chronic and acute stressors, her gastrointestinal health was also improved.

Table 1
Examples of medical conditions that potentially have underlying behavioral causes

Presenting Medical Condition	Possible Behavioral Causes
Foreign-body ingestion	Pica, compulsive disorder, separation anxiety, lack of mental stimulation
Injuries caused by dog or cat fights in the home	Interdog aggression or intercat aggression in the home, interspecies aggression
Chronic hemorrhagic gastroenteritis	Chronic anxiety, generalized anxiety disorder, sound phobias, separation anxiety
Injuries from escape behavior (including broken teeth, nails, and bruising or muzzle abrasions from attempting to escape from confinement)	Separation anxiety, storm or sound phobias
Acral lick dermatitis	Compulsive disorder, situational or generalized anxiety disorder, sound phobias, separation anxiety

BENEFITS OF INTEGRATING VETERINARY BEHAVIOR INTO GENERAL PRACTICE

Besides the benefits of reducing relinquishment/euthanasia rates and enhancing the human-animal bond, integrating behavioral services into general practice provides direct and indirect financial benefits. Direct financial benefits are reflected through the offering of behavioral services and the increased revenue generated by these services. Indirect financial benefits are associated with pet retention, client referrals, increased veterinary visits, and decreased routine examination time and staff assistance (**Table 2**).

Let us consider an example of how pet relinquishment can affect your hospital. It is estimated that about 15% of a veterinarian's clients are lost annually as a result of pet

Table 2
Indirect financial benefits of integrating veterinary behavior into general practice

Behavioral Welfare/Service	Potential Indirect Financial Benefits
Low-stress interactions, handling, and restraint	Less fearful patients and increased client satisfaction equates to an increase in veterinary visits. Clients are more likely to refer friends and family to your hospital
Identifying behavior concerns early through routine screening	Early intervention increases the likelihood of resolution/improvement, thus decreasing the risk of relinquishment. Relinquished pets result in financial losses to the clinic
Offering prevention services such as prepurchase counseling, puppy socialization classes, kitten classes, adolescent pet behavior wellness appointments, training classes, prebaby planning	Client education fosters empathy and understanding of the motivations for behavior; thus decreasing relinquishment. These services allow for preventive training
Puppy socialization classes, kitten classes	Decreased examination-room time attributable to ease of handling and restraint learned in class. Many problems can be prevented with early intervention

behavioral issues[13]; this could be due to relinquishment, rehoming, or euthanasia. A veterinary hospital that loses a conservative 5% of its patients because of unaddressed behavioral concerns can experience a significant financial loss.

For example:
- A hospital has 3000 active patients.
- A loss of 5% of patients equates to 150 patients per annum.
- The average annual veterinary expenses for a pet in 2011 was US$505.[14]
- Therefore, the total annual loss would be $75,750 (150 patients × $505).
- Consider a 10% loss: 300 patients × $505 = $151,500 per year.
- 15% loss: 450 patients × $505 = $227,250 per year.

Early intervention and preventive behavior services likely will increase pet retention and decrease financial loss incurred from unresolved behavioral concerns. In fact, arguably the best driver of owner expenditures is the human-animal bond. Therefore, when the bond is weakened because of behavioral issues, these pet owners are less likely to seek veterinary care and follow veterinary recommendations.[15]

Pet owners whose pets enjoy visiting your hospital will visit more often. Integrating low-stress interactions, handling, and restraint creates a positive experience for the pet and owner. Similarly, satisfied clients will tell their friends and family about the compassionate care received, thus potentially increasing your clientele through referrals.

Dogs and cats are easier to examine when they have had repetitive positive experiences in the veterinary hospital, which can be initiated, for example, by offering puppy socialization and kitten classes in the hospital. Positive experiences associated with handling and restraint decrease examination time and the need for extra staff assistance with restraint.

Providing owner education, counseling, and preventive services can be a niche that trained veterinary staff can fulfill. Opportunities for professional growth and increased responsibilities can lead to increased job satisfaction, thus increasing staff retention rates.

Incorporating behavioral services into general practice helps prevent the emotional toll that pet relinquishment has on the client and the financial impact on the veterinary hospital. These services generate additional revenue for the hospital, improve client and patient welfare, and boost staff morale.

INTEGRATING VETERINARY BEHAVIOR INTO GENERAL PRACTICE
Create a Pet-Friendly Veterinary Practice

Although covered in detail in the article by Herron and Shreyer elsewhere in this issue, providing appropriate social interactions between staff members and patients in a low-stress environment is the first step toward incorporating behavior into the veterinary hospital.

A few vital recommendations include:
- Educate staff on how to provide nonthreatening body language (avoid direct eye contact/look away, approach the pet from the side rather than directly).
- Allow the patient time to acclimate to the environment and solicit attention on the pet's terms.
- Have a variety of easily accessible high-value treats for use in the lobby and examination areas.
- Toss treats to the pet initially rather than approaching and reaching out to deliver a treat, which may induce fear or be perceived as threatening.
- Implement low-stress handling and restraint techniques.

- Be willing to reschedule a wellness appointment if a patient fails to acclimate to the environment.
- Use medications when appropriate to reduce fear and anxiety, and when necessary use chemical restraint to avoid negative associations with physical restraint.

Incorporate Behavioral Questions into Standard History Taking

There are many reasons pet owners may not be forthcoming in divulging behavioral concerns about their pet to the veterinarian.

Common motives for failing to discuss such concerns include:
- They do not realize that help is available.
- They are embarrassed or blame themselves for their pet's behavior. Although owners can sometimes unknowingly condition unwanted behaviors, rarely are they the primary cause of the behavior.
- They previously sought advice and used techniques that failed to remediate the problem(s).
- They think that harsh techniques will be needed to rectify the behavior, and they do not want to subject their pet to inhumane treatment.

By incorporating a few behavior questions into routine wellness examinations, many common concerns can be easily addressed. Inappropriate elimination was the most common behavioral concern reported in pets that were relinquished.[4] Understandably, this is a behavior that is damaging to the human-animal bond. However, many pet owners are unaware of litter-box preferences for cats and/or appropriate techniques for house-training dogs. Consequently, elimination habits (among other behavior topics) should be addressed in puppy and kitten visits as well as being routinely screened for during the adolescent, adult, and senior patient visits.

There is likely a positive correlation between early identification, appropriate intervention, and a successful outcome. The longer the duration of the undesirable behaviors, the less amenable they may be to treatment.

An example of some behavioral topics to be approached at each and every wellness visit can be found in **Table 3**. Questions can be asked either interactively as part of the history taking or via a questionnaire. A trained technician or assistant can aid in the process of history taking, thus decreasing the number of probing questions required by the veterinarian. The use of open-ended questions is suggested whenever possible.

If veterinarians waited for clients to inquire about dental care for their pets, many pets would needlessly suffer. Behavior wellness is of paramount importance because behavior problems are the leading cause of death in young and adolescent dogs and cats. Preventive discussions and inquiries regarding behavior should be the expected standard of care. The American Animal Hospital Association (AAHA) Canine Life Stages Guidelines and the American Association of Feline Practitioners–AAHA Feline Life Stages Guidelines both emphasize the importance of behavioral topic discussions at each life stage.[16,17]

The First Appointment

The first time a pet, whether young, adult, or senior, visits your veterinary hospital it should be as pleasant an experience as possible. If the pet is distressed by the visit, the owner is likely also distressed. Animals are constantly learning about their environment, and negative experiences that induce fear can be difficult to forget. The

Table 3		
Behavioral topics to inquire about at different life stages		
Life Stage	**Dog**	**Cat**

Puppy (<4 mo)
Kitten (<3 mo)
	Age obtained?
	Litter size?
	Where does the puppy spend
	    most of its time?
	House training
	    Routine meals
	    Log of elimination
	    Reward desired behavior
	    Substrate preferences
	    Location preferences
	    Cleaning accidents
	Puppy socialization class
	Any growling, barking,
	    snarling, chewing, or
	    nipping/biting?
		Age obtained?
		Early exposure to other kittens?
		How is or will the kitten be
		    managed (indoor vs outdoor)?
		Litter-box training
		    Reliability of use
		    Number
		    Size and type
		    Location
		    Substrate
		    Cleaning frequency
		Kitten class
		Any growling, hissing, scratching,
		    or nipping/biting?

Juvenile, adolescent,
    adult
Canine: 4 mo to ~7 y
Feline: 3 mo to ~12 y
	Where is the dog managed?
	Attending positive training?
	Walking frequency?
	Training equipment?
	Toys and enrichment?
	House-training status?
	Any signs of aggression
	    (growling, barking,
	    snapping, biting)?
	Any changes in behavior?
		Litter-box questions (same as
		    kitten)
		Any signs of aggression (growling,
		    hissing, scratching, nipping,
		    biting)?
		Toys and enrichment?
		Any changes in behavior?

Senior
Canine: ~7 y+
Feline: ~10–12 y+
	Where is the dog managed?
	Mental stimulation?
	    Training classes
	    Walking frequency
	    Food storage toys
	Changes in behavior DISHA(A)?
	    Disorientation
	    Interactions with people
	        (withdrawn)
	    Sleep-wake cycle
	    House soiling
	    Activity/anxiety
	Mobility?
	Any signs of aggression?
		Litter-box questions (same as
		    kitten)
		Changes in behavior DISHA(A)?
		    Disorientation
		    Interactions with people
		    Sleep-wake cycle (nighttime
		        vocalization)
		    House soiling
		    Activity/anxiety
		Any signs of aggression?

Abbreviation: DISHA(A), cognitive dysfunction: Disorientation, Interactions, Sleep-wake cycle changes, House soiling, Activity (Anxiety) levels.

precedent on which future visits are based should be a positive first visit. Besides following the general recommendations in the pet-friendly hospital as already stated, enact a policy to provide extended-time appointments for new patients, thus allowing the pet adequate time to acclimate to the new environment. Numerous high-value small treats should be used during the visit to provide for a positive association with the clinic (classical conditioning) (**Fig. 3**).

Puppy and kitten appointments
Starting the new puppy and kitten owner on the correct path from the beginning is much easier than trying to repair problems that could have been prevented.

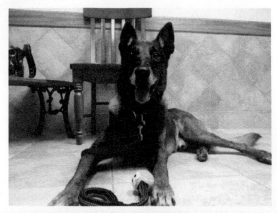

Fig. 3. This dog enjoys playing with his ball while acclimating to the examination room. On arrival at the hospital, it is best to immediately provide the client and patient with a private examination room to avoid unpredictable encounters in more high-traffic areas of the hospital.

During routine puppy and kitten vaccination series visits, discuss preventive topics such as:

- Socialization and environmental habituation (localization)
- Developmental periods and normal behavior
- Body language
- Enrichment, management, and routine
- Risks of punishment and aversive training techniques
- Positive training and appropriate problem-solving methods
  - Some specific puppy topics to address include house training, play mouthing/biting, teaching appropriate play with people, jumping, chewing, digging, barking, countersurfing/stealing objects, food-bowl exercises to prevent resource guarding, handling and restraint, crate and independence training to prevent separation anxiety, and the pros and cons of castration/ovariohysterectomy.
  - Some specific kitten topics to address include litter-box factors, appropriate play with people and toys, scratching, play biting, crate training, harness training, offering a varied diet to avoid finicky eaters, restraint and handling, indoor-only versus outdoor access, surgical declaw, and the benefits of castration/ovariohysterectomy (**Fig. 4**).

Kittens and puppies usually acclimate quickly to novel environments, and a liberal use of treats can foster a positive association. Once acclimated, a short demonstration using lure reward or clicker training with the puppy/kitten encourages the use of positive training methodology and motivates the owner to start training the pet early. Most puppies or kittens can quickly learn to offer a sit or eye contact through positive reinforcement. A veterinary technician or assistant proficient with positive training can demonstrate proper training techniques.

Appointment with the new pet owner

Some newly obtained pets will be out of their puppy or kitten stage and will come into their new home as an adolescent, adult, or senior patient. Because of previous learning experiences (possibly not all positive), it may take longer for these pets to acclimate to the environment. A discussion about positive training, problem solving, and humane training tools are important to give the client the necessary knowledge to address potential concerns that may arise.

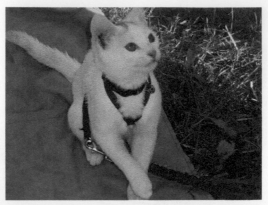

Fig. 4. Acclimating a young cat to a harness can allow for outdoor activities with the owner while providing safe exploration.

Adolescent Behavior Wellness Appointments

More pets are relinquished during adolescence than at any other life stage. Adolescence is also a time when routine veterinary care has a lull. Vaccination series are usually completed around 4 months of age, and many pets are altered between 5 and 7 months of age. The next recommended visit is often at 15 or 16 months, for vaccine boosters. Much is happening behaviorally during this 8- to 11-month window. The adolescent dog is likely larger, stronger, and more independent, and owners are often less tolerant of unruly behavior. The adolescent dog is often more difficult for the owner to walk, control, and confine. The adolescent cat may be marking via urine or scratching, and may be less accepting of other unfamiliar cats.

Screening for behavior problems during adolescence can be accomplished in a variety of ways. One method would be to schedule an adolescent wellness appointment when the pet is between 8 and 12 months of age. Another option is to send a simple behavioral questionnaire via mail/email that helps to identify behavioral concerns. This method may help owners to recognize the importance of addressing behavioral concerns early and to seek veterinary advice.

For example, the announcement might say:

Is Fluffy digging in the garden, having accidents in the house, destructive when left alone, pulling on the leash, or displaying other behaviors that are concerning? If you answered yes to any of these questions, please contact our office today. Our veterinary team can guide you to compassionate and humane ways to improve these behaviors and your relationship!

Identifying how the pet is being housed and managed can provide a clue to possible behavioral concerns. The cat that is confined to a bathroom or laundry room may be displaying inappropriate scratching or elimination. A dog that is being managed in the yard when the owner is away could be suggestive of untreated separation anxiety. Perhaps the dog eliminated or was destructive in the home, and consequently the yard was chosen for management. Digging or destructive behavior in the yard is often more tolerable than destruction in the home. For the welfare of the pet and to prevent escalation of this behavior, a behavior wellness appointment would be recommended and the behavior concerns addressed.

Similarly, for dogs that are not being walked routinely, is it because the dog is overreactive to stimuli on walks by barking, lunging, or biting? Has the dog not been taught how to walk politely on a leash? Does the owner not have time or recognize the benefits of routine exercise in the form of walks off the property?

Senior Behavior Wellness Appointments

Screening for cognitive dysfunction syndrome (CDS) in senior pets is vital because early detection and treatment may improve the quality and quantity of life. Behavior questionnaires designed to identify the DISHA signs (Disorientation, Interaction changes, Sleep-wake cycle changes, House soiling, and Anxiety or activity changes), are available through a variety of companies (Virbac, Pfizer, Hills). A senior screening questionnaire and a cognitive dysfunction questionnaire can be found in *Behavior Problems of the Dog and Cat*, 3rd edition (see Recommended Resources).

Common medical conditions seen in aging patients (such as cardiovascular or liver disease) may exacerbate oxidative damage to the brain. Sex hormones present in unaltered pets may have a protective effect against CDS.[18] Neutered or spayed senior pets with medical ailments should be closely monitored for signs of CDS as well as other anxiety-related conditions.

In a Pfizer study (1998), 48% of pet owners identified at least 1 sign of CDS in dogs older than 8 years. By contrast, veterinarians estimated that 17% of dogs older than 8 years show signs consistent with CDS. This discrepancy suggests that many veterinarians were unaware of the prevalence of the condition. Furthermore, practitioners surveyed reported that only 7% to 12% of pet owners voluntarily mention signs associated with aging. A more recent Internet-based survey estimated the prevalence of CDS to range from 5% in dogs aged 10 to 12 years to 41% in dogs older than 14, with an overall prevalence of 14.2%.[19] However, a diagnosis had only been made in 1.9% of dogs; thus, more than 85% of cases had been missed. In one cat study, 35% had signs consistent with CDS after medical problems were ruled out, which ranged from 28% of 95 cats aged 11 to 14 years and 50% of 46 cats aged 15 and older.[20] Thus it is clear that clients are often not forthcoming with information describing behavior changes in their aging pets, perhaps thinking that they are normal signs associated with aging. Screening for behavior changes and early intervention should be the primary focus. Furthermore, behavioral signs may be the first or only sign of underlying medical problems. In fact, a diagnosis of cognitive dysfunction is made only by identifying behavioral signs and ruling out medical issues that might be causing or contributing to these signs. Another critical issue for the senior pet is to maintain a healthy level of enrichment, both mentally and physically, as this has been demonstrated to help prevent, slow, or improve signs of cognitive dysfunction (**Fig. 5**).[21]

Preventive Behavior Services

In addition to routine behavioral screening and providing a pet-friendly veterinary practice, the practitioner should consider adding ancillary behavior services (**Table 4**). Implementation of these services by a trained veterinary technician or qualified trainer associated with the hospital may keep pets in their home (**Fig. 6**).

Intervention Behavior Services

By incorporating behavior questions into your routine history taking, many potential issues will be identified early before they have become a significant problem. However, even with good screening and preventive care, behavior disorders may still develop. A behavior disorder can be defined as a psychological or behavioral pattern outside the behavioral norms for the species. Behavior disorders often have an affective component.

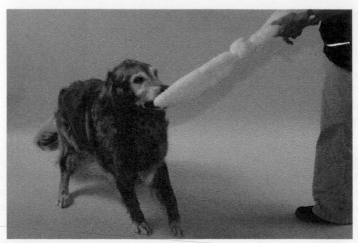

Fig. 5. Mental stimulation in the form of gentle low-impact play and positive training for the senior pet can help improve behavioral well-being.

With a thorough screening process and knowledge of normal behavior for the species, age, sex, and breed, the veterinarian is often able to identify whether a behavior is normal, abnormal, the manifestation of a medical condition, an inappropriately conditioned behavior, or simply related to a lack of training/manners.

Table 4
Preventive behavior services

Behavior Service	Description
Pet selection counseling	Provides guidance through education and preparation to clients contemplating obtaining a new pet
Prebaby counseling	Prepares the pet and owners for changes associated with welcoming a newborn into the house
Kids and pets	Provides clients and children with skills and knowledge to help facilitate a safe and enjoyable relationship between pets and children in the home. Including information on common triggers for aggression toward children
Puppy socialization classes	For puppies in their socialization period. A well-run puppy socialization class provides a safe environment for exploration and preventive exercises. Puppy parents learn positive methods for beginning training and addressing normal canine behaviors
Kitten classes	For kittens <4 mo old. Geared toward educating owners on normal cat behavior, preventive exercises, and positive exposure to novelty
Canine manners training classes	For juvenile, adolescent, and adult dogs. Manners training focuses on useful skills for the pet dog such as settle on a mat, calm greeting with guests, and loose leash walking
Canine senior classes	For dogs >7 y old. These classes focus on mental stimulation, positive training, low-impact exercise, and educating clients regarding senior behavioral concerns
Private prevention/training appointments	Private in-home or in-clinic appointments to address specific normal behavioral concerns; walking on leash, crate training, house training, etc

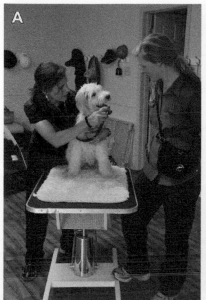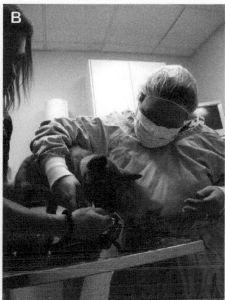

Fig. 6. (A, B) Restraint and handling exercises being practiced by the veterinary technician and client in puppy socialization classes.

Providing clinical behavioral consultations can be a rewarding break from everyday general practice. Consultations are similar to those in other areas of veterinary medicine.

The behavior consultation should include:

- A physical examination
- A thorough evaluation of the patient's behavioral and medical history
- A diagnosis and list of differential diagnoses
- A prognosis
- A treatment plan addressing owner education, the patient's management/housing, patient's temperament, behavior modification/training, environmental modification, and the use of medication when appropriate
- Follow-up and adjustment to the treatment plan based on the patient's clinical response

Referral to a veterinary behaviorist should be considered if a desirable response to treatment is not seen or the presenting issues are beyond the scope of knowledge and expertise of the practice.

DEFINING THE ROLES OF BEHAVIOR TEAM MEMBERS

A mutual understanding of the roles of animal behavior professionals is critical to facilitating a team approach and, thereby, improving case outcomes and client satisfaction. To work together with other paraprofessionals, one must understand each other's roles in improving the patient's welfare. There are potentially 5 categories of qualified individuals that may be involved in the behavior team, each with specific roles and contributions to the therapy (**Table 5**):

- General practitioner (Doctor of Veterinary Medicine)

Table 5 Roles of the behavior team		
Veterinarian, DACVB	**CAAB**	**RVT, Qualified Trainer**
Assess	Assess	Assist DVM or CAAB
Rule out medical disease	Work closely with DVM	Initial assessment or
Diagnose	Behavioral diagnoses	observations/behavioral
Prognose	Develop/change treatment	triage
Develop/change treatment	plan	Help client implement
plan	Unable to prescribe medication	treatment plan
Prescribe/adjust medication		Provide feedback to DVM
		and/or CAAB

Abbreviations: CAAB, Certified Applied Animal Behaviorist; DACVB, Diplomate of the American College of Veterinary Behaviorists; DVM, Doctor of Veterinary Medicine; RVT, Registered Veterinary Technician.

- Veterinary Behaviorist: Diplomates of the American College of Veterinary Behaviorists (DACVB) or European College of Animal Welfare and Behavioural Medicine (Behaviour) (ECAWBM)
- Certified Applied Animal Behaviorist (CAAB)
- Veterinary Technician Specialist in Behavior (VTS-Behavior) or Registered Veterinary Technician (RVT) with advanced education in animal behavior and training
- Qualified professional animal/dog trainer

General Practitioner

The general practitioner determines the hospital's policies and procedures regarding the treatment of behavior cases. The veterinarian is responsible for the clinical assessment of all patients presented to him/her in the veterinary hospital, and should be the first point of contact for the pet owner. A veterinarian with an interest in addressing and treating animal behavior should be a member of the American Veterinary Society of Animal Behavior (www.avsabonline.com), and should also seek to advance knowledge and skills through continuing education in veterinary behavior and training.

When treating behavior problems, the veterinarian's role includes:
- Determining how behavior problems will be addressed in the hospital; which cases will be seen and which will be referred
- Developing behavior consultation history and treatment forms for medical documentation
- Establishing a behavioral diagnosis and a list of behavioral and medical differentials
- Conducting further diagnostic testing, when applicable
- Providing a prognosis
- Developing a treatment plan and modifying the plan as needed
- Prescribing medication and adjusting medication

The general practitioner is responsible for ruling out potential medical causes of behavior disorders, and either providing a comprehensive behavior consultation or referring the client to a specialist. Because animal behavior and training is largely unregulated, anyone can call themselves a behaviorist without meeting a specified set of standards. Veterinary professionals need to be familiar with the qualifications of individuals to whom they refer their clients.

Veterinary Behaviorist: Diplomate of the American College of Veterinary Behaviorists

When possible the general practitioner should refer to a board certified veterinary behaviorist. As defined on the American College of Veterinary Behaviorists (ACVB) Web site:

> Diplomates of the American College of Veterinary Behavior (DACVB) are veterinarians who are specialists in the field [In Europe board-certified veterinary behaviorists are Diplomates of the European College of Animal Welfare and Behavioural Medicine (Behaviour)]. These specialists have completed a residency or training program in the discipline of veterinary behavioral medicine. As part of this program they have studied topics including but not restricted to: sociobiology, psychology of learning, behavioral genetics, behavioral physiology, psychopharmacology, ethology, and behavioral endocrinology. Specialists in veterinary behavioral medicine have both the medical and behavioral knowledge to evaluate cases to determine if there is a medical component and to determine if the patient would benefit from medication. In addition, specialists often determine which medication(s) would be most appropriate as part of an integrated treatment program that includes behavioral modification plans appropriate to the individual patient.

Furthermore, all standards, procedures, training, and professional conduct of the ACVB are under the oversight of the American Board of Veterinary Specialists (ABVS), which is an organization within the American Veterinary Medical Association (AVMA); and those of the ECAWBM are overseen by the European Board of Veterinary Specialists. Specialists in veterinary behavioral medicine are also held accountable to local and state laws of veterinary practice. Members can be found at www.dacvb.org and ecawbm.org.

Certified Applied Animal Behaviorist

The following definition for CAABs has been modified from the ACVB Web site. A CAAB has earned a PhD in biological or behavioral sciences with an emphasis on animal behavior. Associate Certified Applied Animal Behaviorists (ACAABs) have earned a master's degree. Applied Animal Behaviorists are trained in the science of animal behavior and are very knowledgable in subjects such as ethology, learning theory, and psychology. CAABs and ACAABs have the skills to take a detailed behavioral history, and are skilled at implementing behavior-modification programs appropriate to the individual animal.

Unless the CAABs or ACAABs are veterinarians, they will not have the medical background necessary to assess if or how much a medical component is contributing to the problem. Nonveterinary CAABs cannot make an assessment regarding which medication would be most efficacious nor assess which medication would be the most appropriate based on the individual animal's medical history. Only veterinarians can assess the aforementioned.

CAABs and ACAABs earn their certification from the Animal Behavior Society (ABS: http://animalbehaviorsociety.org/), which sets the educational, ethical, experiential, and professional criteria that must be met. Members can be found at www.certifiedanimalbehaviorist.com.

Applied animal behaviorists recognize the importance of working closely with the patient's regular veterinarian as part of an integrated team approach.

Veterinary Technician

The veterinary technician with advanced skills in behavior and training can play an integral role in prevention services and assisting with the implementation of a behavioral treatment plan. The veterinary technician may have a variety of roles in behavior, including:

- Behavioral triage: assess the client's concerns and determine appropriate referral depending on the situation (preventive vs intervention services)
- Client preventive behavior education and services
- Assist the veterinarian with history taking and the clinical behavior consultation
- Coach and assist the client with the implementation of behavior modification and training
- Act as the liaison between all behavior team members (veterinarian, client, qualified trainer, hospital staff)

The aspiring and knowledgable veterinary behavior technician can act as the case manager, relaying important information between the various behavior team members and providing continuity and guidance to the owner.

In 2008 the National Association of Veterinary Technicians in America (NAVTA) recognized the specialty for veterinary technicians in animal behavior. Through the Academy of Veterinary Behavior Technicians, veterinary technicians have the capability of becoming recognized as a Veterinary Technician Specialist (Behavior). Applicants approved to sit for examination will have met stringent criteria reflecting their experience and knowledge in animal behavior. The examination includes assessment of knowledge through a comprehensive written examination, as well as applied demonstrations of clinical skills.

Qualified Professional Trainers

Because the veterinary technician's job is multifaceted in general practice, it may also be beneficial to have a professional dog (or animal) trainer associated with the veterinary hospital. The trainer may be either an employee of the hospital or a referral source for specific services and training.

Because animal training is largely an unregulated profession, anyone can label themselves a dog trainer or animal behaviorist regardless of their education, knowledge, experience, or skills. Several organizations have sought to recognize and certify trainers that have advanced skills and knowledge. A few that bear mentioning are the Certification Council for Professional Dog Trainers, International Association of Animal Behavior Consultants, and the Karen Pryor Academy. These organizations have set standards and criteria to reflect an individual's skill set and knowledge to eventually recognize these individuals with certifications or titles.

However, even with certification and standards, observing a trainer teaching pet owners or attending a class oneself is the best way to determine whether the trainer's methodology and skills meet the standards that the veterinary clinic would want to recommend for their clients' pets.

Characteristics of a qualified professional trainer include:
- Good communication skills; provides information in a positive, nonblaming, and motivational manner
- Calm, patient, open-minded, and polite with people and animals
- Solid understanding of learning theory and applied behavior analysis
- Well versed in normal behavior and communication for the species they work with
- Keeps current on advances in humane training techniques through continuing education
- Recognizes and reinforces desirable behavior in animals and people

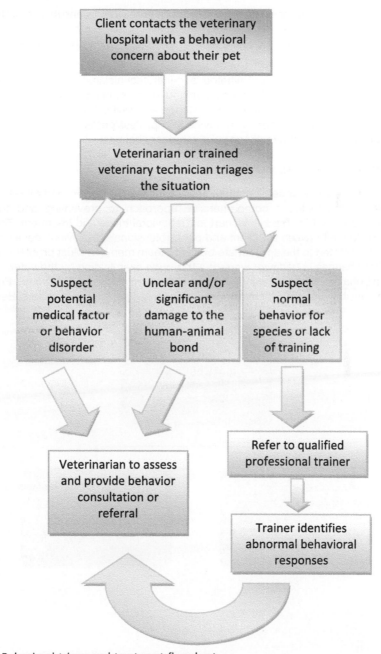

Fig. 7. Behavioral triage and treatment flowchart.

- Avoids the use of choke, pinch, electric collars, or other aversives in training
- Does not adhere to dominance theory as a motivation for most canine behaviors
- Avoids providing guarantees on behavior because it is unethical
- Uses motivational methods such as treats, toys, play, and praise

- Ignores, manages, or redirects undesirable behaviors rather than resorting to correction or aversives
- Collaborates openly with veterinarians, especially when abnormal behavior is suspected

The credentials of an individual, whether a trainer, technician, CAAB, or veterinarian, should not replace the personal assessment and interview of a potential partner associated with your hospital. Individuals' knowledge and skill set will vary depending on their experience and education. The advice and professionalism the individual conveys to others will reflect directly on your veterinary hospital.

INTEGRATION OF THE BEHAVIOR TEAM

As defined in the previous section, there are various team members and roles that can be fulfilled when taking a comprehensive approach to preventing and treating behavior disorders. **Fig. 7** is a flowchart for behavioral triage and treatment. Through an open dialogue between the client and paraprofessionals, behavioral cases can be triaged and directed to the appropriate behavior team member. Most problem behaviors and/or changes in behavior warrant a thorough examination by the veterinarian.

Once a behavior disorder (no longer in the preventive stages) is suspected, **Fig. 8** illustrates possible pathways for treatment utilizing the various team members. Because

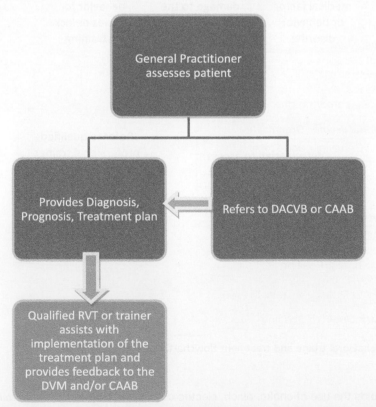

Fig. 8. Behavioral intervention flowchart. CAAB, Certified Applied Animal Behaviorist; DACVB, Diplomate of the American College of Veterinary Behaviorists; DVM, Doctor of Veterinary Medicine; RVT, Registered Veterinary Technician.

DACVBs are not available in all areas, some DACVBs provide phone, fax, or email support to assist practitioners with their client's behavioral concerns with their pet.

SUMMARY

Behavior medicine and triage should be incorporated into all general practices. All behavior problems have medical rule-outs. Behavioral medicine in general practice incorporates preventive care and solicitation of behavior topics, and provides appropriate resources for clients who seek treatment. The behavioral team working together in unison provides the best chance for a successful behavioral outcome. This situation is rewarding for the hospital, the client, and the pet's welfare. The human-animal bond is maintained and enhanced through compassionate and humane behavior practices.

RECOMMENDED RESOURCES
Veterinary Professional Organizations

American College of Veterinary Behaviorists (ACVB) www.dacvb.org
Academy of Veterinary Behavior Technicians (AVBT) www.avbt.net
American Veterinary Society of Animal Behavior (AVSAB) www.avsabonline.org
European College of Animal Welfare and Behavioural Medicine (ECAWBM) www.ecawbm.org
Society of Veterinary Behavior Technicians (SVBT) www.svbt.org

Certified Animal Behavior Professionals

Certified Applied Animal Behaviorists (CAAB) www.certifiedanimalbehaviorist.com
Animal Behavior Society (ABS) www.animalbehaviorsociety.org
Association of Pet Behaviour Counsellors (APBC) www.apbc.org.uk/help/regions
The Association for the Study of Animal Behaviour (ASAB) http://asab.nottingham.ac.uk/accred/reg.php

Professional Trainer Organizations

Animal Behaviour and Training Council (ABTC) http://www.abtcouncil.org.uk/
Certification Council for Professional Dog Trainers (CCPDT) www.ccpdt.org
International Association of Animal Behavior Consultants (IAABC) www.iaabc.org
Karen Pryor Academy (KPA) www.karenpryoracademy.com

Handouts

AVSAB Position Statements (www.avsabonline.org):
  Dominance Position Statement
  Punishment Position Statement
  Puppy Socialization Position Statement
  How to Choose a Trainer Handout

Veterinary Oriented Behavior Books

Gary Landsberg and Debra Horwitz. *Behavior Advice for Clients*. Book and CD of Client Handouts. Lifelearn, 2012.
Gary Landsberg, Wayne Hunthausen, Lowell Ackerman. *Behavior Problems of the Dog and Cat* (3rd edition). Saunders Elsevier; 2013.
Debra Horwitz and Jacqueline Neilson. *Blackwell's Five-Minute Veterinary Consult: Canine & Feline Behavior.* Blackwell Publishing; 2007.
Debra Horwitz and Daniel Mills. *BSAVA Manual of Canine and Feline Behavioural Medicine*, 2nd edition. BSAVA Publishing; 2009.

Steven Lindsay. *Handbook of Applied Dog Behavior and Training* (Vols 1, 2, 3). Iowa State University Press.

Sophia Yin. *Low Stress Handling, Restraint, and Behavior Modification of Dogs & Cats*. Cattle Dog Publishing; 2009.

Karen Overall. *Manual of Clinical Behavioral Medicine for Dogs and Cats*. Elsevier; 2013.

Crowell-Davis and Murray. *Veterinary Psychopharmacology*. Blackwell Publishing; 2006.

Behavior and Training Books

Peggy Tillman. *Clicking with Your Dog*. Sunshine Books; 2000.

American College of Veterinary Behaviorists. *Decoding Your Dog: The Ultimate Experts Explain Common Dog Behaviors and Reveal How to Prevent or Change Unwanted Ones*. Debra Horwitz (editor), John Ciribassi (contributor), and Steve Dale (contributor). Houghton Mifflin Harcourt; 2014.

Kenneth Martin and Debbie Martin. *Puppy Start Right: Foundation Training for the Companion Dog*. Sunshine Books; 2011.

Helen Zulch and Daniel Mills. *Life Skills for Puppies*. Hubble and Hattie; 2012.

Other Resources

Animal Behavior Resources Institute www.abrionline.org

REFERENCES

1. Bergler R. Man and dog. The psychology of a relationship. Oxford (United Kingdom): Blackwell Scientific Publications; 1988.
2. Olson PN. The modern working dog—a call for interdisciplinary collaboration. J Am Vet Med Assoc 2002;221(3):352–5.
3. Serpell JA. Anthropomorphism and anthropomorphic selection beyond the "cute response". Soc Anim 2002;10(4):437–54.
4. Salman MD, Hutchinson J, Tuch-Gallie R, et al. Behavioral reasons for relinquishment of dogs and cats to 12 shelters. J Appl Anim Welfare Sci 2000;3:93–106.
5. New JG, Salman MD, Scarlett JM, et al. Shelter relinquishment: characteristics of shelter-relinquished animals and their owners compared with animals and their owners in U.S. pet-owning households. J Appl Anim Welfare Sci 2000;3:179–201.
6. Godbout M, Frank D. Persistence of puppy behaviors and signs of anxiety during adulthood. J Vet Behav 2011;6:92.
7. Guy NC, Luescher UA, Dohoo SE, et al. Demographic and aggressive characteristics of dogs in a general veterinary caseload. Appl Anim Behav Sci 2001;74:15–28.
8. Guy NC, Luescher UA, Dohoo SE, et al. Risk factors for dog bites to owners in a general veterinary caseload. Appl Anim Behav Sci 2001;74:29–42.
9. Guy NC, Luescher UA, Dohoo SE, et al. A case series of biting dogs: characteristics of the dogs, their behavior, and their victims. Appl Anim Behav Sci 2001;74:43–57.
10. Herron ME, Shofer FS, Reisner IR. Survey of the use and outcome of confrontational and nonconfrontational training methods in client-owned dogs showing undesirable behaviors. Appl Anim Behav Sci 2009;117:47–54.
11. Mariotti VM, Amat M, Ruiz De La Torre JL, et al. Management and environmental influences on owner-directed aggression in dogs. In: Proceedings of the 2009

American College of Veterinary Behaviorists—American Veterinary Society of Animal Behavior Meeting. Seattle (WA): 2009. p. 11–5.

12. Konturek PC, Brzozowski T, Konturek SJ. Stress and the gut: pathophysiology, clinical consequences, diagnostic approach and treatment options. J Physiol Pharmacol 2011;62(6):591–9.

13. Tremayne J. AAFP pens behavior guidelines for DVMs, staff, clients. DVM Magazine 2005. Available at: http://veterinarynews.dvm360.com/dvm/article/articleDetail.jsp?id=155730.

14. AP poll. 2011. Available at: http://ap-gfkpoll.com/uncategorized/ap-petside-com-poll-8-in-10-pet-owners-visited-vet-in-last-year. Accessed date 3 February, 2014.

15. Lue TW, Pantenburg DP, Crawford PM. Impact of the owner-pet and client-veterinarian bond on the care that pets receive. J Am Vet Med Assoc 2008; 232(4):531–40.

16. Bartges J, Boynton B, Vogt AH, et al. AAHA canine life stages guidelines. J Am Anim Hosp Assoc 2012;48:1–11.

17. Vogt AH, Rodan I, Brown M, et al. AAFP-AAHA: feline life stage guidelines. J Feline Med Surg 2010;12:43–54.

18. Hart BL. Effect of gonadectomy on subsequent development of age-related cognitive impairment in dogs. J Am Vet Med Assoc 2001;219(1):51–6.

19. Salvin HE, McGreevy PD, Sachev PS, et al. Under diagnosis of canine cognitive dysfunction; a cross-sectional survey of older companion dogs. Vet J 2010;184: 277–81.

20. Gunn-Moore D, Moffat K, Christie LA, et al. Cognitive dysfunction and the neurobiology of ageing in cats. J Small Anim Pract 2007;48:546–53.

21. Milgram NW, Head EA, Zicker SC, et al. Long term treatment with antioxidants and a program of behavioural enrichment reduces age-dependent impairment in discrimination and reversal learning in beagle dogs. Exp Gerontol 2004;39: 753–65.

Common Sense Behavior Modification: A Guide for Practitioners

Debra F. Horwitz, DVM[a,b,*], Amy L. Pike, DVM[a]

KEYWORDS

- Positive reinforcement • Control devices • Aggression • Behavior modification
- Management

KEY POINTS

- Behavior problems are often given as a reason for pet relinquishment to shelters.
- When presented with any behavior problem, veterinarians should perform a thorough physical examination (including neurologic and orthopedic examination) and a minimum database, including a complete blood cell count (CBC), chemistry panel, and total T4 and free T4 by equilibrium dialysis if the T4 is low, to rule out any medical contributions.
- Veterinarians should be a source of information regarding management, safety, and basic behavior modification for common behavior problems.
- Additionally, various control devices offer pet owners the ability to better manage their pets in difficult situations.

INTRODUCTION

Behavior problems can break the human-animal bond, increasing the likelihood for relinquishment and/or euthanasia. Research has confirmed that behavior problems continue to be a top reason pet owners relinquish their pets to shelters.[1–4] Aggression toward people and other animals is the number one reason given for dogs and the number 2 behavioral explanation given for cats.[1,2] If a veterinary practitioner does not identify problematic behaviors, these pets are left at risk. Yet the opportunity for veterinarians to intervene and help exists only if they use it. One regional shelter study found that 70% of dogs and 50% of cats had visited their veterinarian at least once in the year prior to being relinquished to a shelter.[5] Active behavioral screening and intervention by a veterinarian might have saved these pets from relinquishment. Many resources are available that contain behavior questionnaires and evaluations used for

Conflict of Interest: Dr D.F. Horwitz, Behavior consultant for Ceva Animal Health, Clorox Advisory Panel; Dr A.L. Pike, Nil.

[a] Veterinary Behavior Consultations, 11469 Olive Boulevard, #254, St Louis, MO 63141, USA; [b] Department of Veterinary Medicine and Surgery, University of Missouri, College of Veterinary Medicine, 900 East Campus Drive, Columbia, MO 65211, USA
* Corresponding author. Veterinary Behavior Consultations, 11469 Olive Boulevard, #254, St Louis, MO.
E-mail address: debhdvm@aol.com

> **Box 1**
> **Resources for behavior evaluations and questionnaires**
>
> - Horwitz D, Mills D, editors. BSAVA manual of canine and feline behavioural medicine, 2nd edition. Quedgeley (Gloucester): British Small Animal Veterinary Association; 2009.
> - Landsberg G, Hunthausen W, Ackerman L. Handbook of behavior problems of the dog and cat, 3rd edition. Elsevier Saunders; 2012.
> - Horwitz D, Neilson J. Blackwell's five-minute veterinary consult clinical companion: canine and feline behavior. Ames (IA): Blackwell Publishing; 2007.
> - Overall K. Manual of clinical behavioral medicine for dogs and cats. St Louis (MO): Elsevier Mosby; 2013.

screening purposes (**Box 1**); consequently, this topic is not covered here. Once a practitioner has identified a behavior requiring change, owners need practical guidance and easily implemented solutions for behavior modification. Rather than needing to be skilled in all types of behavioral interventions, practitioners can arm themselves with basic behavioral advice and solutions to help ameliorate many problem behaviors.

What an owner considers an undesirable behavior may be an ethologically normal or adaptive behavior for the pet. For example, urine marking is a normal behavior performed by cats and dogs for signaling purposes[6] yet most pet owners find it highly objectionable. At its most basic motivation, aggression is merely a behavioral strategy that a pet uses in a social interaction to avoid or end an unwanted encounter and to relieve underlying fear or anxiety. It is imperative that veterinarians educate owners on what constitutes both normal and abnormal behavior and how to eliminate an unwanted behavior by teaching and reinforcing desirable behaviors. The focus should be on determining what pets are communicating by their behavior, why they are performing the behavior, and how owners can intervene to help. Most importantly, owners should strive to use humane, force-free, and kind methods when attempting to change behavior. Creating fear or anxiety through the use of inappropriate punishment or painful techniques only serves to damage the human-animal bond, compromise animal welfare, and increase rather than decrease fear, anxiety, and the potential for aggression.

The behavior modification detailed throughout this article can be used in a veterinary practice in a variety of ways. Individual client counseling can be performed by a clinician, skilled technician, or trusted trainer during a regularly scheduled appointment. Clinics can alternatively offer behavior seminars or group classes that focus on problem behaviors. Clinics can create their own handouts on the subjects or use one of the many written handouts commercially available from a trusted resource: a board-certified veterinary behaviorist, a certified applied animal behaviorist, or a positive method trainer. Behavior counseling may be beyond the capacity of what clinicians are comfortable with or even wish to offer as a service. All clinicians should, however, at the least, screen for behavioral problems, rule out medical causes for behavior, and offer some management solutions and referral to a behavior specialist when necessary. It is imperative that clinics use and recommend the use of a positive trainer or behaviorist. Web sites to help locate a behaviorist (Diplomate, American College of Veterinary Behaviorists or Certified Applied Animal Behaviorist) or trainer are found in an article elsewhere in this issue.

PROVIDING SPECIES-APPROPRIATE INFORMATION ON DOG AND CAT BEHAVIOR

Canine aggression is a serious behavioral problem and, when directed toward people, is also dangerous. Inherent in any intervention is the requirement to discard outdated and disproved theories to explain canine behavior. Often canine aggression is attributed to canine aspirations to become "dominant" to the humans in their social group. Although dominance as an explanation for canine behavior is no longer used in applied behavior therapy by either veterinary behaviorists or applied animal behaviorists, the theory has become pervasive in some sectors of the training community, resulting in confrontational and harmful techniques to train dogs. The use of dominance to explain canine behavior was extrapolated from early observations (1940s) and research of captive wolves. These animals engaged in repeated agonistic encounters, which seemed to indicate the existence of dominance hierarchies among the pack members. Unfortunately, this information was put into the prevailing literature of the time and perpetuated for many years. In the 1990s, however, research on wild wolf packs did not reveal any aggressive encounters but rather amicable and cooperative relationships between group members, all of whom were related. Unfortunately, the damage was done, and results in dreadful consequences when these theories are applied in behavior modification or training.[7] Recent observation of a group of unrelated neutered male dogs showed that dominance is truly not a character trait of an individual dog but rather a qualitative description of a contextual relationship of 2 dogs that can vary based on the environmental framework.[7] Dominance theory, as regrettably applied to the human-animal relationship, has caused popular media and uneducated trainers to espouse ideas, such as the alpha roll and gaining authority over pets using physical punishment, threat, and force. The American Veterinary Society of Animal Behavior has a position statement against the implementation of dominance theory and common myths about wolves and dogs, which can be found at their Web site, www.avsabonline.org. It is important to remember that when animals do not behave as expected, they are not exhibiting dominance over us. Their actions are merely a construct of their normal behavioral patterns, a concept discussed throughout this article.

Misconceptions about cats may lead owners astray when attempting to implement behavior modification as well. Cats are considered a social species with many opting to live in groups. There are individuals, however, that choose solitary living, and territory disputes are not uncommon in cats, which often results in the aggression and anxiety demonstrated in a multicat household.

LEARNING PRINCIPLES

In order to change behavior and create behavior modification plans, how learning occurs and the basic principles that guide learning must be understood. Psychologists define learning as the process by which an event or experience produces a lasting change in behavior or mental processes.[8] Learning engages the internal processes of perceiving an event, categorizing the experience, and then creating a memory. Learning takes place at a neurochemical level involving synapses and neurotransmitters and creates a lasting change in the neuroanatomy of the brain. Consequently, learning allows a sentient being to adapt to changing situations and novel environments. In teaching behavior modification, learning principles are capitalized on to produce an efficient and lasting change in behavior.

Constraints on Learning

For learning to take place, several things must be in place. Learning can be compromised in injured, ill, or painful individuals; therefore, good health and sensory health can optimize learning. Learning cannot occur well with distractions. So both human and pet must be in a calm environment without distractions. Other major constraints on learning are fear and anxiety, which generally underlie many of the behavior problems seen in dogs and cats. Learning new things is difficult when a pet is highly emotionally aroused. When dogs are actively performing an unwanted behavior, they are focused on what is happening at the time and unlikely to focus on learning something new, making the situation far from an optimal learning environment. This is why the implementation of management and environmental controls is so important, but if these do not decrease the arousal level so learning can occur, some animals may need medication included in their overall treatment plan, to help reduce excessive arousal and facilitate treatment. Additionally, the ability to learn a new task or association is often dependent on the intensity, frequency, speed, or some other attribute of the stimulus that causes the reaction. Therefore, to be successful, a stimulus gradient must be identified so that a pet is able to learn a new behavior while calm and under threshold limitations.[9] Finally, for learning to occur, a behavior treatment program must be tailored to needs, desires, temperament, and threshold of individual animals.

Definitions

Classical conditioning
- Definition: When a stimulus that produces an innate reflex becomes paired with a neutral stimulus that then, on its own, produces the same response.[8] This is often known as pavlovian conditioning. See **Box 2** for a depiction of Pavlov's classic experiment. In this type of learning, a reflexive response, such as fear, becomes associated with something that for another individual may be neutral. When paired often enough, the stimulus alone can elicit the fearful response.

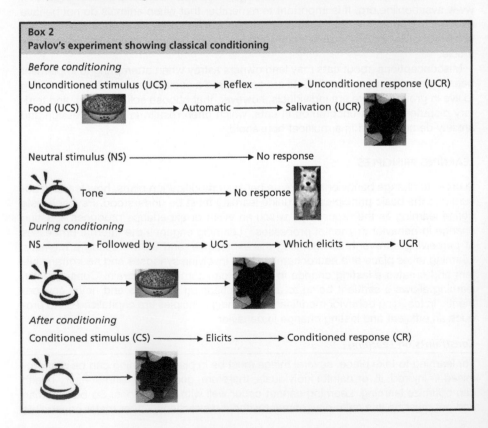

Box 2
Pavlov's experiment showing classical conditioning

Before conditioning

Unconditioned stimulus (UCS) ⟶ Reflex ⟶ Unconditioned response (UCR)

Food (UCS) ⟶ Automatic ⟶ Salivation (UCR)

Neutral stimulus (NS) ⟶ No response

Tone ⟶ No response

During conditioning

NS ⟶ Followed by ⟶ UCS ⟶ Which elicits ⟶ UCR

After conditioning

Conditioned stimulus (CS) ⟶ Elicits ⟶ Conditioned response (CR)

- Example: The doorbell can easily become a conditioned stimulus if a dog is frightened of strangers entering the home. Initially, the doorbell means nothing but, when repeatedly paired with the entrance of fear-evoking unfamiliar people, the doorbell quickly becomes the predictor of bad things and initiates the fear response on its own.
- Advantage: Classical conditioning is a passive process; by repeated pairings, the animal learns new associations
- Disadvantage: Because it can occur passively, unwanted associations are possible.

Operant conditioning
- Definition: Occurs when the consequences (either reward or punishment) of the performance of a behavior influence the maintenance of the behavior.[8] Unlike pavlovian conditioning, which is a passive process, in operant conditioning, an individual can "operate" on the environment in response to the stimulus, resulting in either a favorable or unfavorable outcome. Outcomes that are favorable tend to be repeated; those that are aversive are not.
- Example: If dogs are rewarded for jumping on people entering the home by gaining the attention that they seek, this behavior will be repeated in the future. If they are ignored and attention is given only when dogs are sitting, however, they are less likely to jump and more likely to sit in the future.
- Advantage: Because behavior is continued based on the consequences, the use of operant techniques allows teaching dogs new tasks.
- Disadvantage: If not done properly, different associations may be made. In addition, there is a tendency to rely heavily on the use of aversive outcomes rather than teaching new tasks. Whether an interaction or consequence is considered positive or negative, however, is dependent on the animal that receives it. What motivates one pet may not motivate another and what one pet considers aversive (yelling or knee in the chest) another may not consider aversive.

See **Table 1** for the differences between classical and operant conditioning.

Positive reinforcement
- Definition: An event, stimulus, or condition whose presentation immediately follows a response (or behavior) and increases the likelihood of that response being performed again.[8]
- Example: A dog jumps up and grabs a sandwich off the counter. Obtaining food is positive reinforcement for counter surfing, making it more likely to happen again.
- Advantage: It is always easier to teach what is wanted because usually what an owner wants a pet to do is clear. Even if a behavior is rewarded prematurely or behavior that was not intended to be rewarded is rewarded accidentally, fear or anxiety has not been created.

Table 1
General features of classical versus operant conditioning

Key Feature	Classical	Operant
Muscles involved	Smooth (also glands)	Striated
Behavioral response	Involuntary, passive	Voluntary, active
Training involved	Pairing the neutral stimulus with the unconditioned response	Use of reward or punishment

- Disadvantage: The use of continuous reinforcement may only teach a pet to perform the behavior when the expected reward is present. Although this may not make for a reliable response, however, it does not harm welfare or create fear or anxiety. See schedules of reinforcement and timing for more information. Another disadvantage is that what is rewarding for one individual may not be rewarding for another. Additionally, pets may be rewarded in ways owners are not aware of and the behavior maintained in spite of any attempts to extinguish it.

Negative reinforcement
- Definition: The removal of an aversive condition, which also serves to increase the likelihood of a response being performed again.[8] One type of negative reinforcement is escape—the animal runs away, thus avoiding the consequence.
- Example: This is how a Gentle Leader head collar (PetSafe, Knoxville, Tennessee) can be used to stop barking. When a dog barks, a gentle upward pull on the leash closes the mouth and barking stops. When it does, the pressure is released along with a verbal reward. The dog learns that a pull on the leash closes the mouth and stops barking when the owner approaches to do so.
- Advantage: When properly applied, an animal can learn the correct response.
- Disadvantage: With poor timing, animals may not learn the association between the withdrawal of the aversive stimulus and their behavior. In addition, any use of an aversive is an issue of welfare for a pet if an alternate positive approach could have been used and potentially cause a classically conditioned fearful association with the stimulus or situation.

Punishment
Definition: The application or creation of an aversive condition, which results in a decreased frequency of a response.[8] Punishment can actually be either positive or negative.
- Positive punishment: Something aversive is added to the situation—whether that is a swat on the bottom, a jerk with a collar, or an electric shock. To be a punishment, what is added is something that the animal finds aversive, perhaps even painful.
  - Example: Electronic shock bark collars work on the principle of positive punishment: the dog barks causing the collar to shock the dog and thus the dog is less likely to bark in the future. The authors oppose the use of electric shock for training any animal.
  - Disadvantage: A key quality of positive punishment is that the aversive stimuli have to be painful enough to overcome the desire and innate reward of performing the behavior itself. What is aversive to one animal may not be aversive enough to another.
- Negative punishment: The removal of a rewarding stimulus or condition that serves to decrease the performance of a behavior[8]; in other words, taking something that the animal desires away.
  - Example: Negative punishment can occur several of ways: withholding a treat when it is expected, walking away if a dog does not sit when asked, and ending a play session with a mouthy puppy. By doing so, the likelihood of the behavior occurring in the future is decreased.
  - Advantage: Does not present as much of a danger to a pet as positive punishment and less likely to cause fear or anxiety.
  - Disadvantage: Can be frustrating for a pet, timing is important, and does not teach an animal the correct behavior it needs to perform to get the reward.

See **Table 2** for a visual depiction of the 4 types of reinforcement and punishment contingencies.

Extinction
- Definition: Extinction is the process by which a behavior is eliminated by no longer being reinforced.[9] Extinction is only effective if all reinforcement for the behavior can be identified and removed. Often identifying all reinforcement is difficult. This process is commonly used to eliminate many types of nuisance behaviors, including jumping up on people and whining or pawing for attention.
- Example: When a dog barks at owners for attention, they must withdraw all attention; they must not look at, talk to, or interact with the dog in any way; otherwise, the barking will continue.
- Advantage: Is relatively passive and does not involve anything other than eliminating the reinforcer.
- Disadvantage: In order to be successful, all reinforcement must cease each and every time the behavior occurs. Another difficulty is the appearance of extinction bursts and spontaneous recovery. An extinction burst is an initial increase in the rate and intensity of the behavior prior to being extinguished.[9] In other words, the dog says, "Really, are you serious about this?" and tries harder to get the owner's attention. Spontaneous recovery is a reappearance of the behavior even after being extinguished and without the presentation of the reward but generally at a lower frequency or intensity compared with the original behavior.[9] Extinction bursts and spontaneous recovery can be frustrating to owners and often lead to the incorrect conclusion that the behavior modification is not working. Therefore, owners must be warned that the behavior will get worse before it gets better. Finally, merely extinguishing a behavior is not enough because it does not teach a pet the correct and wanted response.

Counterconditioning
- Definition: Counterconditioning is the endeavor to replace an undesirable response with a favorable one.[8] There are 2 types of counterconditioning: classical and operant.
  - Classical: Uses food rewards to change the underlying emotion associated with a stimulus.
  - Operant: Asking for an alternate behavior as a substitution for the undesirable response.
- Examples
  - Classical: Using meat-flavored baby food smeared on an examination table so a dog associates being on the table and getting vaccinations with a desirable item.
  - Operant: Teaching a dog to sit and focus on the owner when another dog passes by on a leash-walk, rather than lunging and barking.

Table 2		
Contingencies of punishment and reinforcement		
Stimulus, Condition or Event	**Positive**	**Negative**
Reinforcement	Addition of a stimulus ⬆ behavior	Removal of a stimulus ⬆ behavior
Punishment	Addition of a stimulus ⬇ behavior	Removal of a stimulus ⬇ behavior

- Advantage: By teaching another incompatible response, an underlying emotional state can also be changed, thus not only getting a physical change in behavioral patterns but also a physiologic one.
- Disadvantage: When a dog is severely anxious, finding a food reward that is desirable enough to overcome the anxiety may be difficult. Thus, a product or medication intervention may need to be added to decrease the arousal level. In operant counterconditioning, if the stimulus intensity is too high, then the animal may be unable to perform the task.

Desensitization
- Definition: Desensitization is the method of decreasing an emotional response, such as fear or anxiety, associated with an aversive stimulus through repeated controlled exposure. This is a procedure that is commonly paired with counterconditioning, called desensitization and counterconditioning (DSCC), to change the underlying emotion associated with a stimulus and create a new behavioral outcome through either classical or operant conditioning. DSCC must be done in a controlled fashion, keeping pets under their threshold or tolerance level, in order for them to overcome the anxiety and facilitate a lasting change in behavior.
- Example: Slowly getting dogs accustomed to nail trimming by using a high-value food reward, starting with just touching the toe nails, rewarding compliance, and gradually progressing to clipping the nails.
- Advantage: Provides a lasting change in behavior from a previous fear-inducing situation.
- Disadvantage: Can take a prolonged period of time to develop this lasting change, especially if the behavior has been long-standing or the situation produces marked fear.

Implementation of Learning Principles: Timing and Selection of Rewards

For learning to occur and be long lasting, the frequency of reinforcement, the timing of the reward or punishment, and the value of that reinforcement must be considered.

When teaching a new behavior, the timing of the reward is important. Unless a reward is given within 5 seconds, it is likely that the pet is already performing another behavior and that is what has been rewarded. If the pet begins another behavior within the 5-second window, the opportunity to reward the desired behavior has been missed. Consider teaching a dog to sit on a verbal command. If dogs are asked to sit and they place their rear end on the floor but stand up when the reward is handed to them, then "sit and stand up" has just been rewarded. Additionally, the type of reward is important: although one dog or cat might work for kibble, another may only work for chicken—to get the best responses, what that animal finds rewarding must be used. It is also useful to pair a food reward with a verbal one. Sometimes an owner needs a pet to comply and does not have food, so the pet may be satisfied with a "good dog" on occasion.

The same timing parameters are necessary for punishment to be effective—it must be immediate, controlled, and effective. If a pet has destroyed something in an owner's absence, then punishment when the owner returns is for the owner and the pet being present with trash on the floor but not for the act of putting trash on the floor, which is the target behavior that is wished to change.

The schedule at which reinforcement is delivered is also important. If a food treat is given every time a dog sits when asked, then there likely will be a high rate of responding. If, however, an owner stops giving a food treat, sitting on request may go away. To make a behavior more reliable without rewarding every time, rewards need to be given in a variable way. Once a dog learns to sit on command, then the rewards come every third time, then every fifth time, then twice in a row, and so on. The goal is to keep the dog guessing about when the food treat will appear, so that the rate of compliance stays high.

Finally, the trap of repeating a request several times must be avoided. Each request should be given once wait for the pet to comply. If a pet does not comply (and the owner is sure the pet knows the request), then the reward is withheld. It often helps to walk away, take a break, and come back and try again. Once a pet learns that compliance means do it right away or no reward, then the behavior should be performed more quickly.

GENERAL PRINCIPLES TO GUIDE INTERVENTIONS
How to Get Started and Questions to Ask

Veterinary practitioners need to identify key information from owners prior to being able to set forth a behavior modification plan that will work for each individual patient.[10]

- o What exactly is the behavior they want to change?
- o What will the "correct" behavior look like?
- o In what situations or circumstances does the problem behavior occur?
- o Is this a normal behavior for the pet but an unwanted response for the owner?
- o What management would be useful and can the owner handle?
- o Are the owners willing and do they have the time to change an unwanted behavior?
- o Do they need more guidance or one-on-one help from a behaviorist or trainer?
- o What are their expectations for change, and are they realistic?

It is also important to ascertain the underlying emotion driving the undesirable behavior. Most behavior problems are the result of fear, anxiety, high arousal, and excitement. And these emotions can be changed with consistent, predictable interactions and structured environments that encourage a dog to choose an alternate desirable behavior. Finally, to make interventions more successful and help the owner move forward, it is essential that an intervention move beyond "stop this behavior" to "do this behavior," a task that is actually easier to achieve.

Medical Diagnostics

Veterinarians' first obligation is to perform a physical examination and diagnostics, including laboratory analysis and imaging studies, if warranted, on any patient. This is especially important if a behavioral change is truly sudden in onset (although most are not, once the behavior history is delved into) or occurs in an older animal as a very new behavior. Many behavioral changes can stem from primary medical concerns like pain, endocrine disorders, organ dysfunction, or malignancies. A standard minimum database for any behavioral assessment should include a CBC, chemistry panel, total T4 and free T4 by equilibrium dialysis if the T4 value is low, urinalysis, physical examination, orthopedic examination and basic neurologic examination (**Box 3**). This minimum database is also useful if psychotropic medication is determined to be an additional part of therapy. Once any concurrent medical diagnoses have been treated appropriately, it is important to remember that learning may contribute to the maintenance of any unwanted behavior[11] and behavior modification may still need to be implemented for resolution.

Helping owners manage unwanted behaviors is actually not difficult. Several simple steps and management tools can facilitate enormous changes in behavior. The

| Box 3 |
| Minimum database for behavioral assessment |

Examination	Laboratory Analysis
Physical examination	CBC
Cranial nerve function	Chemistry panel
Basic neurologic and orthopedic assessment	Total T4
	Free T4 by ED/TSH
± Imaging studies if warranted	Urinalysis

following interventions combined or alone can help create lasting changes in a pet and each is discussed in more detail:

- Avoidance of trigger stimuli
- Reward-based training and predictable interactions and consequences
- Behavior tools and products
- Behavior modification
- Ancillary products

Avoidance of Trigger Stimuli

When obtaining a behavioral history, it is important to identify all the triggers for a problem behavior. Although avoidance does not teach an animal a new behavior, it is an essential intervention. Avoidance can provide safety in cases of known aggressive triggers, prevent escalation of problem behavior, decrease the ability of a pet to practice and perfect problematic behavior, diminish a pet's reactivity associated with that situation, and facilitate learning in a low-arousal setting. It may be useful to compile a list of each triggering situation and triage that list from the most to the least dangerous or fear-evoking situation so that owners can clarify which ones require their maximal attention.

Avoidance strategies include:

- Confining a pet away from certain individuals or other pets
- Avoiding large crowds of people
- Leash walking in low-traffic areas and during low-traffic times
- Setting up privacy fencing in the yard

Other strategies may need to be implemented depending on the environment, family composition, and needs of individual families. Some clients find it easiest to simply avoid the triggers and do not wish to proceed with further modification. If an owner is able to safely manage a pet and implement stimulus-avoidance techniques, many problematic situations become tolerable and even resolved.

Reward-Based Training and Predictable Interactions and Consequences

Often owners have already attempted behavior modification on their own with guidance from books, television, the Internet, or a trainer.[12] Unfortunately, these are punishment-based confrontational techniques that put people at risk for owner-directed aggressive responses,[10] damaging the human-animal bond and creating fear and confusion for the pet. Numerous studies have shown confrontational and punishment-based techniques worsen fear, anxiety, and aggression[10–12] and a decrease in playful behaviors,[11] all of which damage the human-animal bond and may lead to relinquishment and euthanasia. Positive reward-based training has been shown to increase performance in a novel training task[11] and facilitate better responses to obedience tasks[13] that may equate to a better overall ability to learn. One study of 140 dogs also found that reward-based training rarely elicited aggression, regardless of presenting complaint.[12] Positive reinforcement training is essential to creating lasting changes in behavior without increasing anxiety or aggression or damaging the human-animal bond.

Clients who have not previously been educated on the clear benefits of reward-based training may be reluctant to change, especially in light of the popularity of media figures that advocate the use of punishment under the auspices of dominance theory. Owners may also think that punishment is effective, because they have witnessed it can stop an undesired behavior from being performed. When questioned, however, the onset of the undesirable behavior has not changed, but the ability to stop the ongoing behavior may be the effect. One of the risks of using punishment is that although outward manifestations of the behavior may diminish, the underlying motivation may remain. When the problem is aggressive responses, which are often due to fear or anxiety, a dog may no longer signal through lower-level aggressive threats but may bite if put in the same situations repeatedly. In effect, the dog has suppressed early warning signals of aggression, making the aggression seem more unpredictable, random, and severe in nature.[12]

To help restore the damage done by these types of training techniques and create lasting change, pet and owner must learn to communicate in a manner that is clear, predictable, and rewarding. This type of interaction has been called many things over the years: "nothing in life is free" (Victoria Voith), "learn to earn" (William Campbell), and many others, including "doggy please." The authors of this article use the "doggy please" concept to help owners understand the goal: predictable consequences for requested behaviors. This can help to re-establish trust between owner and pet and create clear communication. At its simplest, a dog or cat is taught a basic response, such as "sit" or "wait," using positive reinforcement training. Then, when pets ask for something they want—to be fed, to go outside, or to jump on the couch—the owner requests the pet to perform the task. The request is given one time and the owner waits for the appropriate response. If it is not given (and the pet normally performs the task), then the requested item is withheld. So, for example, a dog goes to the owner and paws for attention (or so the owner thinks). The owner response is to ask the dog to "sit." The dog complies; the owner pets the dog a few times and stops. Alternately, if the dog does not sit, then the owner does not pet the dog. The goal is to accomplish 3 things: first, it teaches the pet that when the owner wants something, the pet needs to comply with a command and sit quietly; second, it helps the pet learn to look to the owner for what to do in any situation; and third, it begins a form of communication that is clear and predictable, setting up a foundation for stable, anxiety-free interactions. A fourth, often unintended, consequence is that the owners learn that what the dog wants is information (ie, "What should I do?"), and when that is provided, the dog is calmer.

Behavior Tools and Products

There are a multitude of products available to help owners not only control their pet but also redirect their behavior to more acceptable outlets. An owner's ability to control a pet is an essential first step in providing safety, avoiding triggers, and applying behavior modification. There are many ways in which an owner can have positive control over a pet in a way that is nonconfrontational and safe for all involved.

Leashes
Set length leashes are always recommended over flexible extendable leashes. Extendable leashes are cumbersome and make it difficult to quickly bring a dog

back toward the owner when necessary. The line used on an extendable leash is thin and easily broken if a pet lunges forward or can wrap around appendages, causing serious injury. A set length leash of 4 to 6 feet is ideal to have constant positive control over a dog. The flexible leash is a device that might not make sense for training or walking but rather to allow dogs, especially small breeds for which the cord is sufficiently strong, the freedom to explore an environment while maintaining a means of physical control.

Collars

- Flat collar: Traditional collars that are useful for holding identification tags but do not provide control for walking if the dog pulls on lead.
- Martingale collar: Originally designed for sight hounds, like greyhounds, whose necks are larger than their heads. A martingale allows better control and prevents escape by tightening the small loop when the dog pulls, thus tightening the larger loop around the neck. It lies loosely around the neck when the dog is not pulling.
- Choke collar: A nooselike collar that tightens down and chokes a pet when tension is applied. This type of collar is not recommended due to the pain and injury possible when continually applied.
- Pinch collar: Also known as a prong collar. It is a series of sharp metal interlocking links, which forcefully grab into a dog's skin when tension is applied by the leash. The authors do not advocate the use of pinch collars because they are painful and have caused serious puncture wounds (**Fig. 1**).
- Shock collar: These collars apply an electronic shock to a pet when activated, either remotely or directly as a result of behavior performed by the pet (barking or boundary). Shock collars are punishment tools that are inhumane, can increase fear and anxiety, and are never recommended.

Head collars

Head collars provide a humane and effective alternative to commonly used neck collars—pinch, prong, or choke collars—that rely on punishment to achieve control. Head collars (or head halters as they are sometimes referred to) derive their effectiveness from the control of the head. An appropriately fitted head collar (**Figs. 2** and **3**) works through the ability to move the muzzle of the dog in the desired direction, causing its body to follow. They also work on a dog's oppositional reflex—the desire to pull against pressure, so that by pulling forward and upward the dog opposes by

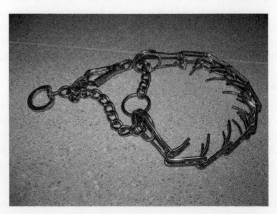

Fig. 1. Pinch collar.

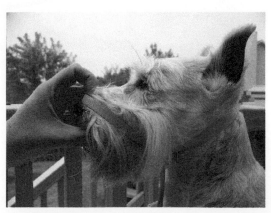

Fig. 2. Properly fitted nose piece on Gentle Leader reaches near the end of the nose but cannot be pulled off.

going backward and down (into a sit). Head collars provide an effective means of walking a dog without pulling, the ability to redirect the dog away from a stimulus, and a training tool for problematic behaviors, such as barking or jumping. There are many head collars commercially available including the Gentle Leader, the Halti (The Company of Animals, Surrey, United Kingdom), the Snoot Loop (created by Dr Peter Borchelt: http://snootloop.com/), and the Walk'n Train! Head Collar (Coastal Pet Products, Alliance, Ohio) (**Figs. 4** and **5**). Some head collars are made in 2 parts and, even if the nosepiece comes off, they remain on the dog (Gentle Leader). Others are 1 unit and, if the head collar comes off the dog, the dog is loose (Halti). These types of head collars require an additional short line clipped to the neck collar for safety.

Head collars are useful for dogs that pull when on a leash and especially for situations where good control of the head is necessary. They can also help with other unruly behaviors, such as jumping and barking. If an owner cannot safely handle a dog around the face and neck, head collars may not be suitable.

Proper fit and conditioning are essential when using a head collar. See **Box 4** for instructions on how to accomplish these 2 things.

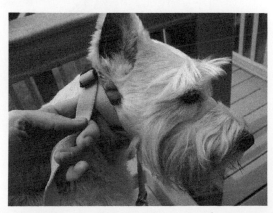

Fig. 3. Properly fitted neckpiece on a Gentle Leader; only 1 finger space between neck and collar.

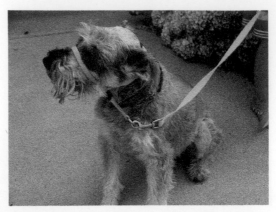

Fig. 4. Gentle Leader on a dog.

Body harnesses

If dogs are brachycephalic or do not have behaviors where a head halter is necessary, body harnesses offer a good alternative to punishment devices to gain better control and reduce pulling. A body harness is not appropriate for dogs that show aggression on walks or in other situations where control of the head increases safety. Body harnesses allow better owner control, especially for a well-muscled dog that pulls on lead, and can offer an easy alternative to head collars. Use of either a front clipping body harness, such as the Easy Walk harness (PetSafe), or one with dual control (front and back clips), like the Freedom No-Pull harness (Wiggles, Wags and Whiskers, Monroe, North Carolina), can provide an owner with better control and ability to redirect a

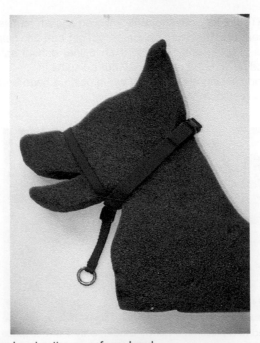

Fig. 5. Gentle Leader head collar on a foam head.

Box 4
Muzzle training

When animals are properly conditioned to the use of a muzzle, they accept wearing it and remain calm. Forcing a muzzle on a fearful and anxious dog creates an unpleasant association not only with the situation but also with the tool.

- Use a high-value reward like peanut butter or braunschweiger (liverwurst) smeared on the inside of the basket muzzle to entice dogs to voluntarily stick their nose inside the muzzle.

- Once dogs are comfortable placing their nose inside to retrieve the treat, work up to clipping the muzzle in place for short periods of time.

- For some dogs, this may take many sessions, and others are comfortable very quickly. This is especially true if the muzzle has been used inappropriately in the past.

- It is important to continue to associate the muzzle with positive things, rather than only when some procedure needs to be performed.

- Dogs should always view the muzzle as a positive situation.

- Emphasize to owners that muzzles should NEVER be used as punishment tools.

- The muzzle should be placed on dogs preemptively to prevent a bite incident and not after a bite has already occurred.

- Use of a muzzle does not mean that dogs should then be allowed to be placed in provocative situations. It does not allow subsequent complacency about avoidance.

---

dog away from a stimulus. Body harnesses often take less conditioning for proper wear and can also be worn indoors with a light dragline so that the owner has a physical means to redirect problematic behavior inside the home as well. As with head collars, retractable leashes are not recommended because they do not allow for swift or reliable owner control and can cause owner injuries. Body harnesses can also be used with cats to allow them safe outdoor access. The Come with me Kitty harness (Pet-Safe) is often well tolerated by cats and easy to fit.

Muzzles

There are many styles of muzzles (**Fig. 6**), including basket, cloth, or mesh. Basket-style muzzles are preferred for dogs needing to wear them for extended lengths of time because they can pant, drink water, and even take treats through the slots for counterconditioning exercises. For cloth muzzles to be most effective at inhibiting biting, they must be tight enough that a dog is unable to open its mouth making it impossible for the dog to pant or take treats (**Fig. 7**). A mesh muzzle provides good safety, but dogs are unable to take treats although they can often pant and perhaps drink water (**Fig. 8**).

Muzzles are a valuable tool that can be used when the owner needs to perform body care tasks, including bathing, nail trimming, or medicating ears on a dog that is aggressively aroused when handled in these situations. They also can provide safety in certain contexts or with certain individuals, including veterinary and grooming professionals.

Proper conditioning to wearing a muzzle is fundamental for comfort and welfare. Instructions are listed in **Box 5**.

Crates and confinement tools

Confinement training can be an essential tool for controlling, avoiding, and providing safety from unwanted behaviors once a dog or cat is comfortable being confined.

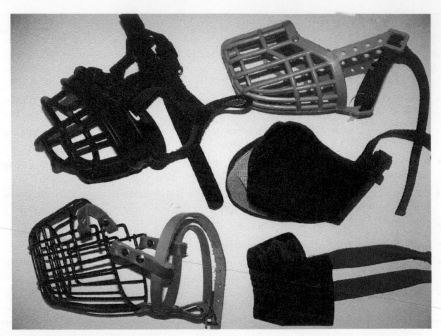

Fig. 6. Different types of muzzles.

There are soft-sided crates (**Fig. 9**), wire crates, or the airline-approved plastic Vari Kennel (Petmate, Arlington, Texas) available commercially, although the wire or plastic crates offer the best safety for aggressive patients. If a pet is small, does not jump, or is not aggressive, an open-top exercise pen, a child gate across a doorway, or a screen door can be used for confinement. Even cats can and should be crate trained not only for needed confinement but also so transportation to a veterinary hospital is easier and less stressful. A crate should be located out of high-traffic areas in the home and preferably also behind a closed lockable door if aggression is a concern. See **Box 6** for crate training tips. The type of confinement used should depend on the problem behavior; aggressive animals should be behind secure confinement where the ability

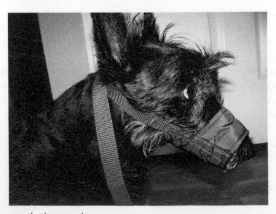

Fig. 7. Dog wearing a cloth muzzle.

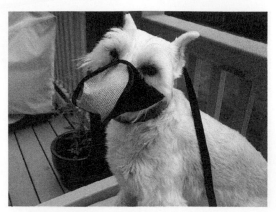

Fig. 8. Dog wearing a mesh muzzle.

to interact with and touch the pet is impossible. Large dogs that become aggressively aroused at the sight of people or other pets may plunge right through the screening, making this a nonviable option.

Behavior Modification

The ultimate goal of behavior modification is to replace undesirable behaviors with new, desired ones. For that to occur, both clinician and owner should have a clear idea of what that new behavior would look like. Once an alternate behavior has been determined, training can take place using positive reinforcement (food rewards).

Box 5
Crate training tips

- Proper conditioning is necessary prior to usage.
- Ensure the crate is used preemptively and not for punishment purposes.
- A crate should always be viewed as a positive place.
- Teach the dog or cat to go into and come out on command—use clicker training or food rewards thrown into and outside the crate.
- Wet food smeared on the back wall of the crate lures an animal inside.
- Both actions need to be associated with a word or phrase of the owners choosing (for example—"kennel up" and "come on out").
- Once an animal is sufficiently comfortable going in and out, the door can be shut for brief periods of time and then opened.
- Only release an animal when it is calm and quiet, so keep initial confinement times very short.
- Time spent in the crate should be pleasant: use of food dispensing toys can facilitate calm, pleasant activity inside.
- Use food dispensing toys, like a Kong (The Kong Company, Golden, Colorado) stuffed with peanut butter or canned food to facilitate a positive experience.
- Owners can progressively move further and further away from the crate until pets are able to be comfortable in their absence.

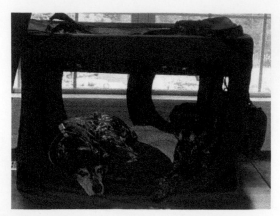

Fig. 9. Dogs in soft-sided crate.

As discussed previously, creating the proper environment for learning is essential to be successful. The following new behaviors are useful for many of the problematic behaviors that dogs and cats perform. To have the greatest utility, each of these tasks should be taught and practiced with minimal distractions and over time progress to different locations and circumstances.

The combination of "sit" and "stay" can be useful to keep a pet away from an aggressive provoking trigger. A "sit" command is easily taught by using a high-value food reward and luring a pet's nose up and back, resulting in the dog falling into a seated position, which then is coupled with the word (sit) and rewarded. Once repetition produces a robust sit, the lure can be phased out. "Stay" is taught by gradually increasing the distance the owner steps away from the pet and lengthening the time of each immobile interval. Initially a tether and body harness may be

---

Box 6
Retrieving stolen items

- First, try trading the dog for a high-value reward, such as a turkey hotdog.
- Never trade directly in front of the dog and the object; many dogs quickly eat the food item and quickly grab the stolen object, possibly resulting in a bite.
- Show the dog the delectable food and then toss several of them across the room and encourage the dog to follow them.
- If the dog goes far enough away, it may be safe to pick up the item.
- Otherwise, the dog should be lured with the food away from the stolen item and into a safe location.
- Lure the pet by holding onto the food and using a series of "come" and "sit" commands until the dog is at a safe distance.
- For additional safety, lure the dog into a secure room or crate and close the door before picking up the item.
- If another person is in the home, he or she can go and pick up the item and dispose of it properly.
- In some cases, "changing the subject," such as ringing the doorbell and retrieving the stolen object after the dog drops it and while its focus remains on the door, may distract a dog.

useful to physically restrain the pet in a set location but can be phased out unless necessary for safety purposes.

A "watch me" or "look" command teaches a dog to focus on the owner. At its simplest, this task allows a pet to change attention from other possibly provocative stimuli to the owner, who can then praise calm and quiet behavior. Several methods are used to teach this behavior to dogs and cats. Initially, show the pet a highly valued food item, close the palm, and bring it up to eye level. The pet naturally will look at the owner's eyes because the food item is located there. Pair this action with the command and reward the look with the food. Gradually increase the held length of the gaze and phase out continuous food rewards.

Often it is necessary to quickly but calmly remove a dog from an approaching stimulus that might trigger an unwanted response. When outdoors, a reverse of direction can be linked with a verbal phrase so the dog and owner can leave the situation. A 180° turn in the opposite direction can be taught to a dog using a head collar and food reward and luring the dog in the direction the owner wants it to travel. This task can become associated with a verbal prompt—"let's go," "follow me," or whatever the owner chooses to use. At the heart of this intervention is increasing the distance between the pet and the stimulus and can be accomplished by crossing the street. Once a task has been reliably learned, when owners see the stimulus approaching from afar they can cross the street to increase the distance between the dog and the stimulus, which should diminish the reactivity and fear.

Training a pet to go to a safe place on command can provide owners with the safety needed to allow people into the home. This safe place should be selected based on the behavior problem and the household needs. The place can be a dog bed in a low-traffic spot in the living area (with or without a tie-down/tether which are only used under supervision), a separate room that can be closed off using a baby gate or door, or a crate. The dog can be coaxed onto a dog bed or into a room by tossing treats and pairing it with a "go to place" command. Alternately, the dog can be walked to the spot using a head collar and leash and rewarded with treats for correct placement. Pair the "go to place" command with confinement training if using a room or crate. These same techniques can be used with cats.

Ancillary Products

Fear and anxiety are underlying components of many aggressive or problematic behaviors exhibited by companion animals. A pet's heightened arousal level can prevent the learning of a new task or alternate behavior, making management or modification nearly impossible. In these cases, it may be necessary to use ancillary products to decrease a pet's anxiety level first, prior to successful implementation of behavior modification.

Pheromones

The use of Adaptil pheromone products (for dogs) (Ceva, Lenexa, Kansas) in either a collar, diffuser, or spray format has been shown to decrease anxiety in puppies,[14] diminish noise and storm phobias,[15] decrease anxiety in the veterinary setting,[16] reduce stress of dogs in a shelter environment,[17] and help in the treatment of separation anxiety. These products are clinically useful to decrease arousal level in dogs to facilitate learning. A diffuser can be plugged into a confinement room or next to a crate and in rooms where dogs spend a majority of their time. The collar can be worn at all times, allowing a pet to have pheromone effect even when not inside the home environment. The spray can be used on a bandana, body wrap, or calming cap or sprayed in an examination room or on the hands of veterinary staff.

Feliway (Ceva) (for cats) is the synthetic analog to the feline facial pheromone and is available in a diffuser or spray format. Studies have shown efficacy in using Feliway to alleviate stress-induced behaviors,[18] decrease urine spraying,[19] and calm cats in the veterinary setting[20] and is anecdotally useful for the introduction of new cats to a household.

NurtureCALM collars for cats and dogs (Meridian Animal Health, Omaha, Nebraska) are also commercially available pheromone collars. At the present time these products have no studies supporting their efficacy in anxiety-producing situations in dogs and cats.

Nutraceuticals and herbal supplements

Anxitane (Virbac Animal Health, Fort Worth, Texas) contains L-theanine, an amino acid found naturally in green tea. L-theanine increases concentrations of γ-aminobutyric acid and levels of both serotonin and dopamine.[21] When tested in a laboratory setting, L-theanine decreased anxiety-related behaviors associated with fear of people.[22] The product labeling suggests twice-daily administration with additional doses prior to stressful events, such as thunderstorms, fireworks displays, or travel. The product is formulated as a highly palatable chewable tablet that is anecdotally well tolerated even by cats.

Harmonease (Veterinary Products Laboratories, Phoenix, Arizona) is an herbal supplement containing the active ingredients *Magnolia officinalis* and *Phellodendron amurense*. Harmonease has been shown in a laboratory setting to reduce anxiety-related behaviors from noise phobias[23] and may be useful for other situational anxiety-based behaviors as well. For noise phobias, the product manufacturers recommend starting the product 1 week prior to an event.

There are many senior supplements available that may be able to help with early cognitive decline and dysfunction, including Novifit (Virbac Animal Health, Fort Worth, Texas), Senilife (Ceva, Lenexa, KS), and Neutricks (Quincy Animal Health, Madison, Wisconsin).[24] Because cognitive dysfunction is a diagnosis of exclusion, these supplements may be useful when a behavior problem is a new manifestation in an older pet.

Food

Royal Canin recently introduced the Calm diet (Royal Canin, St Charles, Missouri), which is available in a dry formulation for both cats and dogs under 33 lb. Calm contains alpha-casozepine, a bovine derived casein milk protein, and L-tryptophan, which is an amino acid precursor for serotonin. On a single-blind crossover study of 44 owned dogs, Calm was effective in reducing owner-reported anxiety-based behaviors.[25] Alpha-casozepine (Zylkène, Vétoquinol, Fort Worth, Texas) is also available as a separate supplement in some countries and recently has become available in the United States. Many cat and small dog owners find difficulty in administering medication or supplements to their pets, making the Calm diet a beneficial adjunctive therapy for relieving anxiety, simply by providing the product as the sole source of caloric intake. Anecdotally, the diet is highly palatable and seems well tolerated gastrointestinally after a proper changeover period.

When cognitive dysfunction is suspected, dietary modification may be warranted. Hill's Prescription Diet B/D (Hill's Pet Nutrition, Topeka, Kansas) and Purina Vibrant Maturity formula for senior dogs (Nestlé Purina, St Louis, Missouri) both offer diets that help to delay age-related cognitive changes and reduce the toxic effects of free radicals.[26,27]

Environmental Enrichment and Exercise

Many pets live in environments that are deprived of enrichment and many do not receive adequate daily exercise. Lack of environmental enrichment and exercise can contribute to or exacerbate many behavior problems. Addressing enrichment in dogs and cats is an imperative step in the behavior modification process and more information is found in the chapter on enrichment by Heath and Wilson elsewhere in this issue.

SOME COMMON PROBLEMS AND INTERVENTIONS
Basic Underlying Tenets of Changing Behavior

The initial goal in any behavioral intervention is to begin with management and creating predictability to decrease underlying anxiety so learning can begin. Once anxiety is diminished and management strategies put in place for safety purposes, basic behavior modification can be implemented. Average pet owners have a limited knowledge of animal behavior and what they know may be inappropriately influenced by popular media sources. Dogs and cats live more in the present moment and respond to what is in front of them at the time. Two common areas of misunderstanding must be addressed to go forward with change. The first is the perception that a pet feels "guilty" for misbehaviors when the owner is not present. Canid appeasement body postures often foster this misunderstanding (**Fig. 10**). Rather than their guilt over the act, the dog assumes these postures because of the angry responses of the owner when they encounter destroyed property or house soiling that occurred in their absence. The dog does not look this way when home alone with the damage. Once an owner is able to conceptualize how the dog or cat really looks at the world, it makes the implementation of the behavior changes more reasonable. By understanding the underlying emotions that fuel the behavior, an owner can then clearly see what needs to be done to change the emotion to one where the acceptable behavior is easily performed.

The owners' job is not only to care for pets by providing food, water, a safe home, and veterinary care but also to protect them from things that make them feel frightened

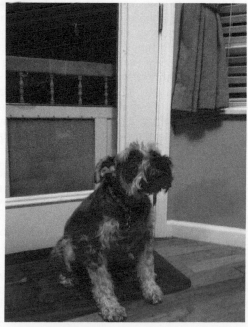

Fig. 10. Dog showing typical "guilty" look.

or anxious. Therefore, veterinarians must help pet owners understand that all animals come with limitations and that as sentient beings they should have the right to say "no." If a dog or cat is resting and a human approaches and the animal gives an appeasing or go away signal, this should be respected. Animals do not like to be disturbed when resting any more than humans do. If an animal is not comfortable greeting new and unfamiliar people, then owners should be their guardians and not make them interact when they clearly signal that they do not wish to socialize. If an animal is not comfortable in settings with many other animals (dog parks, play groups, or outdoor cafes), then owners should respect their need to remain at home. Naturally, some animals can be taught new behaviors, but it is always important to assess if a situation is something that pets "want" to do or "need" to do and decide, based on their response, how necessary it is to make them comply.

Below are some clinical examples of how these behavior principles might be applied for a variety of problems. Examples are selected for problem behaviors that are not discussed elsewhere in this issue.

Intraspecific Aggression Toward Familiar Dogs

Why it happens
Intraspecific aggression between 2 familiar dogs is often centered over resources, which include food, toys, resting spots, human attention, and access to confined spaces. These dogs often get along for the majority of time and play well, with fights occurring when access to a preferred resource is challenged or denied or the humans in the home artificially manipulate access order. Fights may begin when one or more dogs reach social maturity, when an elderly dog no longer reacts appropriately to social signals, or when health issues arise.

Owner involvement
In a multidog home, owners can play a crucial role in the development and maintenance of aggression. Feeding dogs in close proximity to one another and verbal admonishment for normal species signaling over resources can increase rather than decrease anxiety and heighten reactivity. Owners often give rawhides or pig ears to each dog in the other's presence, wrongly assuming they will not fight if each has its own. Owners may attempt to make things fair among all the dogs by trying to pay attention to all dogs equally and at the same time, despite signaling between dogs that they find this uncomfortable. An owner's verbal admonishment for low-level aggressive threats, such as lip-lifting and growling, which are often appropriate and clear to the recipient dog, can often exacerbate the problem by causing the other dog to continue pursuing the resource, thus leading the aggressor to escalate.

What to do
Avoiding stimuli Because severe injury can occur to either dog or any person attempting to intervene, safety is of primary importance. Dogs should never be left unattended and must be confined when owners are unable to supervise interactions. If dogs need to be separated during a fight, spray the dogs with a water hose, use a loud air horn to distract them, or have 2 people pick up each dog's back legs and wheelbarrow them backward away from one another. Never attempt to grab either dog by the collar or get in between them.

Resource allocation in a multidog household is key for harmony. Each dog should be fed separated from one another with no visual or physical access to other dogs during meal times. Treats need to be small and quickly consumed. If long-lasting food items are given, such as rawhides or stuffed rubber toys, the dogs should be confined away from one another through the use of baby gates, closed doors, or crates. In some cases, each dog may have a preferred resource, which another dog does not care about. Therefore, it can help to give each dog preferential access to the resource they most desire. Ultimately, regardless of the resource, the owner must be in control of access to any resource and of the dogs so that all resources can be given safely and calmly.

Behavior modification After fighting episodes, dogs can be reintroduced using head collars and leashes to prevent any unwanted behavior. Muzzle conditioning and confinement training can add an additional layer of safety to interactions. Each dog should also be under excellent verbal control, including being able to wait for the other dog to preferentially exit a doorway or go down a hallway, waiting for another dog to get human attention, and being sent away when it is no longer its turn for owner interaction. Tie-downs (under owner supervision and so that the dogs cannot reach each other) at a comfortable safe resting spot can be used for each pet and each dog should be taught to go to its spot on verbal command.

Fear-Based Aggression Toward Unfamiliar Dogs Outside

Why it happens
Like any fear-based aggression, there can be contributions from personality, genetics, and lack of socialization to other dogs or even traumatic experiences with other dogs.

Owner involvement
When addressing this problem, veterinarians need to emphasize that in many cases this is a problem for the owners and not necessarily the pets; therefore, they need to manage the expectations of the owners. Although dog parks and doggie daycare provide busy owners an easy outlet for their dog's energy, there are just some dogs who do not, and will not ever, tolerate being around other dogs, especially dogs they do not know. One of the issues with dog parks and doggie daycare situations is that there are often different dogs there each time a dog attends. This can be stressful for some dogs, because they have to continually gauge the behavior of the other dogs and determine how each dog tolerates interaction or play. Additionally, many owners think taking their dog to places with other dogs socializes them and forces them to accept and enjoy the company of other dogs. Leash walking can be especially problematic for dogs with fear-based aggression to unfamiliar dogs but is exacerbated by owners who take these dogs to parades, crowded parks, and public events.

What to Do

Avoiding stimuli
The easiest management comes in realizing and accepting a dog's limitations and avoiding the situations that cause it fear and aggression. A fearful or fearfully aggressive dog does not need to go to dog parks, doggie daycare, or the annual canine event. Often this advice is difficult for owners to hear, but it can also give them the empowerment to do what is truly best for a pet. Often a dog has 1 or 2 "doggy friends," however, and social interaction with these individuals can be arranged and may be satisfying for both owner and dog.

Behavior modification
When leash reactivity is the main concern, modification similar to fear-based aggression to unfamiliar people can be used. Commands to be used include an emergency exit command, "sit", "stay," or "watch me," or simply crossing the street to increase the distance to the stimulus.

Nocturnal Activity in Cats

Why it happens
Wild felids are typically nocturnal[6] and domesticated cats can often retain this crepuscular daily rhythm. This may manifest as excessive play behavior at night, fighting with other household cats overnight, excessive vocalization, or desire for food consumption. If this behavior manifests in an older animal, cognitive dysfunction should be considered.

Owner involvement
Owners may inadvertently reinforce this behavior by paying attention to the cat or feeding the cat in an attempt to quickly quiet the problem at that moment. This intermittent reinforcement can lead, however, to exacerbation of the nighttime activity. Owners may also not ensure adequate exercise and play and mental stimulation during the daylight hours.

What to do
Tools Owners can simply confine a cat away in a room alone at night or confine it out of the sleeping rooms to minimize disruptive behavior and eliminate possibility for inadvertent positive reinforcement. Timed feeding devices can be used to go off at regular intervals throughout the night to satisfy the cat's need for a midnight snack. Food dispensing toys can also be left throughout the home for the cat to eat and play as needed. Motion-activated toys can be useful so that the cat directs its playful energy toward an object rather than attempting to garner owner interaction.

Behavior modification Confinement training needs to take place so that management is successful. Ensure that all owner interactions are predictable and under verbal control so the cat understands when and how it is appropriate to interact.

SUMMARY

Veterinarians can help clients through many behavior problems by first understanding the basics of learning theory. Outlining a management and safety plan that keeps the family, other household pets, and any visitors safe can go a long way to solving even the most troubling of problems.[28] Many owners are satisfied once safety is addressed and provisioned for. Behavior modification can also be undertaken to curb and change unwanted behaviors, and there are many experts in the field available to assist clients if needed.

REFERENCES

1. Salman M, Hutchison J, Ruch-Gallie R, et al. Behavioral reasons for relinquishment of dogs and cats to 12 shelters. J Appl Anim Welf Sci 2000;3(2): 93–106.
2. Kass P, New J, Scarlett J, et al. Understanding animal companion surplus in the United States: relinquishment of nonadoptables to animals shelters for euthanasia. J Appl Anim Welf Sci 2001;4(4):237–48.
3. Miller D, Staats S, Partlo C, et al. Factors associated with the decision to surrender a pet to an animal shelter. J Am Vet Med Assoc 1996;209:738–42.
4. Shore E. Returning a recently adopted companion animal: adopters' reasons for, and reactions to, the failed experience. J Appl Anim Welf Sci 2005;8:187–98.
5. Scarlett J, Salman M, New J, et al. Exploring the bond: The role of veterinary practitioners in reducing dog and cat relinquishments and euthanasias. J Am Vet Med Assoc 2000;220(3):306–11.

6. Bradshaw J, Cameron-Beaumont C. The signalling repertoire of the domestic cat and its undomesticated relatives. In: Turner D, Bateson P, editors. The domestic cat: the biology of its behaviour. 2nd edition. Cambridge (United Kingdom): Cambridge University Press; 2000. p. 67–95.

7. Bradshaw J, Blackwell E, Casey R. Dominance in domestic dogs- useful construct or bad habit? J Vet Behav 2009;4(3):135–44.

8. Zimbardo P, Johnson R, McCann V. Learning and human nurture. In: Psychology core concepts. 7th edition. Upper Saddle River (NJ): Pearson Education, Inc; 2012. p. 132–69.

9. Malott R, Whaley D, Malott M. Extinction and recovery. In: Elementary principles of behavior. Upper Saddle River (NJ): Prentice Hall; 1997. p. 91–108.

10. Hsu Y, Liching S. Factors associated with aggressive responses in pet dogs. Appl Anim Behav Sci 2010;123:108–23.

11. Rooney NJ, Cowan S. Training methods and owner-dog interactions: links with dog behaviour and learning ability. Appl Anim Behav Sci 2011;132:169–77.

12. Herron M, Shofer F, Reisner I. Survey of the use and outcome of confrontational and non-confrontational training methods in client-owned dogs showing unde-sired behaviors. Appl Anim Behav Sci 2009;117:47–54.

13. Hiby E, Rooney N, Bradshaw J. Dog training methods- their use, effectiveness and interaction with behaviour and welfare. Anim Welf 2004;13:63–9

14. Denenberg S, Landsberg G. Effects of dog-appeasing pheromones on anxiety and fear in puppies during training and on long-term socialization. J Am Vet Med Assoc 2008;233(12):1874–82.

15. Sheppard G, Mills D. Evaluation of dog-appeasing pheromone as a potential treatment for dogs fearful of fireworks. Vet Rec 2003;152(14):432–6.

16. Mills D, Ramos D, Estelles M, et al. A triple blind placebo-controlled investigation into the assessment of the effect of Dog Appeasing Pheromone (DAP) on anxiety related behaviour of problem dogs in the veterinary clinic. Appl Anim Behav Sci 2006;98:114–6.

17. Tod E, Brander D, Wran N. Efficacy of a dog appeasing pheromone in reducing stress and fear related behaviour in shelter dogs. Appl Anim Behav Sci 2005;93: 295–308.

18. Griffith C, Steigerwald E, Buffington T. Effects of a synthetic facial pheromone on behavior of cats. J Am Vet Med Assoc 2000;217(8):1154–6.

19. Mills D, Redgate S, Landsberg G. A meta-analysis of studies of treatments for fe-line urine spraying. PLoS One 2011;6(4):1–10.

20. Kronen P, Ludders J, Erb H, et al. A synthetic fraction of feline pheromones calms but does not reduce struggling in cats before venous catheterization. Vet Anaesth Analg 2006;33:258–65.

21. Nathan P, Lu K, Gray M, et al. The neuropharmacology of L-theanine (N-ethyl-L-glutamine): a possible neuroprotective and cognitive enhancing agent. J Herb Pharmacother 2006;6:21–30.

22. Araujo J, Rivera C, Ethier J, et al. Anxitane tablets reduce fear of human be-ings in a laboratory model of anxiety-related behavior. J Vet Behav 2010;5: 268–75.

23. DePorter T, Landsberg G, Araujo J, et al. Harmonease chewable tablets reduces noise-induced fear and anxiety in a laboratory canine thunderstorm simulation: a blinded and placebo-controlled study. J Vet Behav 2012;7:225–32.

24. Landsberg GM, Nichol J, Araujo JA. Cognitive dysfunction syndrome: a disease of canine and feline brain aging. Vet Clin North Am Small Anim Pract 2012;42: 749–68.

25. Kato M, Miyaji K, Ohtani N, et al. Effects of prescription diet on dealing with stressful situations and performance of anxiety-related behaviors in privately owned anxious dogs. J Vet Behav 2012;7:21–6.
26. Milgram NW, Head EA, Zicker SC, et al. Long term treatment with antioxidants and a program of behavioural enrichment reduces age-dependant impairment in discrimination and reversal learning in beagle dogs. Exp Gerontol 2004;39: 753–65.
27. Pan Y, Larson B, Araujo JA, et al. Dietary supplementation with medium-chain TAG has long-lasting cognition-enhancing effects in aged dogs. Br J Nutr 2010;103:1746–54.
28. Horwitz D, Neilson J. Blackwell's five-minute veterinary consult clinical companion: canine and feline behavior. Ames (IA): Blackwell Publishing; 2007.

Canine and Feline Enrichment in the Home and Kennel:
A Guide for Practitioners

Sarah Heath, BVSc, CCAB, MRCVS[a],*,
Clare Wilson, MA, VetMB, CCAB, MRCVS[b]

KEYWORDS

- Enrichment • Behavior • Welfare • Canine • Feline • Environment

KEY POINTS

- Enrichment of the home and kennel environments should aim to maximize quality of life.
- Ensure that the environment supports natural species-specific behaviors.
- Remember that the environment is both social and physical.
- Encourage owners, and staff at boarding or research facilities to consider social and physical enrichment of the environment as a priority.

INTRODUCTION
Definition of Enrichment

Enriching a captive animal's environment, whether the creature is captive in a zoo, a laboratory, or a home, should involve enhancing their quality of life by making life more rewarding and meaningful. This should be done in accordance with their natural behavioral needs so as to increase behavioral choices and encourage species-appropriate behavior.[1]

Goals of Enrichment

The goals of enrichment are to enhance mental and physical development in young animals through the provision of a complex environment, and to ensure good welfare in adult animals by providing them with a complex environment that meets all their behavioral needs.

It is the role of the general veterinary practitioner to safeguard the welfare of animals and to ensure that the requirements of their 5 freedoms[2,3] are met. In addition to the

[a] Behavioural Referrals Veterinary Practice, 10 Rushton Drive, Upton, Chester CH2 1RE, UK;
[b] Behaviour Veterinary Practice, Bramley House, Coventry Road, Church Lawford CV23 9HB, UK
* Corresponding author.
E-mail address: heath@brvp.co.uk

Vet Clin Small Anim 44 (2014) 427–449
http://dx.doi.org/10.1016/j.cvsm.2014.01.003
0195-5616/14/$ – see front matter © 2014 Elsevier Inc. All rights reserved.
vetsmall.theclinics.com

traditional veterinary role of safeguarding health and advising on appropriate nutrition, it is important for the veterinary practitioner to also consider their contribution to ensuring that animals have freedom from fear and distress and freedom to express their natural behavior. To this end, veterinarians need to engage with owners and with those caring for dogs and cats in boarding kennels or research facilities and in their own veterinary facilities to offer appropriate and practical advice regarding the issue of environmental enrichment. This term is perhaps more closely associated with zoos and other wild animal facilities but it is important to remember that our companion animal species also deserve to live in environments that enhance their quality of life and ensure good welfare.

CONSIDERING ENRICHMENT IN THE HOME ENVIRONMENT

When owners take on a pet, they may be prepared for the financial commitment in terms of veterinary care, food, and equipment, and may also have considered time input in terms of training, especially when they are taking on a dog. However, very few owners have seriously considered the possibility of adapting their household to meet the behavioral needs of their new family member and are at a loss to know what is important in terms of environmental enrichment. In order to better understand the environment that their pet requires they must first understand their species-specific requirements. This is of particular importance to cat owners, who have very little in common with their new pet in terms of social behavior and behavioral requirements. That does not mean that education of dog owners is not also important; in fact, better education regarding social interactions with dogs and their requirements in terms of play, exercise, and training would go a long way to preventing many of the behavioral problems encountered by the general veterinary practitioner.

MAKING A CAT-FRIENDLY HOME

Creating a cat-friendly home is a vital part of responsible ownership, but it is also a rewarding process and one that can be great fun for kitten owners at the start of their new relationship. It is also crucial that owners are educated regarding understanding of cat communication and body language so that they can accurately interpret signs of stress, relaxation, and pleasure in their cats. Providing an enriching home environment involves paying attention to the home itself but also needs to consider the outdoor environment immediately around the home.[4] Cats have a fundamental requirement for a safe core zone within their environment to eat, sleep, and play.[5,6] Within this core zone, provision of access to 3-dimensional (3D) space can help to provide for natural feline coping strategies of elevation and hiding (**Figs. 1** and **2**).[7] Cats need to fill their time budget with normal feline behaviors, such as marking and hunting[8]; therefore, access to the outdoor environment is preferable wherever possible. When cats do need to be confined to the home, there is additional responsibility for owners to ensure that the indoor environment makes sufficient provision for the performance of normal feline behaviors.[9,10] Confining cats primarily in an indoor environment is extremely challenging in terms of providing both appropriate mental and physical stimulation, and is not suitable for all cats. The domestic cat has descended from solitary wild cats and, although as a species they are highly flexible in terms of social organization[6,11–13] and many individuals can adapt to group living, they are very sensitive to stress caused by social factors. Therefore, modifying the environment to ensure feelings of security is crucial, particularly in multicat households or in neighborhoods with high cat densities.[4,14]

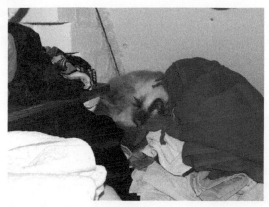

Fig. 1. Providing hiding places for cats is important.

Enrichment of the indoor environment
- Space
- Resources
- Privacy
- Ability to perform normal behaviors

Space

Access to 3D space can significantly increase the size of the home in feline terms, and cats should be given lots of opportunity to climb and explore. Elevation and hiding are

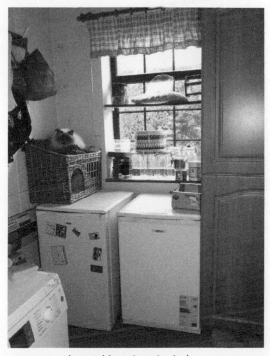

Fig. 2. Allowing cats access to elevated locations is vital.

important feline coping strategies that help in the regulation of stress. Therefore, provision of access to safe havens is an important feature of the cat-friendly home.[4,7,15] The use of shelves, cat furniture, tops of cupboards, and wardrobes can all be effective. It is important to keep these areas clear for access at all times (**Fig. 3**).

Resources

Cats have a requirement for free and immediate access to resources and these include the following:

- Food
- Water
- Litter facilities
- Resting places
- Safe points of entry and exit from the territory

It is not just the number of resources but also the distribution that is important. Cats need to be able to select locations that offer privacy when they are eating, drinking, toileting, and resting and ideally they should not be forced to be in visual contact with any other cat when engaging in these activities. They also need to be able to access these resources without running the gauntlet of members of other feline social groups within the household or neighborhood.

Privacy

Offering a better distribution of resources increases the possibility of privacy within the home, but offering specific sources of privacy can also be helpful. It also may be

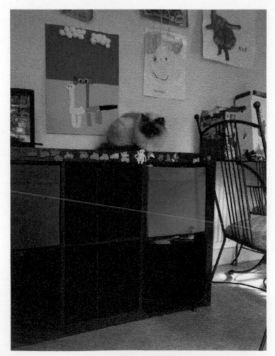

Fig. 3. Elevated locations should be kept clear at all times.

helpful to use pheromone therapy to ensure that the available core territory is recognized as a safe and secure location.[16]

Privacy from outside cats is also vitally important and potential visual access from other cats into the home is a significant factor. It is important to position essential resources away from windows and glass doors (**Fig. 4**) and it may also be helpful to modify the outdoor environment to remove vantage points (eg, to prevent unfamiliar cats from staring in through a window). Ensuring the core territory is protected from physical invasion is essential. Free access flaps are very stressful because of the risk of invasion by other cats. Instead, owners should consider installing the microchip-operated flaps that provide enhanced security.

When multiple cats are restricted to the indoors, litter boxes must be located throughout the environment in such a way as to allow cats to access them without being forced into close contact with other household cats. Ideally, if litter boxes are placed in confined spaces, they should be accessible by separate entrances and exits so that cats can avoid each other whenever possible and litter boxes do not become a location in which one cat may lie in wait to ambush another cat.

Ability to Perform Normal Behaviors

Cats have some fundamental behavioral requirements that need to be met, including the ability to hunt, play, and scratch. Although social play between kittens is seen, play in adult cats is usually object or prey-target based and involves practicing hunting behaviors.[17–19] If cats are given access to the outside world, many of these behaviors will be easily available in ways that do not cause any tension with owners or require any active effort on the part of owners. However, when cats have restricted outdoor access, whether part-time (such as being kept in overnight or while owners are at

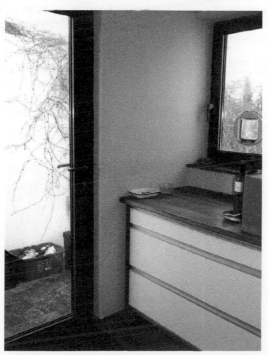

Fig. 4. This is a poor arrangement of resources, leaving the cat to feel vulnerable.

work) or full-time, it can be important for owners to realize that these natural behaviors may need to be specifically catered for within the home environment.

There is a misperception among many cat owners that their cat needs a feline companion to ensure good welfare. Normal feline social groups consist of related females and are highly dependent on resource availability,[11] and inappropriate introductions of unfamiliar cats can cause significant stress,[15] particularly if individuals lack appropriate intraspecific socialization. Socially bonded cats can hugely enrich each other's lives by allogrooming, allorubbing, and sleeping together (**Fig. 5**), but owners must manage introductions carefully for this to be a successful form of enrichment.

Enrichment of the Outdoor Environment

When cats have access to the outdoors, it is important to advise owners about ways in which they can enrich their gardens (yards) and surroundings and ensure that their cat's freedom from fear and distress and freedom to express normal behavior is protected when they are out and about, as well as when they are at home.

- Providing accessible and significant scratching places
- Blocking access by other cats, both visual and actual
- Providing hiding places and vantage points
- Providing outdoor toilets

Editors Note: The authors of this article are British, and in the United Kingdom (as well as much of Europe), it is uncommon for cats to be restricted to the indoors, as is commonly done in the United States. Nevertheless, all of the basic principles of feline enrichment detailed in this article can and should be applied to the indoor environment, and, in fact, doing so should be considered even more critical for the welfare of the domestic cat confined to the indoors. Special fencing, specifically intended to keep resident cats inside of a yard and prevent access by stray cats, is widely available and can be used to provide cats with a safe and enriched environment in areas in which unrestrained outdoor access can be very dangerous.

Providing Accessible and Significant Scratching Places

Scratching is an important marking behavior in establishing a buffer zone for cats in multicat neighborhoods, and scratching sites should be provided at the edge of the garden for this purpose. Softwood posts are easy to install and owners can encourage cats to use them by rubbing the post against already-established scratch posts to gain

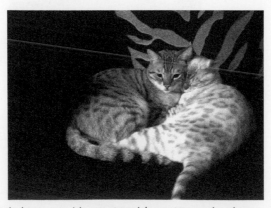

Fig. 5. Socially bonded cats provide great enrichment to each other.

familiar scents and scratching them with a wire brush to simulate scratch marks and attract attention.

Blocking Access by Other Cats, Both Visual and Actual

Traversing the territory of others is a normal feline behavior and is not particularly stressful, but when cats from another social group lurk in the territory or spend time resting within it, then stress levels rise considerably.[15] If the intruder cat uses vantage points within the territory to observe and threaten the resident cat, more overt behavioral issues may arise, such as indoor marking.[20] It is therefore beneficial to identify any vantage points used by other cats and block the view from these places into the home. This can be achieved by using a combination of plants, shrubs, sheds, and trellises. It can also be beneficial to make vantage points uncomfortable for cats to settle and rest within the garden. The use of long (8–10-cm) flat-headed nails that are spaced 4 to 6 cm apart along fences can help to stop other cats from resting, while still giving them the opportunity to traverse the garden while they are patrolling their own environment. Alternatively, spiky plastic door mats or intruder-deterrent plastic spikes can be used. Obviously, it is essential that owners do not use anything that could be dangerous for, or cause injury to, other cats.

Providing Hiding Places and Vantage Points

The resident cat needs easily defended resting places within its outdoor environment from which it can observe its surroundings and monitor the behavior of other neighborhood cats. It can be beneficial to fix shelves to fences or walls or even to place wooden platforms in trees so that the cat has elevated locations in which to rest.[21] It can also help to clear shelves in an open garden shed so that cats can sit by windows and look out. The provided vantage points must face away from the house and into the garden so as to prevent other cats from using them to intimidate the resident when it is in the house. They should also be positioned in locations that prevent the resident cat from intimidating his neighbors in their houses. For cats living in very densely populated feline neighborhoods, it may be beneficial to provide hiding places and vantage points, which can be achieved by investing in planters, pots, and patio furniture. When cat flaps are being installed, they should be positioned so that the cat has shelter and privacy as it leaves the safety of the house. This can be achieved by the strategic use of patio furniture and potted plants and by ensuring that the cat flap does not open onto visually vulnerable locations (**Fig. 6**). Outdoor enclosures for confined cats should make use of the valuable 3D space to provide elevation and hiding places and also have visual barriers to prevent intimidation by other cats outside the enclosure (**Fig. 7**).

Providing Outdoor Toilets

In situations in which there is social tension among cats in the neighborhood, some cats can feel intimidated, making it difficult for them to access suitably secluded locations in which to toilet. For other cats, the garden simply does not afford suitable locations in which to site latrines, because of minimalistic garden design and lack of border areas with suitable top soil or as a result of the weather, which may result in flooding or freezing of appropriate sites. In these situations, it can be beneficial for owners to provide outdoor latrines that are positioned in safe and easily accessible locations. Preferably, these latrines should be at the periphery of the garden and in sites that are obscured by shrubs so as to offer privacy. When there have already been incidents of intercat aggression or where levels of intercat tension are very high, the latrines should be sited nearer to the house and the use of hooded litter trays can also be considered, although these may be too conspicuous for other cats. An alternative is to

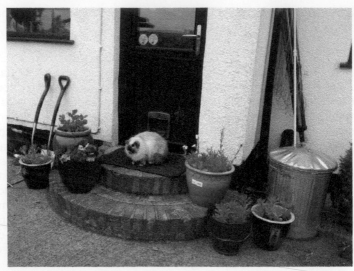

Fig. 6. Using plant pots around the entry/exit point can provide important security for cats.

make a sunken latrine by digging a hole 60 to 90 cm deep and 60 to 90 cm square, and filling the bottom two-thirds with pea-sized gravel for good drainage. Top up with soft white sand (playground type) and once the latrine is being used, start to scatter top soil over the sand. Use a litter scoop to remove feces and dig out and refresh the sand every 2 months.[21] Sand latrines do not get waterlogged or frozen, so are available all year round. This is particularly relevant to cats who suffer from idiopathic cystitis, in which frequent urination is to be encouraged, in addition to controlling exposure to stressful situations (**Fig. 8**, **Table 1**).[22]

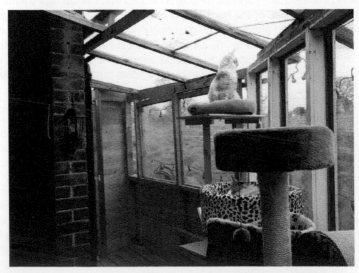

Fig. 7. An example of an outdoor enclosure with elevated resting places.

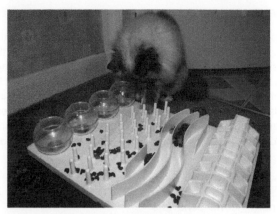

Fig. 8. Activity feeders can offer valuable enrichment for cats.

Table 1
Summary of making a cat-friendly home

Feline	Requirements and Examples	Conditions
Social	Cats can form social bonds but they are not dependent on social interaction for survival. Multicat household owners must be aware that their cats may be tolerating each other rather than being in the same social group.	The level of social interaction required by individual cats will vary and is dependent on socialization, experience, and genetics.
Physical	Three-dimensional space is highly important to cats that use elevation as a coping strategy when frightened. The environment should allow cats to climb, use vantage points, and to hide. Cats with access to outdoors will naturally exercise physically, but owners of indoor cats may need to provide opportunities for physical exercise, such as chasing toys.	The environment may need to be altered if older cats become less physically capable. Owners should remember that the 3-dimensional outdoor environment is just as important as the 3-dimensional indoor environment.
Mental	Predatory behavior is highly innate and can provide excellent mental stimulation for cats. Outdoor cats will find these opportunities themselves, provided the outdoor environment is suitable, but indoor cats need to be provided with appropriate prey targets, such as fishing rod toys. Activity feeders can enhance the life of indoor or confined cats.	If introducing mental stimulation as a new activity, ensure the cat is set up to succeed and then gradually make the challenge more difficult.
Natural behaviors	Marking (urine, feces, scratching, facial and flank marks), litter facilities, hunting, avoidance of threats through hiding and elevation, avoidance of other cats, vocalization, and so forth.	Owners may need reminding that their pet still has strong innate natural behaviors that need to be catered to.

MAKING A DOG-FRIENDLY HOME

Creating a suitable environment for dogs should be examined in a very different manner from that for cats. Dogs are social creatures, and for them the structure and layout of the physical environment is relatively less significant than the social environment (**Figs. 9** and **10**). Physical and mental stimulation should be met though provision of appropriate outlets for exercise and interaction with both the environment and social stimuli. It is also crucial that owners are educated regarding understanding of dog communication and body language, so that they can accurately interpret signs of stress, relaxation, and pleasure in their dogs (**Fig. 11**). **Table 2** summarizes these requirements.

Enrichment for indoor environment
- Space
- Ability to perform normal behaviors
  - Social interaction
  - Mental stimulation
  - Appropriate opportunities for natural feeding strategies
  - Toileting opportunities
- Freedom from fear and stress
- Training

Space

Space requirements in the indoor environment will vary depending on size and activity level, which will be influenced by the breed and age of the individual dog. However, in general terms, dogs should be given access to as large an area as possible. Particular consideration should be given to choice. For example, with regard to resting areas, dogs may choose different locations to rest during the day and night depending on activity in the house or on temperature. Dogs also should have the opportunity to eat meals or chews/treats without being disturbed by passing traffic. This could be achieved by feeding them when the family is seated for a meal, or by allowing them access to an area where people will not be passing through at that time. Some owners choose to crate or kennel their dogs when they are unsupervised, and although strict rules exist for licensed establishments, pet owners are left to make their own judgments. Depending on the reasons for using such measures, dogs should be confined

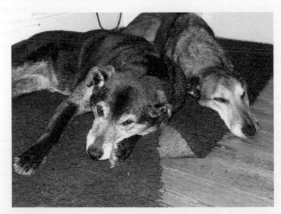

Fig. 9. For socialized dogs, canine companionship is essential.

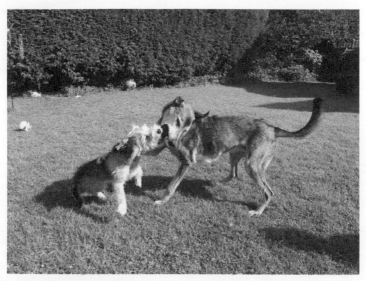

Fig. 10. Canine companions at play.

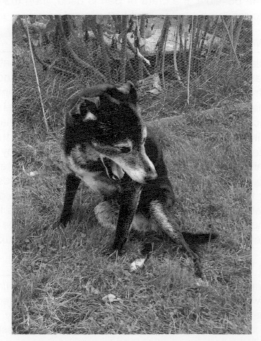

Fig. 11. This dog is showing mild signs of stress and owners must learn to recognize such signals.

Table 2 Summary of making a dog-friendly home		
Canine	Requirements and Examples	Conditions
Social	Dogs are an obligate social species and do not cope well with isolation. Opportunities for interaction with humans and canines should be provided. Humans must learn about dog body language to be able to effectively understand and communicate with their pets.	Dependent on socialization and experience.
Physical	Access to large safe areas to allow free running are important. Training a recall cue from an early age can allow owners to give their dogs plenty of freedom.	Dependent on breed, age, health status, and so forth.
Mental	Sniffing, social encounters, choice, reward-based training, problem solving (such as searching games, activity feeders, operant conditioning training).	If introducing mental stimulation as a new activity, ensure the dog is set up to succeed and then gradually make the challenge more difficult.
Natural behaviors	Scavenging, chewing, digging, vocalization, toileting, marking, social needs, physical exercise, and so forth.	Owners may need reminding that their pet still has strong innate natural behaviors that need to be catered to.

for the minimum time possible. If a crate or pen is used, then there must be ample space for the dog to reach up, stretch, and turn around.

Ability to Express Normal Behaviors

Dogs are highly social, and unfortunately many owners enforce unnatural expectations onto their pets by expecting them to cope with long periods of social isolation from both humans and from conspecifics. There is no ideal requirement in terms of how long dogs should be left alone, and the recommendation for this should be the minimum that is realistically achievable.[23] Full-time working owners may wish to employ a pet sitter, dog walker, friend, or neighbor to visit their dog during the day and, if their dog is well socialized to other dogs, considering canine company is also desirable Dogs are also social eaters and it is normal for eating to be facilitated in the company of their social group, but this may need to be modified in households in which there is interdog tension or food guarding.[24] Rules, such as ensuring the dog eats after the people in the household, are outdated and are not advised. Dogs that are appropriately socialized to humans, other dogs, and other species should be given ample daily opportunities to interact. Social enrichment is a necessity, not a luxury.

Mental Stimulation via Play

There is individual variation between dogs in the types of toys they find motivating and enjoyable. Some owners may say that their dogs are not interested in toys, but it is possible that they have not offered the dog sufficient variety. Novelty, particularly olfactory novelty, is an important factor in whether dogs show interest in toys.[25] Other owners may say that they stopped giving their dog toys because the dog destroys them. Many dogs gain enormous enrichment by chewing and dissecting soft toys, and if owners prefer not to spend money replacing these, they can provide their dogs with easily disposable enrichment, such as cardboard boxes or tubes with treats hidden inside. Appropriately socialized dogs will also gain significant enrichment through engaging in play with other dogs and with their owners. For dog-dog play, it is preferable for the dogs to be familiar with each other, so that they have mutual trust, to play in pairs, and be supervised to ensure fair play.[26] Younger dogs may more readily engage in play with unfamiliar dogs[27] and it is particularly important in this context that experienced supervisors intervene if one dog starts to intimidate another. Dog-dog play and dog-owner play appear to have different motivations, and it is therefore important in multidog households for owners to still ensure that they play with their dogs.[28]

Feeding

Dogs became domesticated many thousands of years ago as they learned to scavenge for human leftovers around early village settlements.[29] They have retained this omnivorous scavenging nature, and therefore an excellent way of providing enrichment is to feed dogs in a manner that requires exploration rather than from a simple bowl. This can be as basic as scattering kibble over the lawn or kitchen floor or can be more complex, involving homemade or commercial activity feeders (**Fig. 12**). Research on laboratory dogs in kenneled situations shows benefits of using activity feeders[30] and it is therefore likely that similar benefits can be gained for dogs during confinement in a home situation. Meehan and Mench[31] suggested that providing appropriate problem-solving opportunities to captive animals improved welfare. Dogs show social facilitation of eating, so eating at the same time as the family can be beneficial to their welfare, provided that there are no coexisting issues over food resource guarding.[24]

Access to Toileting Facilities

Dogs that have been effectively house trained may become stressed if they are not given access to outdoors when they need to eliminate. It is therefore important that dogs have regular opportunities to access a suitable outdoor environment where they feel comfortable to urinate and defecate. Owners who are working full-time should be particularly aware of this requirement, and, as advised previously regarding social isolation, the help of a pet sitter or neighbor can be used. Some owners may choose to fit a dog flap, which allows their pet access to the garden or yard when needed.

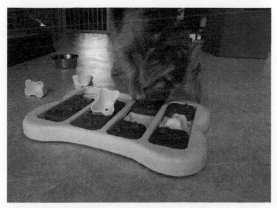

Fig. 12. Activity feeders are a great way to provide mental stimulation.

Freedom from Fear and Stress

Depending on the history of the individual dog, in terms of genetics and experience, certain situations may cause fear or stress to that individual. Dogs may seek reassurance from their owners or they may seek hiding places. It is important that the individual dog's coping strategy is recognized and supported. Owners with dogs that are experiencing fear or stress on a regular basis should be encouraged to seek referral to an appropriately qualified behavioral counselor (see further resources). Possibly most importantly those breeding and rearing puppies should be well educated about ways in which they can minimize development of fear-related behavioral responses with gentle human handling and good maternal care during the early weeks of the puppies' lives.

Training

Training a dog is an excellent form of enrichment for improving welfare, particularly if operant conditioning methods are used that allow the dog a degree of control and encourage problem solving.[31] Working with the dog to teach tricks, basic obedience, or higher-level tasks, such as agility or tracking, is also highly beneficial to the owner-dog relationship (**Fig. 13**). Owners should be actively encouraged to begin the training process early and to use reward-based methods and avoid aversives, which can be damaging to the pet-owner relationship and animal welfare, and increase the risk of aggression.[32–34] Every case needs to be assessed on an individual basis, and if large gatherings, noisy environments, or close proximity of other dogs are sources of negative stress for an individual dog, the advice about training should be modified appropriately. Repeatedly attending stressful training situations can be detrimental and may even increase the risk of negative behavioral change.

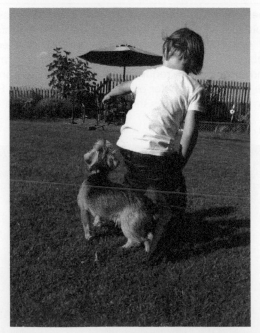

Fig. 13. Reward-based training provides enrichment and enhances the owner-dog relationship.

Enrichment for outdoor environment
- Physical exercise
  - Reliable recall training
- Mental stimulation
- Toileting opportunities

Exercise and Mental Stimulation

Physical exercise is important for the general state of health and fitness but it also provides an important opportunity for mental stimulation for dogs. The type of exercise that dogs require will vary considerably between breeds and individuals and should be tailored to each situation. Leash walking alone may not be sufficient for the more active dog types, which generally require greater opportunities for more vigorous exercise, such as running. Some of the smaller dogs that have been bred purely as companion animals may be better able to cope with leash-only exercise but this is not ideal. Sniffing and investigation are highly driven natural dog behaviors and exercise must involve the opportunity for these activities. Simply taking a dog jogging or alongside a bike will provide for physical exercise but will not give these exploratory opportunities or appropriate opportunities for social interaction with conspecifics. Many owners choose to tire their dog out by repetitive ball throwing, which again results in physical fitness but does not provide the mental stimulation that could be gained from the dog exploring his own surroundings and can also create problems of excessively high arousal levels. Social interaction with other dogs can be a highly enriching activity for dogs that are appropriately socialized and this is particularly important for dogs in single-dog households.

The Garden or Yard

The garden or yard will vary in its importance for dogs depending on the level and type of exercise they are given out of the home and also the amount of time they spend in the garden. For dogs that are not regularly walked off lead, a safely fenced garden can provide a very important area for physical and mental stimulation. A visible boundary fence must be used, as unseen buried electric fences that activate shock collars can have serious adverse consequences (Karen Overall, unpublished case study discussion at IVBM Lisbon 2013).[35]

Some breeds show a greater tendency for digging behavior than others, but for individuals that are highly motivated to dig (**Fig. 14**), owners should consider providing an area of the garden that allows this activity. There are many causes of digging, including to bury and store food, as part of the hunting sequence, to create a cozy resting or cooling place, as part of play or exploratory behavior, or due to frustration or anxiety.[36]

The amount of foliage present in a garden has been shown to be correlated with the amount of investigatory behavior seen in dogs, so increasing planted areas in a barren garden could provide improved enrichment.[37] Different surfaces, such as grass, paving, gravel, and sand, can provide further enrichment. If dogs are left outside while the owner is out at work, then provision of appropriate shelter is essential, and issues of potential noise pollution in residential areas must be considered. Providing areas of safety for the resident dog and preventing exposure to repetitive challenges, in the form of people or other dogs approaching or passing the property, must be considered.

Play behavior has been seen to occur more when people are present in the garden, even in multidog households, so it is important for owners to spend time in the garden with their dogs.[37] In fact, some dogs have little or no interest, and may even be more anxious when confined to the garden, unless accompanied by owners or other family

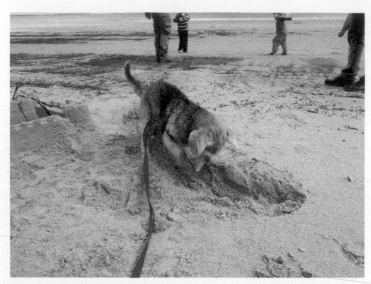

Fig. 14. Digging is important for some dogs.

pets. Excessive barking and escape attempts are a cause for concern for the owners, neighbors, and the dog.

Feed and chewing opportunities can also greatly enhance the time a dog spends in the garden. Bones have been shown to keep a dog's interest for longer (hours) than dry food dispensers (minutes) (**Fig. 15**, see **Table 2**).[37]

CONSIDERING ENRICHMENT IN THE KENNEL ENVIRONMENT

To assist in designing boarding or research kennel facilities, and maximizing the benefits of existing premises, it is useful to consider the following criteria:

- Space
- Toileting facilities
- Provision for appropriate species-specific stimulation

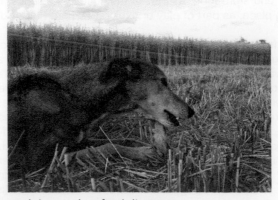

Fig. 15. Bones last much longer than food dispensers.

- Freedom from fear and stress
- Ease of management and maintenance of hygiene

In addition to the preceding list, for dog and cat rehoming shelters it is important also to consider how the environment can affect rehoming potential through influencing the behavior of those animals. Although good welfare during their stay is clearly crucial, rehoming provides the most appropriate long-term welfare option for these animals.[38]

Spatial Requirements

The space requirements vary according to the species, the breed, and the individual, as well as on the duration of stay and the animal's health status. There are written guidelines regarding housing of animals in both research and boarding establishments, and these must be adhered to. However, it should be remembered that these are the minimum standards and where possible exceeding these guidelines will be beneficial. Increasing pen size has been shown to increase activity in shelter and laboratory dogs.[39–41]

The amount of available space can be significantly improved for long-stay cats by providing variation of height within the pen, which also allows the cats to use their natural stress-coping strategy of elevation. Dog kennels need to be large enough for the dog to stand up, lie down, turn around, and sit comfortably, and when they are boarding for long periods or are in long-term research facilities, provision of larger areas that allow physical exercise also should be considered. Outdoor housing has been shown to increase activity in laboratory dogs and should be considered a beneficial enrichment.[42]

Toileting Facilities

When cats are confined in catteries or research facilities, it is important to provide them with toileting facilities that favor normal elimination behaviors. For boarding cats, it is also important to take into account the normal toileting facilities for that particular individual when it is at home.[43] For this reason, the following criteria need to be considered:

- Adequately sized litter tray
- Suitable soft and rakeable litter (preferably one that is familiar to the cat)
- Sufficient depth of litter to allow for natural toileting behavior
- Provision of privacy where possible
- Adequate cleaning regimen

For dogs, it is important to ensure sufficient access to elimination sites that the individual considers acceptable. House-trained dogs may be very distressed if "forced" to eliminate "indoors" during their stay in kennels and may retain urine or feces for prolonged periods in an attempt to avoid soiling indoors. Dogs will learn substrate and location preferences for toileting and, depending on their individual experiences, may prefer to toilet on grass, paving, or gravel, for example.

Provision for Appropriate Species-Specific Stimulation

Both dogs and cats require physical and mental stimulation during their time in confined accommodation, and care must be taken to provide adequate and appropriate stimulation in relation to the species and the individual's clinical condition. Visual access may be important for dogs by providing stimulation in the kennels,[44] whereas the ability to hide is a prerequisite for cats, and visual access should be minimized.

Dogs are social creatures, and provision of human interaction is likely to be benefi-cial, although obviously this will be subject to the level of socialization and resulting fear responses of the individual. It also can be beneficial for dogs to be group housed rather than individually housed to enhance their welfare, provided they are socially compatible.[45] If aggression arises only at feeding times, this might be the only time that access needs to be restricted (eg, tie down, cage feeding). Cats, on the other hand, are not obligate social creatures, and provision of stimulation that is not people dependent may be preferable,[46] particularly depending on their socialization history.[47] Cats that are appropriately socialized with other cats[17] may find interactions with their own species enriching, but this must be done with great care to provide a variety of heights and hides and sufficient space.

Stimulation opportunities should take into account natural species-specific behav-iors and time budgets. Therefore, provision of opportunities for chewing, digging, and engaging in social interaction will be relevant for dogs, whereas for cats it is important to ensure opportunities for observing, patrolling of territory (by ensuring routes are passable), and climbing. Benefits also have been found through providing appropriate enrichment toys to individually housed cats in terms of increased physical activity.[48]

Freedom from Fear and Stress

Frightened animals will often prefer to hide and, as long as it does not impair moni-toring, offering a shelter within the enclosure may provide comfort for the frightened animal.

Segregation of species can be important in reducing fear and stress and this may be total, by using species-specific areas in catteries and boarding kennels, or partial, by using strategic use of barriers.

Sensory challenges should be evaluated in light of species-specific behavior to minimize freedom from fear and stress. Factors, such as metal pen doors, dogs bark-ing within kennels, and cat transportation across the site, will need to be considered. On the other hand, appropriate auditory stimulation, such as classical music, has been shown to have beneficial effects on dogs in the kennel environment.[49]

The use of pheromones within the veterinary and kenneled environment, both boarding and research, has been shown to be beneficial in terms of reducing anxiety in both dogs and cats.[50,51]

Ease of Management and Maintenance of Hygiene

There is often a compromise to be made between the demands of the staff and those of the animals. Management necessitates clear visibility of the animals, but this must be balanced with freedom from fear and stress. Housing needs to be easily cleaned, but materials also need to offer comfort and low levels of auditory stress. Cost also must be taken into account, but animal needs, such as sufficient volumes of cat litter,[43] should not be compromised.

Personnel Requirements

To maximize welfare in kenneled environments, it is important to pay attention to phys-ical criteria relating to the pen sizes and structure, but the human element is also important, and ideally the personnel working within hospitalization wards should offer the following:

- Predictable temporal routine
- Unambiguous communication
- Appropriate handling and restraint

Predictable temporal routine

For animals undergoing medium-term to long-term stays in the kennel environment, the development of a predictable routine is important. Cats have been shown to have elevated physiologic and behavioral indicators of stress as a result of unpredictable management routines, and research has shown that unpredictability significantly increases the impact of negative experiences.[7,52,53]

Unambiguous communication

Consistency and predictability are important factors in controlling the negative effects of stressful situations, and consistent communication with animals being kept in confined environments is essential.

Try to avoid rushing interaction with the animals because of human time constraints, and remember that routine jobs, such as feeding and cleaning, are important activities that must be adequately addressed.

Appropriate handling and restraint

Most animals in the research environment require some type of restraint at some point during their time in the facility, but restraint can be easily misinterpreted as confrontation. Therefore, it is important to consider how we can ensure that every handling experience is as positive as possible.[54,55] The requirements will vary according to whether the animal is healthy or is undergoing some procedure, but in either case, the methods of handling and restraint should aim to minimize suffering, both physical and mental.

Regardless of the species, chemical restraint should be considered if the animal is severely distressed, the procedure is painful, or the staff are at risk.

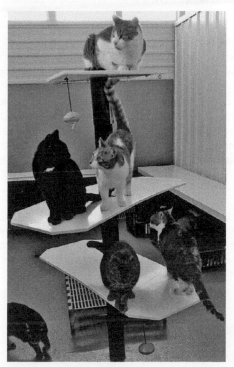

Fig. 16. Increasing 3D space in confined facilities.

Table 3 Summary of enhancing welfare in confined cats and dogs		
Confined Animals	Canine	Feline
Routine	Predictable routine and interaction are essential to reduce stress.	
Procedures	Animals in research facilities that are undergoing regular procedures, such as blood sampling, should be trained to accept such procedures using reward-based methods.	
Social	If appropriate, dogs should be housed in groups. Human interaction must be given regularly to dogs that are appropriately socialized.	Cats within the same social group can be group housed but must still be given opportunities for privacy and ample access to resources.
Physical	Access to large areas for free running must be provided on a regular basis, at least daily but preferably more often.	Three-dimensional space is very important.
Mental	Provision of novel toys, activity feeders, social interaction, opportunities for olfactory exploration, reward-based training.	Provision of novel toys, activity feeders, social interaction if appropriate, opportunities for olfactory exploration, reward-based training.
Natural behaviors	Sniffing, digging, social interaction, scavenging, and so forth.	Scratch posts, appropriate litter facilities, opportunities to express hunting behavior, hiding, and so forth.

Note that the information in **Tables 1** and **2** is also applicable to confined animals.

With the availability of short-acting, safe anesthetic agents and reversible sedative agents, there is no excuse for brute force or animal suffering in place of appropriate chemical restraint. Medication must be appropriate. For example, the use of acepromazine alone for the purposes of handling and restraint does not address fear and anxiety. Time should be taken to acclimatize animals to necessary procedural interventions, reward training, and counterconditioning for procedures, such as carrier transport for cats, nail clipping, blood sampling (if required regularly), or otoscopic examination, and tolerance of the proximity of specific equipment should be instituted at an early age and carried out on a regular basis (**Fig. 16, Table 3**).[56]

SUMMARY

As general veterinary practitioners, we have a duty of care that applies not only to the physical health needs of the animals in our care, but also to their mental well-being. Advising clients about how to enrich their home and kennel environments is an important part of fulfilling that duty of care and will also enrich the relationship between the veterinary practitioner and client.

REFERENCES

1. Young RJ. Environmental enrichment: an historical perspective. In: Environmental enrichment for captive animals. Universities Federation for Animal Welfare, Wheathampstead: Blackwell publishing; 2003. p. 1–2.
2. Dramboll report. London: HMSO; December, 1965. ISBN 0 10 850286 4.

3. Farm Animal Welfare Council press release December 1979. Accessed October 2013 at www.fawc.org.uk/pdf/fivefreedoms1979/pdf.
4. Ellis S, Rodan I, Carney H, et al. AAFP and ASFM Feline Environmental Needs Guidelines. J Fel Med Surg 2013;15:219–30.
5. Bernstein PL, Strack M. A game of cat and house: spatial patterns and behaviour of 14 domestic cats (Felis catus) in the home. Anthrozoos 1996;9:25–39.
6. Liberg O, Sandell M, Pontier D, et al. Density, spatial organisation and reproductive tactics in the domestic cat and other felids. In: Turner DC, Bateson P, editors. The Domestic Cat; The biology of its behaviour. 2nd edition. Cambridge (UK): Cambridge University Press; 2000. p. 119–47.
7. Carlstead K, Brown JL, Strawn W. Behavioural and physiological correlates of stress in laboratory cats. Appl Anim Behav Sci 1993;38:143–58.
8. Turner DC, Bateson P, editors. The Domestic Cat; The biology of its behaviour. 2nd edition. Cambridge (United Kingdom): Cambridge University Press; 2000.
9. Rochlitz I. A review of the housing requirements of domestic cats (Felis silvestris catus) kept in the home. Appl Anim Behav Sci 2005;93:97–109.
10. Jongman EC. Adaptation of domestic cats to confinement. J Vet Behav 2007;2: 193–6.
11. Crowell-Davis SL, Curtis TM, et al. Social organisation in the cat: A modern understanding. J Fel Med Surg 2004;6:19–28.
12. Natoli E. Spacing pattern in a colony of urban stray cats (Felis catus I.) in the historic centre of Rome. Appl Anim Behav Sci 1985;14:289–304.
13. MacDonald DW, Yamaguchi N, Kerby G. Group-living in the domestic cat: its sociobiology and epidemiology. In: Turner DC, Bateson P, editors. The Domestic Cat; The biology of its behaviour. 2nd edition. Cambridge (United Kingdom): Cambridge University Press; 2000. p. 95–118.
14. Ramos D, Arena MN, Reche-Junior A, et al. Factors affecting faecal glucocorticoid levels in domestic cats (Felis catus): a pilot study with single and large multi-cat households. Anim Welf 2012;21:285–91.
15. Levine ED. Feline fear and anxiety. Vet Clin North Am: Small Anim Pract 2008;38: 1065–79.
16. Pageat P, Gaultier E. Current research in canine and feline pheromones. Vet Clin North Am: Small Anim Pract 2003;33:187–211.
17. Mendl M. The effects of litter-size variation on the development of play behaviour in the domestic cat: litters of one and two. Anim Behav 1988;36:20–34.
18. Barrett P, Bateson P. The development of play in cats. Behaviour 1977;66:106–20.
19. Caro TM. Predatory behaviour and social play in kittens. Behaviour 1981;76(1): 1–24.
20. Herron ME. Advances in understanding and treatment of feline inappropriate elimination. Top Companion Anim Med 2010;25(4):195–202.
21. Bowen J, Heath S. Appendix 3, Advice Sheet 1, Improving the outdoor environment for cats. In: Behaviour Problems in Small Animals: practical advice for the veterinary team. City: Elsevier Saunders; 2005. p. 265–6.
22. Buffington CAT. Idiopathic cystitis in cats – beyond the lower urinary tract. J Vet Intern Med 2011;25:784–96.
23. Rehn T, Keeling LJ. The effect of time left alone at home on dog welfare. Appl Anim Behav Sci 2011;129:129–35.
24. Case LP, Daristotle L, Hayek MG, et al. Feeding regimens for dogs and cats. In: Canine and Feline Nutrition. 3rd edition. MO: Mosby Elsevier; 2011. p. 192–3.
25. Pullen AJ, Merrill RJN, Bradshaw JW. Preferences for toy types and presentations in kennel housed dogs. Appl Anim Behav Sci 2010;125:151–6.

26. Adler C, Mackensen-Friedricks I, Franz C, et al. Social play behaviour of group housed domestic dogs (Canis familiaris). J Vet Behav 2011;6:98.

27. Rezac P, Viziova P, Dobesova M, et al. Factors affecting dog-dog interactions on walks with their owners. Appl Anim Behav Sci 2011;134:170–6.

28. Rooney NJ, Bradshaw JW, Robinson IH. A comparison of dog-dog and dog-human play behaviour. Appl Anim Behav Sci 2000;66:235–48.

29. Coppinger R, Coppinger L. Wolves Evolve into Dogs. In: Dogs: a new understanding of canine origin, behaviour and evolution. Chicago: The University of Chicago Press; 2001. p. 39–67.

30. Schipper LL, Vinke CM, Schilder MB, et al. The effect of feeding enrichment toys on the behaviour of kennelled dogs (Canis familiaris). Appl Anim Behav Sci 2008;114:182–95.

31. Meehan CL, Mench JA. The challenge of challenge: can problem solving opportunities enhance animal welfare? Appl Anim Behav Sci 2007;102:246–61.

32. Rooney NJ, Cowan S. Training methods and owner-dog interactions: links with dog behaviour and learning ability. Appl Anim Behav Sci 2011;132:169–77.

33. Hsu Y, Sun L. Factors associated with aggressive responses in pet dogs. Appl Anim Behav Sci 2010;123:108–23.

34. Herron ME, Shofer FS, Reisner IR. Survey of the use and outcome of confrontational and non-confrontational training methods in client-owned dogs showing undesired behaviours. Appl Anim Behav Sci 2009;117:47–54.

35. Millsopp S. The ethics of shock-collar containment fences for dogs and cats. Association of Pet Behaviour Counsellors; 2011. Available at: www.apbc.org.uk/blog/ethics_of_pet_containment_fences. Accessed August 2013.

36. Odendall JS. An ethological approach to the problem of dogs digging holes. Appl Anim Behav Sci 1996;52:299–305.

37. Kobelt AJ, Hemsworth PH, Barnett JL, et al. The behaviour of Labrador retrievers in suburban backyards: the relationships between the backyard environment and dog behaviour. Appl Anim Behav Sci 2007;106:70–84.

38. Wells DL, Hepper PG. The influence of environmental change on the behaviour of sheltered dogs. Appl Anim Behav Sci 2000;68:151–62.

39. Normando S, Salvadoretti M, Marinelli L, et al. Effects of pen size on old shelter dogs' behaviour. J Vet Behav 2009;4(2):86.

40. Hetts S, Clarke JD, Calpin JP, et al. Influence of housing conditions on beagle behaviour. Appl Anim Behav Sci 1992;34:137–55.

41. Hubrecht RC, Serpell JA, Poole TB. Correlates of pen size and housing conditions on the behaviour of kennelled dogs. Appl Anim Behav Sci 1992;34:365–83.

42. Spangenberg EM, Bjorklund L, Dahlborn K. Outdoor housing of laboratory dogs: effects on activity, behaviour and physiology. Appl Anim Behav Sci 2006;98:260–76.

43. Neilson JC. Pick of the (cat) litter. Proceedings, 82nd Western Veterinary Conference. 2010.

44. Wells DL, Hepper PG. A note on the influence of visual conspecific contact on the behaviour of sheltered dogs. Appl Anim Behav Sci 1998;60:83–8.

45. Mertens P, Unshelm J. Effects of group and individual housing on the behaviour of kennelled dogs in animal shelters. Anthrozoos 1996;9(1):40–51.

46. Ellis S. Environmental enrichment: practical strategies for improving feline welfare. J Fel Med Surg 2009;11:901–12.

47. McCune S. The impact of paternity and early socialisation on the development of cats' behaviour to people and novel objects. Appl Anim Behav Sci 1995;45:109–24.

48. De Monte M, Le Pape G. Behavioural effects of cage enrichment in single-caged adult cats. Anim Welf 1997;6:53–66.
49. Wells DL. A review of environmental enrichment for kennelled dogs, Canis familiaris. Appl Anim Behav Sci 2004;85:307–17.
50. Tod E, Brander D, Waran N. Efficacy of dog appeasing pheromone in reducing stress and fear related behaviour in shelter dogs. Appl Anim Behav Sci 2005;93: 295–308.
51. Mills DS, Ramos D, Estelles MG, et al. A triple blind placebo-controlled investigation into the assessment of the effect of Dog Appeasing Pheromone (DAP) on anxiety related behaviour of problem dogs in the veterinary clinic. Appl Anim Behav Sci 2006;98:114–26.
52. Stella JL, Lord KL, Buffington CA. Sickness behaviors in response to unusual external events in healthy cats and cats with feline idiopathic cystitis. J Am Vet Med Assoc 2001;238(1):67–73.
53. Gottlieb DH, Coleman K, McCowan B. The effects of predictability in daily husbandry routines on captive rhesus macaques (Macaca mulatta). Appl Anim Behav Sci 2012;143:117–27.
54. Rodan I. Understanding feline behaviour and application for appropriate handling and management. Top Companion Anim Med 2010;25(4):178–88.
55. Moffat K. Addressing canine and feline aggression in the veterinary clinic. Vet Clin North Am: Small Anim Pract 2008;38:983–1003.
56. Landsberg G. Handling the difficult cat: From clinical examination to blood sample. In: Proceedings of the 9th International Veterinary Behaviour Meeting. Lisbon: 2013. p. 18–22.

The Pet-friendly Veterinary Practice: A Guide for Practitioners

Meghan E. Herron, DVM[a],*, Traci Shreyer, MA[b]

KEYWORDS

- Low-stress handling • Patient welfare • Staff safety • Handling tools • Safe restraint
- Chemical restraint • Pheromones

KEY POINTS

- Low-stress handling is important both for the safety of the veterinary staff and for the welfare of the patient.
- Before handling animals it is essential to assess the environment and the patient's response to it.
- Taking the time to create a behavior handling plan makes future visits easier and bonds clients to the practice.
- Understanding how and when to use handling tools is key to making patient visits safer, more humane, and more efficient.

INTRODUCTION
Why Low-stress Handling?

Low-stress handling may be a new concept for many practitioners, but the basic principles follow the oath taken by every veterinarian on graduation to further the prevention and relief of animal suffering.[1] The commitment to ensuring the emotional well-being of the patient should be equal to that shown toward the physical well-being of the animals under a veterinarian's care. Furthermore, because dog and cat bites are a substantial cause of injury in a veterinary practice setting,[2–4] handling animals in a safe and effective manner is essential in reducing the costs associated with personnel injury. Many clinicians groan in anticipation of a stressful appointment when they see a difficult dog or cat on their schedules, but they should consider how the animal, as well as the client and their staff, are feeling. Recent reports suggest that the perceived fear and distress an animal feels as a result of a veterinary visit is a major

[a] Department of Veterinary Clinical Sciences, The Ohio State University College of Veterinary Medicine, 601 Vernon L Tharp Street, Columbus, OH 43210, USA; [b] Veterinary Medical Center, The Ohio State University College of Veterinary Medicine, 601 Vernon L Tharp Street, Columbus, OH 43210, USA
* Corresponding author.
E-mail address: meghan.herron@cvm.osu.edu

Vet Clin Small Anim 44 (2014) 451–481
http://dx.doi.org/10.1016/j.cvsm.2014.01.010
0195-5616/14/$ – see front matter © 2014 Elsevier Inc. All rights reserved.
vetsmall.theclinics.com

reason why owners avoid bringing their pets to see the veterinarian.[5] This article helps veterinarians to change such problematic visits into the positive encounters they can be, as well as preventing problems from developing in the first place. All of this can be accomplished without taking much extra time during the appointment, and saves time and stress during future visits. **Box 1** lists the goals of this article.

BENEFITS OF LOW-STRESS HANDLING

- Enhance patient welfare
- Increase job satisfaction
- Bond clients to the practice
- Reduce time and resources spent on subsequent visits
- Prevent stress-induced aberrations in physiologic parameters
- Avoid personnel/owner injury and associated costs and liability

BEFORE HANDLING

Before touching an animal, several assessments should be made, including assessing the environment, assessing the patient, and self-assessment by the clinician. From this information, clinicians can create a successful handling plan and proceed in a safe and effective manner.

ASSESSING THE ENVIRONMENT AND MAKING IT COMFORTABLE FOR THE PATIENT

When assessing the environment, clinicians must consider how the animal perceives and interprets the associated stimuli. What an animal sees, smells, feels, tastes, and hears can strongly affect its well-being and emotional state.[6] Animals with previous frightening or painful veterinary visits may be classically conditioned to associate any or all of the surrounding stimuli with a negative emotional response (fear).[7,8]

MAXIMIZING ENVIRONMENTAL COMFORT

- Visual stimuli
  - Bright and/or constant light can be stressful for animals.[6,9,10] The presence of a tapetum lucidum allows dogs and cats to perceive light in greater abundance than humans, making what people consider soft lighting seem brighter and aversive.[11,12] Consider 60 W bulbs in examination rooms and treatment areas to provide softer lighting.

Box 1
Article goals

- Foster a better understanding of canine and feline body language
- Show how human body language affects the behavior of animal patients
- Learn techniques to ease animal stress and fear associated with the veterinary setting, thereby reducing arousal and aggression
- Promote safety for clinicians and staff
- Increase confidence in handling dogs and cats
- Provide tools for safe and effective restraint of fractious patients

- ○ Keep quick and sudden movements to a minimum, because animals may startle or suddenly feel threatened. If animals are not tolerating subtle movement, it may help to restrict their visual intake through the use of towels or other visual blocking aids, such as a CalmingCap (ThunderWorks, Durham, NC). Towels can be used to cover a cat's head during all parts of the examination and procedures that do not involve the head.
- ○ Cover cat carriers in the clinic with a towel until you are ready to work with the cat. If housing cats in a cage, provide a hiding option, such as a box or a partially covered cage front (**Fig. 1**) so that they can remove themselves from visual stimuli and have the perception of being concealed.[13,14] The sight of dogs or other cats in the lobby or treatment area can be highly stressful.
- ○ Admit fearful or fractious dogs and cats through a side or back entrance to reduce visual contact with other animals and strangers.
- ○ Take off your white coat. Animals may make visual associations with stimuli in the veterinary clinic, including the attire of the veterinary clinicians and staff, with a frightening experience (ie, the white-coat effect).[15] These animals may respond better without exposure to this fear-eliciting stimulus.[16]
- Auditory stimuli
  - ○ Speak softly and sparingly around animals to help them stay calm. Because animals begin to show symptoms correlated with increased stress when ambient sounds approach 85 dB,[17] keeping noise levels at or less than 60 dB is preferable.
  - ○ Avoid reprimands or using harsh or punitive tones of voice, regardless of the animal's behavior, because this is likely to increase stress and may exacerbate aggression.[18]

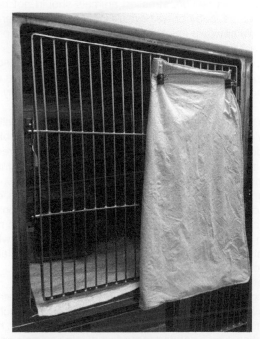

Fig. 1. A towel can be draped over part of the cage to provide a hiding option for the hospitalized cat while allowing visual observation.

- Avoid hard rock or heavy metal music because these stimuli have been shown to cause behaviors associated with stress in animals.[19,20] Staff members who prefer this music when working in a kennel environment should use personal sound devices and wear headphones.
- Play classical music or commercial recordings that might be calming such as Through a Dog's Ear (Sounds True, Inc, Louisville, CO). Classical music has been shown to increase behaviors associated with relaxation in animals.[19-22]
- Use sources of noise cancellation, such as white noise, to mask extraneous and potentially stressful sounds, such as barking dogs and people talking or moving in the adjacent hallway or rooms.
- Olfactory stimulation
  - Allow time for the chemical smell of cleaning agents to dissipate after disinfecting an examination room between patients. A similar period is also important for cage cleaning because placing an animal in a cage that has not fully dried after cleaning exposes it to harsh chemical scents.
  - Use alcohol sparingly during procedures because the strong scent is potentially aversive to animals. If an animal has had a previous frightening experience associated with the smell of alcohol, it may have a conditioned negative emotional response when exposed to this smell at subsequent visits.[7,8] Olfactory processing in the brain has a direct and widespread influence on the parts of the forebrain that affect odor discrimination, emotion, and memory,[23] making the degree of negative emotional association potentially more powerful than for other sensory stimuli.
  - Wipe down exposed surfaces, such as the floors, walls, and cabinets, after stressed animals because they have likely deposited scents and pheromones associated with fear and alarm[24-26] that may indicate that the environment is dangerous. For this reason, stressed animals should not be left in common areas, such as the lobby or waiting area, for prolonged periods. Be sure not to share towels between animals because the scents and pheromones associated with fear and alarm can transfer between patients.
  - Minimize exposing cats to canine odors by having designated cat examination rooms and/or wiping down and airing out rooms between canine and feline patients, because the smell of a potential predator may induce a stress response.[27]
  - Use calming pheromones (Feliway; Adaptil [Ceva Animal Health, Lenexa, KS]) in examination rooms and treatment wards, and on towels, tables, and your own clothing to provide a signal of safety for the animal and to reduce stress. Synthetic pheromone products have been shown to reduce signs associated with fear and anxiety in the veterinary setting.[28-31] Animals are sensitive to the pheromones of animals within their same species[32] and, as such, do not respond to pheromone products based on other species. This distinction makes it possible to use both canine and feline pheromone products in the same vicinity.
  - Use calming scents such as lavender and chamomile[33,34] when handling animals. Essential oils can be dabbed on bedding and handlers can use mildly scented lotions on their hands before handling.
- Tactile stimulation
  - Avoid placing animals on cold, slippery surfaces. Cover metal examination tables with towels; nonslip mats; or soft foam covering, such as Comfort Pet Exam (Comfort Pet Exam, Tampa, FL) to provide a warmer, more comfortable tactile sensation. Use a padded mat when placing animals into recumbency on the floor.

- ○ Place soft bedding inside the cage or kennel to promote rest, to provide warmth, and to prevent cats from resting in their litter boxes.[35] Cats seem to prefer polyester fleece bedding rather than towels and other mat types,[36] which is easily washable between patients.
- ○ Avoid overstimulating touch with animals. Although some pets enjoy petting, others may find it frightening or uncomfortable. For pets that solicit or appear comfortable with petting, pet with a light touch and in the direction of hair growth. Limit petting of cats to the head and neck because long strokes down the back and abdomen may increase arousal and aggression.[37]
- Gustatory stimulation
  - ○ Palatable food is a powerful means of mitigating stress and changing the underlying emotional state of the animal from one of fear to a state of pleasure. Offering food may help keep patients from feeling stressed or fearful and from displaying undesirable, defensive behaviors. Use food for counterconditioning when possible and safe, keeping in mind that the more palatable the food is from the animal's perspective, the greater the effect at conditioning a positive emotional response.
  - ○ Disguise bitter-tasting medications with a coating of food before administration, especially for cats. Use a pill administrator or pill gun so that contact with the tongue is minimized.
- Owner presence
  - ○ Many animals are less anxious and tolerate veterinary handling better with a familiar person present,[38] likely because animals feel safer in proximity to familiar members of their social group. It is also import to be sensitive to owner requests about not being present. A fearful, agitated, or punishing owner may escalate the animal's fear and aggression.
  - ○ Owner presence can be mindfully manipulated, because some animals show less aggression away from their owners. Keep in mind that pets that show less aggression when separated from their owners are not necessarily less fearful or less stressed. Without social group facilitation, stressed animals often cope by retreating or freezing, rather than engaging in a fight, despite still feeling threatened.[13,39] Although an animal that freezes may be easy to handle at that particular visit, if the animal learns that freezing does not end the negative interaction, it may be less apt to use this coping strategy at subsequent visits and may become increasingly difficult to handle. Avoid taking advantage of animals in this emotional state and mitigate stress as you would for animals with more fractious coping mechanisms.
  - ○ Pet owners may feel better being present for procedures and be more apt to agree to the use of other handling tools, such as muzzles, restraints, and sedation, if they perceive the animal's stress level and the clinician's willingness to keep it at a minimum.

ASSESSING THE ANIMAL'S COMFORT LEVEL AND INTENT

Understanding how to read and interpret the body language of the patient is the first step in recognizing and reducing stress, as well as keeping handlers safe. Animals communicate with each other, as well as with humans, through changes in body posture, eye contact, movement, and vocalization. This communication is different from interhuman communication and understanding the difference requires experience and skill. Human caretakers must recognize the intent of the animal and react appropriately in order to effectively handle it, minimize its fear and anxiety, and remain safe. This requires a continuous observation of patient information and adjusting to those data as aspects, such as procedure location, patient position, invasiveness, or restraint, change. Descriptions of canine[40–43] and feline[37,44] body language with regard to intent and handling safety are listed in **Boxes 2** and **3**, according to a green, yellow, and red scale with green being the most relaxed, meaning the patient feels safe and is safe to handle, and red being the most threatened, most dangerous animal to handle. Keep in mind that these are behavioral indicators of an animal's current emotional state in response to the surrounding stimuli and not a static reflection of the animal's underlying personality or temperament.

ASSESSING YOUR OWN BODY LANGUAGE AND BEHAVIOR AND ITS EFFECTS ON THE PATIENT

Your body language can strongly affect an animal's stress and comfort levels. What humans perceive as a friendly, benign interaction may be threatening from the animal's perspective. As primates, humans use forward and ventral approaches, direct eye contact, and outstretched hands to convey friendliness and affection. In contrast, dogs and cats rarely use forward, ventral contact in their communication and tend to take on more of a lateral, indirect approach, avoiding direct eye contact, and they therefore may feel threatened by direct, frontal approaches.[40–42] This reaction is especially evident when greeting a conspecific outside the familiar social group. For example, a dog that greets another, unfamiliar dog with a direct stare, putting its face in the other dog's face, or putting its head on top of the other dog's head or neck is perceived as threatening, causing the other dog to either retreat, freeze, or show aggression.[40,41] This means that there is a miscommunication between human displays of affection and animal perception of threat. Animals become frightened and humans get hurt. **Boxes 4** and **5** present information on how handlers can alter their own body language and behavior to be perceived as less threatening toward the patient.

ASSESSING HANDLER LANGUAGE AND ATTITUDE TOWARD THE PATIENT

The language people use affects their actions as well as the actions of others. Studies in livestock facilities show that the attitude of the handler directly relates to the manner in which the animals are handled, as well as the stress levels of the animals.[45] This concept is directly applicable to small animal handling and those in the small animal veterinary profession should strive to use language and portray attitudes that are appropriate and that promote safe and humane handling.

COMMONLY USED TERMS IN REFERENCE TO PATIENTS THAT RESULT IN POOR HANDLING

- Dumb
- Stupid
- Stubborn
- Spiteful
- Evil
- Mean

| Box 2 |
| Canine body language |

Green: this patient feels safe, is relaxed in the environment, and is safe to proceed with handling

- Posture

  - Weight carried evenly between all 4 limbs

  - Muscles are soft and relaxed throughout the body

  - May see a play bow or a loose body "wag" or "wiggle"

- Tail

  - Held in a relaxed, neutral position

  - May see a loose wag of the tail[a]

- Eyes

  - Steady, relaxed gaze without intense focus

  - Pupils are normal size for the light level of the room

  - Eyebrows and eyelids are soft and neutral, and may be partially closed

- Ears

  - Soft and neutral without being pressed or flattened back

  - May be facing different directions without alerting to anything specific

- Mouth

  - Long, loose lips

  - Mouth may be open with a loose tongue relaxed and lolling

  - Mouth may be closed with lips relaxed over the teeth

- Vocalization

  - Typically none

Yellow: this patient perceives danger and is alert, on the defensive, and would prefer to retreat rather than progress to a fight. This patient may proceed to aggression if provoked further. Note that the displacement behaviors may occur before other postural changes and are good early indicators of stress. Make a handling plan to mitigate the threat that this animal perceives.

- Posture

  - Muscles tense, weight shifted toward the back limbs

  - May crouch low to ground, holding one paw up

  - May roll over slightly to expose belly with or without urination

  - Postural displacement behaviors: shaking off an interaction (wet dog shake), holding one paw up, hind-end checking

- Tail

  - Stiff, held lower to the ground or tucked up against the body

  - May have a low wag,[a] which can be fast or slow

- Eyes

  - Fully open, alert, and scanning or darting

  - Pupils are dilated; may see whites of eyes (whale eye)

  - Eyebrows furrowed and shifting; may be averting gaze to avoid eye contact

- Ears
  - Pressed back and flattened against the head
  - Floppy ears may be pinched and tense
- Mouth
  - Lips pulled back to expose teeth or tensely held over teeth
  - Oral displacement behaviors: excessive or harsh panting, lip licking, chewing, yawning, grooming
- Vocalization
  - Excessive whining or whimpering
  - Low growl

Red: patient perceives a high risk of life-threatening danger and is ready and willing to use an offensive aggression to protect itself with little additional provocation. This animal is not safe to handle. Consider chemical restraint if the procedure is essential, or send the animal home and create a handling plan for the next visit if it is nonessential.

- Posture
  - Muscles are hard and with stiff movements
  - Weight shifted to the front feet
  - May freeze or shut down
  - Frantic attempts to escape, such as climbing walls, rolling, and flipping when handled (gator rolling)
  - Sudden release of urine, feces, and anal gland secretions
- Tail
  - Raised high above the back
  - May be wagging[a] in a slow and stiff manner
- Eyes
  - Hard, direct stare with eyelids wide open or squinted
  - Pupils fully dilated
- Ears
  - Held erect and forward
  - Little movement
- Mouth
  - Top lip retracted, showing front teeth only
- Vocalization
  - Growling, snarling, barking

[a] Tail wag indicates that a dog is ready to interact and must be interpreted with the dog's body language to understand the type of interaction intended.

Box 3
Feline body language

Green: this patient feels safe, is relaxed in the environment, and is safe to proceed with handling

- Posture
  - Head resting on body or flat surface with little movement
  - May roll onto side with limbs outstretched
  - May rub cheeks on people or other objects in the room (bunting)
- Tail
  - Extended away from body or loosely down when standing
  - Minimal twitching
- Eyes
  - Steady, relaxed gaze without intense focus
  - Pupils are normal size for the light level of the room
  - Eyelids may be partially closed
- Ears
  - Turned slightly forward
  - May be erect and face forward or back when alerted by sound
- Vocalization
  - May purr or give a soft meow

Yellow: this patient perceives danger and is alert, on the defensive, and would prefer to retreat rather than progress to a fight. This patient may show defensive aggression if provoked further. Make a handling plan to mitigate the threat that this animal perceives.

- Posture
  - Muscles tense, head held over the body or pressed to the body
  - Limbs retracted and held close to the body in ventral recumbency
  - May see slinking
- Tail
  - Held close to the body
  - Tense and pointing downwards or curled forward
  - Mild to moderate twitching at a slow rate
- Eyes
  - Wide open, alert, and scanning
  - Pupils are partially to fully dilated
  - Slow eye blinks
- Ears
  - Fully erected forward or partially flattened back
- Vocalization
  - None, plaintive meow, hissing, lip licking, stress purring

Red: patient perceives a high risk of life-threatening danger and is ready and willing to use an offensive aggression to protect itself. It is not safe to proceed with handling this animal. Consider chemical restraint if the procedure is essential, or send the animal home and create a handling plan for the next visit if it is nonessential.

- Posture
  - Head is lowered and still
  - May arch back with piloerection
  - Rapid, shallow breathing
  - Frantic attempts to escape or to climb
  - Striking with front paws
- Tail
  - Curled under the body, held low
  - Fast twitching
  - Piloerection
- Eyes
  - Wide open
  - Pupils fully dilated
- Ears
  - Fully flattened toward the back of the head
- Vocalization
  - Spitting, growling, yowling, hissing, shrieking
  - Open-mouth vocalizations

Box 4
Nonthreatening body language and behavior toward dogs

- Turn your body to the side, rather than facing the dog directly.
- Avoid prolonged direct eye contact, averting your gaze when possible.
- If safe, squat by bending at the knees, rather than at the waist, keeping your torso upright, still keeping yourself turned to the side (**Fig. 2**).
- Avoid squatting down with animals whose body language (red on the body language scale) indicates that they may come forward in an aggressive display because this puts you at risk of being bitten in the face or knocked over.
- Avoid bending over or leaning forward toward the dog; as you lean in, the image you project becomes larger and more threatening (**Fig. 3**).
- Hold your hand at your side, patting your leg gently and holding your palm open if the dog approaches, and allow the dog to sniff and investigate. If the dog shows green body language and comes closer, you can gently pet under the chin and neck area and slowly move into the desired examination position. If the animal does not approach, despite your nonthreatening approach, the animal may not be safe to handle and further approach may lead to an aggressive response.
- After the dog shows positive interaction, approach the side of the dog, rather than directly approaching the front of the dog. It may help to start your examination at the middle or rear end of the animal and move toward the head last, facing the same direction as the animal, working behind the point of the shoulder as much as possible.
- Avoid reaching out, petting on top of the dog's head, or suddenly grabbing for the collar. Make your movements more subtle and soft. Be aware that handling of the feet, ears, tail, and underbelly are socially invasive from the animal's perspective and may be as aversive as a physically painful procedure.

Box 5
Nonthreatening body language and behavior toward cats

- Avoid direct eye contact or staring.

- Use toys or food to encourage the cat to approach you first. If the cat approaches and sniffs your hand, you can gently scratch under the chin and pet the side of the head if the cat shows green body language and appears to enjoy this type of touch.

- Pet along the sides of the head, neck, and body if the cat appears to enjoy it. Avoid petting caudal to the waist.

- Avoid looming over, reaching for, or putting your face into the face of a fearful cat.

- Stand to the side of the cat or approach from behind, rather than directly in front of the head, unless you are able to allow the cat to hide its head.

- Minimize hand gestures and move slowly and deliberately.

- Speak softly and sparingly.

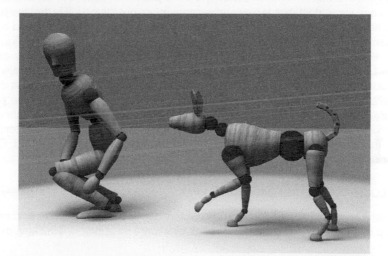

Fig. 2. Nonthreatening human body language encourages the dog to approach.

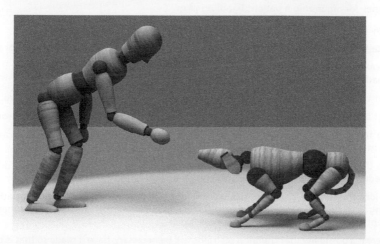

Fig. 3. Threatening human body language elicits fearful posturing from the dog and prevents approach.

TERMS THAT ARE A MORE ACCURATE REFLECTION OF ANIMAL BEHAVIOR AND PROMOTE APPROPRIATE HANDLING

- Fearful
- Threatened
- Inadequately socialized
- Does not understand what is required
- Painful

MAKING A HANDLING PLAN

Once an assessment of the environment, patient, and handler comfort levels is complete, a careful handling plan can be designed and implemented. Keep in mind that each handling plan should be unique to the individual patient and working environment and may require adjustments depending on the patient's response. Often the initial planning and implementation is more time consuming, but the payoff is that the patient is more at ease, the owners leave with a sense of satisfaction and trust, and subsequent visits should be more efficient. After implementing a successful handling plan, keep a record in each patient's chart of what worked well and how things can be improved. That way there is no reason to repeat tasks each visit. This record also promotes communication within the practice. Most handling plans start with a critical consideration of what procedures need to be performed at the visit. If some procedures are not essential, it may be best to plan multiple visits of shorter duration with fewer procedures. Once the itinerary is established, then the plan for counterconditioning, the level of restraint, and the needed handling tools can be instituted. Guidelines for organizing a handling plan can be found in **Box 6**.

USING COUNTERCONDITIONING

Unfamiliar smells, sounds, and sights, and potentially threatening animals and people, assault patients the moment they enter clinicians' care. In addition, clinicians perform

---

Box 6
Guidelines for organizing a patient handling plan

Critically consider what needs to be done:

- Critically consider what needs to be performed: must the procedure be done today, or at all?
- Determine whether and what the patient can eat so that a plan for counterconditioning can be made that is appropriate and safe for the animal.
- Select the appropriate level of restraint for the individual patient and the procedure.
- Select any handling tools that increase safety and decrease the patient's fear and arousal.
- Place the required procedures in order of most important to least important in case the patient is unable to tolerate some of the procedures.
- Place those procedures in order of least offensive to most offensive so that early difficult procedures do not inhibit the ability to complete later ones.
- Consider the level of pain, invasiveness, number of procedures, and how the patient is coping with minimal handling and consider chemical restraint when it is unlikely that the patient will be able to tolerate all the procedures.
- If there is a possibility that chemical restraint will be necessary, have it ready so that it can be implemented before the animal becomes too aroused.

unpleasant, sometimes painful, procedures, often by force. As a result, many animals have been inadvertently conditioned to fear the veterinary setting.[8] This fear often leads to dangerous and undesirable behavior toward the humans in this setting.

Fear is Not Voluntary

To combat the development of this fear or to alter an already established fear of the veterinary clinic settling, animal handlers can rely on counterconditioning.[8] Counterconditioning is a form of classic conditioning whereby an animal's negative emotional response (fear) to a given stimulus (the veterinary setting) is changed to a positive response (pleasure).[8,46] To create this positive emotional response, clinicians pair veterinary experiences with something that naturally elicits a positive emotional response in the animal: food. Palatable food is the easiest and most powerful means of establishing this association because it is a natural and automatic elicitor of a positive emotional response.[7,8,46] This natural emotional makeup is what motivates animals to eat and to survive. Counterconditioning is most effective in the clinic setting when the food is offered while the animal is still in a relaxed (green) state, just before and during the procedure, particularly for aversive procedures.[7] Particularly stressed (yellow) animals may need to be fed for the duration of the time they are handled to prevent escalation of fear and arousal. The palatability of the food needs to be high to maximize the animal's interest in eating and to increase the power of the positive emotional response. Although petting and praise may be enjoyable to some animals, they do not serve as primary or automatic reinforcement of a positive emotional state in the way that palatable food does. **Box 7** lists answers to commonly asked questions regarding the use of food in counterconditioning.

PROCEDURES IN WHICH COUNTERCONDITIONING SHOULD BE USED

- Injections
- Restraint by a stranger
- Toenail trims
- Rectal temperature/palpation
- Otoscopic examinations
- Microchip placement
- Fine-needle aspirates
- Placement onto a cold table

EXAMPLES OF PALATABLE FOODS THAT ARE EASY TO ADMINISTER TO DOGS

- Chicken or turkey baby food
- Peanut butter
- Squeeze cheese
- Kong Paste (The Kong Company, Golden, CO)
- Braunschweiger (liverwurst)
- Canned dog food
- Pill Pockets (Greenies, Franklin, TN)

EXAMPLES OF PALATABLE FOOD THAT IS EASY TO ADMINISTER TO CATS

- Chicken or turkey baby food
- Canned tuna or chicken
- Squeeze cheese
- Canned cat food
- Pill Pockets (Greenies, Franklin, TN)

Box 7
Commonly asked questions regarding the use of food for counterconditioning in a veterinary clinic setting

Question: what if the patient will not eat the food offered?

Answer: try increasing the palatability of the food. Be sure to try many different options. Many animals only eat the food they find most palatable when stressed. Pet owners can help identify preferences and/or bring the animal's favorite treat to the appointment. Rejecting food that the animal typically prefers indicates significant stress in the patient. Some animals, especially cats, may avoid the food receptacle (cup, bowl, hand, and so forth) and may need to have food placed directly onto the table.

Question: what if the patient cannot eat because of impending anesthesia, specific diagnostic testing, or gastrointestinal upset?

Answer: some animals have strong emotional associations with specific toys. Squeaky toys and balls that can be held in the patient's mouth may provide a positive emotional response. For cats, play with toys may be as reinforcing as food. If the patient does not find toys reinforcing, then the handler must rely on maximizing the environmental comfort and/or using chemical restraint. In some cases, the scent of food may be enough to change an emotional state. Smearing and then removing strongly scented foods may be most effective.

Question: what if the patient has food allergies or is on a specialized diet?

Answer: care must be taken when feeding these animals and owners should always be asked about dietary restrictions before starting counterconditioning. Animals on food trials can be offered the canned version of their exclusionary diet, pieces of their kibble, or fresh-cooked meat that matches the dietary source (eg, venison, duck). Many of these diets are also manufactured with a companion complementary treat that can be used as well. Animals with restricted protein or fat needs can safely be tempted with something sweet, such as mini marshmallows; baby carrots, peas, or sweet potatoes; or crispy homemade treats created from the canned diet food.

Question: if I feed an animal that is showing undesirable behavior, am I rewarding it for being bad?

Answer: because owners are not rewarding something that is under the patient's voluntary control (like a sit), the food is not reinforcing bad behavior. Instead, the offering of food is changing the animal's underlying emotional response to the clinic setting and procedures, which is what triggers the undesirable behaviors. Once the food reduces the fear, the motivation to use aggression or other undesirable behavior diminishes.

- Soft cat treats
- Catnip (first ask the owner whether the cat is calmed or aroused by it)
- Whipped cream

SAFE AND EFFECTIVE RESTRAINT

Once the itinerary of procedures has been organized, a restraint plan should be coordinated for each procedure. Less invasive procedures tend to require less restraint, whereas more invasive and aversive procedures may require heavier restraint for safety purposes and so that the animal feels secure. There is often a tendency to over-restrain animals. Much of their stress then revolves around the restraint rather than the procedure. The American Veterinary Medical Association' policy on the physical restraint of animals recommends the use of the least restraint required to allow the specific procedure(s) to be performed properly (**Box 8** for the full policy). Scruffing and stretching cats should not be automatic and should be reserved only for cats that are comfortable with this handling and when the procedure requires the animal to be still in lateral

> **Box 8**
> **American Veterinary Medical Association policy on physical restraint of animals**
>
> The method used should provide the least restraint required to allow the specific procedure(s) to be performed properly, should minimize fear, pain, stress and suffering for the animal, and should protect both the animal and personnel from harm. Every effort should be made to ensure adequate and ongoing training in animal handling and behavior by all parties involved, so that distress and physical restraint are minimized.
>
> *Data from* American Veterinary Medical Association's policy on the physical restraint of animals. 2012. Available at: https://www.avma.org/KB/Policies/Pages/Physical-Restraint-of-Animals.aspx. Accessed August 1, 2013.

recumbency. Lateral recumbency for dogs should be reserved only for procedures that require this positioning, such as orthopedic and neurologic examinations. Most procedures can be performed with the dog in a standing or sitting position.

GUIDELINES FOR RESTRAINT

- Use the least restraint that is necessary to safely perform the procedure. If you are able to use counterconditioning with food, less restraint is often needed.
  - Venipuncture from a lateral saphenous vein in a standing dog is typically better tolerated than placing a dog into lateral recumbency.
  - Many cats tolerate gently being turned into lateral recumbency for a medial saphenous venipuncture without being scruffed. Use a towel that wraps and covers the head and neck and/or keep a hand gently on the neck so that greater restraint can be provided if necessary.
- When greater restraint is needed, support the animal well.
  - Provide firm, balanced restraint with global support around the patient. Prevent flailing by keeping control of head and rear end at all times.
  - When lateral recumbency is needed, move the patient slowly and steadily with full body support.
  - When you need to move your hands or adjust your own position, keep a firm hold of the animal and slide your hands along the patient's body, rather than releasing and grabbing.
- If the pet struggles in response to restraint for longer than 3 seconds, stop, reposition, and try again. Wait until the pet has relaxed, and preferably has started eating, before beginning the procedure. If after 2 to 3 attempts the patient does not relax and/or becomes fractious, stop and consider whether the procedure is essential.[47]
  - If it is essential, make a plan for chemical restraint.
  - If it is nonessential, send the animal home and create a plan for a more successful visit the following day.
  - Creating a successful subsequent visit may require having the pet visit the hospital at a low-traffic time, merely to enter the clinic, be offered food for counterconditioning, and then leaving. This type of visit is often termed a happy visit. These visits can be repeated and, as the animal tolerates it, more contact and handling can be applied in a systematic manner until the pet is comfortable enough to handle the restraint. This systematic desensitization is best accomplished if you can prevent the patient under the threshold of becoming fearful or stressed at each step. Proceeding too quickly or allowing the patient to go over the threshold and become fearful can lead to sensitization, creating an even worse association.

CHEMICAL RESTRAINT

Chemical restraint allows safe and effective handling without causing the patient emotional distress. Avoid waiting for the animal to become fractious and highly agitated before considering the use of chemical restraint. Not only does this reduce the effectiveness of the medication, it also allows for learning to occur, making the fear in that setting more advanced. For cases that require immediate chemical restraint, it is best to create a plan to administer the injection on entrance to the hospital or, in some cases, the parking lot. Allowing the pet to wait in the lobby is likely to increase agitation and arousal and minimize the effectiveness of the medication. Injectable forms of sedation/anesthesia administered intramuscularly are typically the most effective means of rendering a fractious or highly fearful patient safe to handle. The clinician should use sound medical judgment to determine appropriate dosages and protocol selection based on age, temperament, and degree of health/disease. **Tables 1–3** show chemical restraint and reversal protocols. Once the injection has been administered, tools to block visual and auditory stimuli, such as the CalmingCap (ThunderWorks, Durham, NC) over the eyes and cotton balls in the ears, help to maintain the animal on an even plane of sedation. Keep these animals in a quiet area, rather than the open treatment room, because this is more conducive to a full sedation response. For patients that show mild to moderate fearful or fractious behavior in a veterinary clinic setting, oral administration of a sedative/anxiolytic medication before coming into the clinic may be useful. Oral premedication may also be useful for animals that are to undergo injectable forms of chemical restraint so that lower doses of injectable medications can be used. **Table 4** provides drug and dosing information for oral premedication drugs.

HANDLING TOOLS

Animal handling tools are designed to expedite veterinary procedures and increase safety, which in turn reduces patient stress, reduces staff stress, and increases owner satisfaction. The key to successfully integrating handling tools into the veterinary practice is using them correctly, using them often, and using them early. Handling tools are most helpful if integrated early in the handling plan. Owners should be encouraged to expose their pets to these tools at home, away from the presence of noxious stimuli, so that the tools do not become predictors of stressful events.

Table 1
Chemical restraint protocols for young, healthy dogs and cats

	Fractious	Painful
Dog	Dexmedetomidine (10 μg/kg) + opioid (butorphanol 0.2–0.4 mg/kg) IM ± ketamine (3 mg/kg) IM	Acepromazine (0.05 mg/kg) + opioid (butorphanol[a] 0.2–0.4 mg/kg) IM
Cat	Dexmedetomidine (10–20 μg/kg) or acepromazine (0.1 mg/kg) + ketamine (3–5 mg/kg) + opioid (butorphanol 0.2 mg/kg) or morphine 0.2 mg/kg) IM	Dexmedetomidine (10 μg/kg) or acepromazine (0.1 mg/kg) + opioid (butorphanol[a] 0.2–0.4 mg/kg) IM

Avoid dexmedetomidine in animals with cardiovascular abnormalities.
Abbreviation: IM, intramuscular.
[a] When available, a full mu opioid agonist, such as morphine (0.2 mg/kg), hydromorphone (0.05–0.1 mg/kg), or oxymorphone (0.1 mg/kg) is superior for pain management.
(*Courtesy of* Richard Bednarski, Columbus, OH.)

Table 2
Chemical restraint protocols for geriatric dogs (more than 7 years of age) and cats (more than 10 years of age)

	Fractious	Painful
Dog	Acepromazine (0.05 mg/kg) or dexmedetomidine[a] (5 µg/kg) + opioid (butorphanol 0.2–0.4 mg/kg) IM	Midazolam (0.2 mg/kg) or acepromazine (0.02 mg/kg) + opioid (butorphanol[b] 0.2–0.4 mg/kg) IM
Cat	Acepromazine (0.05 mg/kg) or dexmedetomidine[a] (5–10 µg/kg) + ketamine (3–5 mg/kg) + opioid (butorphanol 0.2 mg/kg) IM	Midazolam (0.2 mg/kg) or acepromazine (0.02 mg/kg) + opioid (butorphanol[b] 0.2–0.4 mg/kg) IM

[a] Dexmedetomidine should be used with caution in geriatric patients and reserved for especially fractious patients that cannot be safely handled otherwise.
[b] When available, a full mu opioid agonist, such as morphine (0.2 mg/kg), hydromorphone (0.05–0.1 mg/kg), or oxymorphone (0.1 mg/kg) is superior for pain management.
(*Courtesy of* Richard Bednarski, Columbus, OH.)

Table 3
Reversal protocols for chemical restraint in young and geriatric dogs and cats

	Dexmedetomidine	Mu Agonist (Oxymorphone, Morphine, Fentanyl)	Benzodiazepine
Complete reversal	Use equal volume of atipamezole to dexmedetomidine administered IM	Naloxone (0.01 mg/kg) IM or IV	Flumazenil (0.001 mg/kg, then work up to 0.01 mg/kg) IV
Partial reversal	Use half volume of atipamezole to dexmedetomidine administered IM	Naloxone (0.001–0.002 mg/kg) or butorphanol (0.2 mg/kg) IM or IV	—

Abbreviation: IV, intravenous.
(*Courtesy of* Richard Bednarski, Columbus, OH.)

Table 4
Medications that can be administered orally 90 minutes before veterinary visits to relieve mild to moderately fearful/fractious behavior in a veterinary clinic setting

Drug	Dog	Cat
Trazodone	4.0–12.0 mg/kg PO, not exceeding 300 mg per dose	No published dose
Clonidine[a]	0.01–0.05 mg/kg PO	5–10 µg/kg PO
Acepromazine[b]	0.55–2.2 mg/kg PO	1.1–2.2 mg/kg PO
Lorazepam[c]	0.05–0.5 mg/kg PO	0.05–0.25 mg/kg PO
Diazepam[c]	0.5–2.2 mg/kg PO	Avoid

Always have owners perform a drug trial at home to determine response and appropriate dose.
Abbreviation: PO, by mouth.
[a] Can be used alone or in combination with trazodone. Limited studies in cats.
[b] Should be used in combination with trazodone and/or diazepam or lorazepam for added tranquilizing effect. When used as a sole agent it does not provide anxiolysis.
[c] Use caution in fractious patients because disinhibition of aggression is possible. Avoid in patients that display aggression at home.

Canine Handling Tools

- Muzzles
  - Sleeve style: this style of muzzle fits tightly over the nose and mouth, holding the mouth closed (**Fig. 4**).
    - Pros:
      - The muzzle can be placed quickly if it is the stiffer, leather type.
      - The animal can lick food from the open front of the muzzle.
    - Cons:
      - The muzzle prevents the dog from panting and should only be worn for brief procedures because the patient may overheat if the muzzle is worn for a prolonged period.
      - The dog can still bite with the exposed incisors.
  - Basket style: this type of muzzle is an open plastic or metal cage or basket that encloses the nose and mouth.
    - Pros:
      - The muzzle allows for some level of panting, making it safer to be worn for long procedures and when a dog is kenneled.
      - Food can easily be smeared along the inside of the muzzle, which may encourage the dog to place its nose into the muzzle without a struggle (**Fig. 5**).
      - Dogs can more easily accept and chew food.
  - Proper placement:
    - Stand to the side of the dog.
    - Place the muzzle on the animal from behind and from the side, scooping the muzzle under the chin of the dog, rather than over the head (see **Fig. 5**).
    - Prevent the dog from backing up, using a wall or a person.
    - Be quick and deliberate because there may not be multiple opportunities for placement once the animal realizes the intention of the handler.
    - Offer food if safe and appropriate.
    - Allow the owner to place the muzzle if safe and appropriate (**Box 9**).

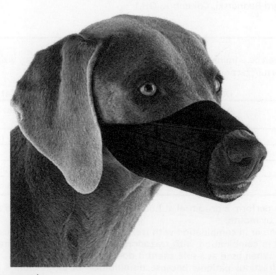

Fig. 4. Sleeve-style muzzle.

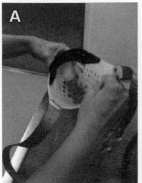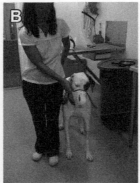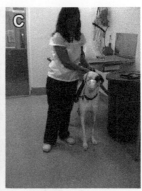

Fig. 5. Food can be smeared inside a basket muzzle (*A*) before the muzzle is placed from below and from the side of the dog (*B*) and the buckle fastened while the dog eats (*C*).

- Dog-appeasing pheromones (Adaptil; Comfort Zone)
  - Available in a spray, body heat–activated collars, and plug-in diffusers.
  - Analogue of the appeasing pheromone produced by the bitch from the sebaceous glands in the intermammary sulcus and that serves as a signal of food, comfort, and safety for the puppies.[48,49]
  - Has been shown clinically to have a calming effect in puppies and adult dogs.[29–31,50–52]
  - The spray can be applied to a bandana that can then be placed on the dog or applied to a towel and placed on the examination table.
  - Never spray directly on a dog. Allow a brief time for an application to air out before placing the bandana on a dog.
  - Diffusers can be plugged into outlets in examination rooms, treatment areas, and kennel areas where dogs are housed.
- CalmingCap (ThunderWorks, Durham, NC) (**Fig. 6**)
  - Soft, semiopaque fabric that covers the dog's eyes in order to limit the intake of visual stimuli.
  - Helps reduce the stress associated with the anticipation of procedures. When dogs do not witness the events before the procedure, the chances are greater they will remain calm.

Box 9
How to determine whether it is safe to allow owners to place a muzzle on their own dogs

1. Ask whether the dog has any history of owner-directed aggression (ie, ask whether the dog has ever growled, nipped, snapped, or bitten, even once, when it was approached at rest, had its mouth or face handled, or its food bowl or toys were handled).

2. Ask what the owners think about placing a muzzle on the dog. Do they feel comfortable? Are they safe or capable?

3. Describe how you would like the owner to place the muzzle on the dog and make sure they do not have any questions or concerns before proceeding.

4. Supervise the owner's placement of the muzzle as well as the patient's body language and, if you sense a problem, you can ask the owner to stop.

5. Pay attention to the owners' nonverbal communication signs when asking these questions and, if you sense that they are uncomfortable despite their verbal consent, it may be best not to proceed with having them muzzle the dog.

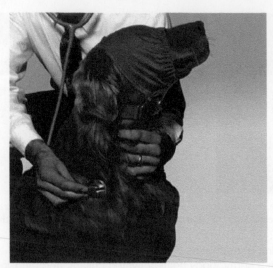

Fig. 6. Calming Cap is used to minimize visual stimuli. (*Courtesy of* ThunderWorks, Durham, NC; with permission.)

- ○ Helpful for dogs with aggression issues associated with the sight of unfamiliar dogs or people when moving them from the car to the lobby, through the treatment area, or from one part of the hospital to another. Hospitalized dogs with dog aggression issues can wear this cap when confined to prevent agitation from the sight of other passing or hospitalized dogs.
- ○ Can be sprayed with dog-appeasing pheromones before placement for added comfort.
- ○ Does not serve as a muzzle, although it can be placed over or under a muzzle.
- • Thundershirt (ThunderWorks, Durham, NC) (**Fig. 7**)
  - ○ Body wrap that swaddles the dog, providing firm, balanced pressure around the chest and torso. The design is based on evidence that evenly applied pressure on the body may reduce anxiety and fear.[53–55]

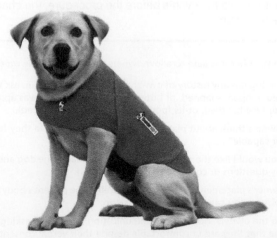

Fig. 7. Thundershirt provides anxiety relief through firm, balanced pressure on the chest and torso. (*Courtesy of* ThunderWorks, Durham, NC; with permission.)

- o For dogs that are calmed by this pressure, the shirt can be applied before entering the veterinary clinic and/or applied before the examination begins.
  - o Can be sprayed with dog-appeasing pheromones before placement for added comfort.
- Squeeze cage
  - o For dogs that are not safe to muzzle, the squeeze cage can be used to administer an injection for chemical restraint. Once the chemical restraint has been administered and has taken effect, the dog should be muzzled before handling for added safety.
  - o The dog can be placed into the cage by the veterinary staff or by the owner, depending on which option is safer and easier for the dog. Once the dog is contained, the back wall is gently pulled forward, pushing the dog up against the front of the cage. After the injection is administered, the back wall is released and the dog can remain in the cage until responding to the sedation (**Fig. 8**).
  - o Alternatives to the squeeze cage may include a chain-link panel that swings out from the wall. The panel can be held open at a 90° angle or greater while the dog is walked into the corner between the wall and open panel and the leash pulled through the crevice between the wall and panel. The panel can then be gently closed toward the wall, securing the dog between the wall and the chain-link panel. The injection for chemical restraint can then be administered through the panel.
- Towel restraint
  - o For dogs that cannot be muzzled because of brachycephalic conformation or intense fear of the muzzle, towels can be used to provide control of the head (**Fig. 9**).
  - o To restrict head movement, a towel can be rolled and wrapped around the neck and chest and held tightly. The towel should be thick and pressure applied evenly from just below the chin down to the chest. Apply just enough pressure to restrict movement but not restrict breathing (**Fig. 10**).
- Elizabethan collar restraint
  - o For dogs that cannot be muzzled because of brachycephalic conformation or intense fear of the muzzle, Elizabethan collars can be used to provide control of the head.

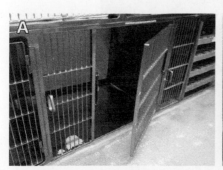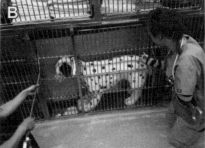

Fig. 8. Squeeze cage allows for chemical restraint administration for fractious dogs. The back panel remains in place to allow the animal to enter the cage (*A*) and then pulls forward (*B*) to keep the dog at the front of the cage for intramuscular injection.

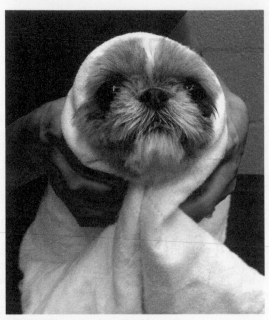

Fig. 9. Use of a towel to control the head of a small dog.

- If safe for the owners to place the collar, it may be best to have them place it at home, before entering the clinic.
- The head can be controlled, using 2 hands behind the collar to grasp the neck and head firmly, but gently.

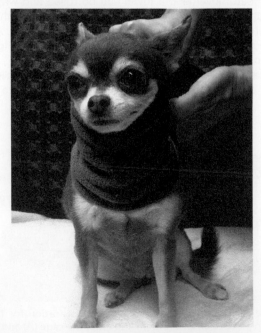

Fig. 10. Use of a towel neck wrap to control the head of a small dog.

FELINE HANDLING TOOLS

- Muzzles
  - In cats, muzzles are typically used to cover both the mouth and the eyes, which provides safety to the handler as well as minimizing visual stimuli that may be stressful for the cat.
  - Soft nylon muzzles are useful if visual stimulation blocking is the primary goal (**Fig. 11**).
  - Stiff leather or plastic muzzles are preferable for fractious cats because the cats are unable to bite through the tougher material (**Fig. 12**).
  - Standing with the cat facing away from you, apply the muzzle while keeping your hands behind the head and, using one swift motion, place the muzzle by coming up from under the chin of the cat. One handler should place pressure on the muzzle, holding it in place while a second handler secures the ties or Velcro straps. A third handler may be needed to prevent the cat from backing out of the muzzle if the other handlers are unable to do so.
- Towels
  - Head control and reduction of visual stimuli are the primary purposes of towels when handling cats.
  - For fleeing or fearful cats, it is often enough to place the towel over the head, then push the towel under to include the head and feet. Any movement forward is inhibited by the pressure of the towel and many cats then calm down. The clinician then has access to the rear end of the cat for auscultation, abdominal palpation, and medial saphenous venipuncture (**Fig. 13**).
  - For access to the head of the cat, or for cats that are stressed by having the head covered, low-stress immobilization can be performed using a towel wrap (half-burrito wrap).[56] In this method the cat is first placed on the center of the towel and the front of the towel is pulled up around the neck to keep control of the head. While holding the towel in place with one hand, the other hand is then used to wrap the sides of the towel around the body of the cat. Be sure

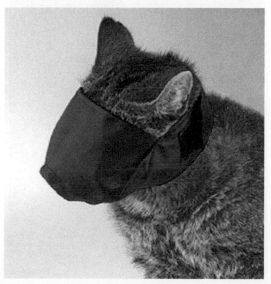

Fig. 11. Soft muzzle for a cat blocks visual stimuli while also covering the mouth.

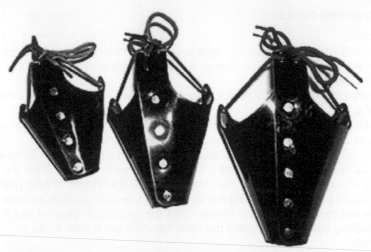

Fig. 12. Hard plastic muzzle prevents biting in a fractious cat.

that the wrap fits snuggly to provide firm, balanced lateral support. This method prevents flailing and helps the cat remain calm, while preventing scratching with the front or rear claws (**Fig. 14**).

- Feline facial pheromones (Feliway; Comfort Zone)
  - Available in a spray and plug-in diffuser.
  - Analogue of the facial pheromone released from the perioral gland of cats when cheek rubbing (bunting)[44,57] on prominent objects, people, and other animals. Cats typically perform bunting behaviors when in an environment they perceive to be safe and comforting.

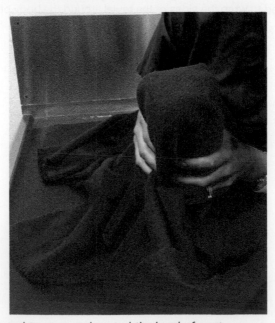

Fig. 13. Use of a towel to cover and control the head of a cat.

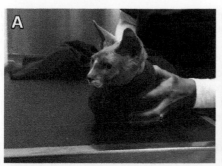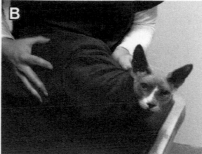

Fig. 14. (*A*, *B*) Use of a towel wrap (half burrito wrap) to control movement in a cat and give access to head examination.

- ○ Placing synthetic facial pheromones in the hospital environment may help cats eat faster[58] and be more tractable with handling.[28] These pheromones may be useful in treating aggressive behavior between cats[59] and to reduce stress-related marking behaviors,[60–63] suggesting a general calming effect that is highly applicable to the veterinary clinic setting.
  - ○ Pheromones should not be directly sprayed onto the cat. Instead, spray the examination table towel, cage padding, and/or the inside of a cage cover. Often a towel or blanket can be draped over half of the cage door to give the cat the ability to feel hidden as well as to hold sprayed pheromone product (see **Fig. 1**).
  - ○ Another synthetic feline facial pheromone is the F4 analogue Felifriend, which is associated with familiarization and allomarking in cats. At present, the product is in limited distribution in Europe. The product is applied to the hands to facilitate introduction to unfamiliar people, including veterinarians and staff.[64,65]
- • Clipnosis (KVP International, Irwindale, CA)
  - ○ Clipnosis is performed using the proprietary Clipnosis Gentle Calming Clips (**Fig. 15**) or other tools such as binder clips that provide firm, steady pressure when placed on the scruff of a cat's neck. The pressure provided is greater, more evenly distributed, and more consistent compared with hand scruffing. Scruffing a cat typically does not provide equivalent behavioral calming. Once the pressure is applied, there is a resulting pinch-induced behavioral inhibition.[66] Cats reach a trancelike state, becoming calm, semi-immobile, and relaxed, without activation of a stress response.[66]
  - ○ This tool allows hands-free, stress-free restraint in cats that are responsive to it.

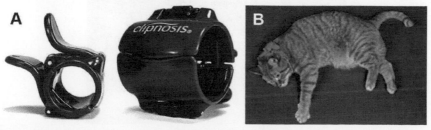

Fig. 15. Clipnosis Calming Clips (*A*) applied to induce calm, hands-free restraint in a cat (*B*). (*Courtesy of* KVP International, Irwindale, CA; with permission.)

- o Not all cats are responsive to the clips. Cats that are averse to pressure on the scruff or that are fractious with handling are not candidates for Clipnosis.
  - o Some veterinarians have reservations regarding the clipping procedure and its effects on behavioral inhibition through freezing versus calming. The authors' experience, and supporting evidence,[66] point toward the latter.
  - o Clips should be placed on cats that are calm and relaxed. An explanatory video can be viewed at www.clipnosis.com
- The carrier
  - o The cat's own carrier can be a valuable handling tool, especially for fearful cats. Carriers should be of the type that allows the cat to easily exit on its own or have a removable/movable top that allows the cat to remain in the bottom portion during examination. A towel can then be slid under the top and over the cat as the top half of the carrier is slowly lifted and removed.
  - o This method allows the cat to remain in a familiar area and tends to prevent fleeing because the sides of the carrier provide some sense of concealment (**Fig. 16**).
  - o Soft-sided carriers are useful for cats in need of intramuscular injections for chemical restraint. In this case, the cat remains in the familiar carrier while the soft side is pressed up against the animal at the injection site.
  - o Allowing hospitalized cats to have their own carrier within their cage also provides a sense of familiarity and stress relief. Keeping the familiar carrier within the cage has been shown to help hospitalized cats begin eating sooner during recovery.[58]
  - o The carrier is an effective tool for cats that have been conditioned to feel comfortable entering on their own and remaining calm in it during car travel. **Box 10** lists tips on teaching owners how to help their cats to be more comfortable with the carrier and car travel.
  - o Another option is clicker training the cat to use the carrier (see http://catalystcouncil.org/search/search.aspx).
- Thundershirt for cats (**Fig. 17**)
  - o Body wrap that swaddles the cat, providing firm, balanced pressure around the chest and torso. It is based on evidence that evenly applied pressure on the body may reduce anxiety and fear.[53–55]

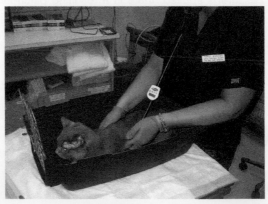

Fig. 16. Use of the cat's own carrier during the physical examination helps provide a sense of security and familiarity.

Box 10
Tips for helping cats be more comfortable with the carrier and car travel

1. Keep the carrier in a familiar area of the home so that it becomes a familiar piece of furniture.

2. Toss treats, toys, and/or catnip into the carrier daily to condition a positive emotional response with entering the carrier.

3. Teach the cat to enter the carrier on a verbal cue, using treats or clicker training.

4. Place familiar, soft bedding inside the carrier.

5. At least 30 minutes before having the cat enter the carrier, spray the bedding with feline facial pheromones.

6. If needed, remove the top of the carrier to allow the cat easy access to the carrier and replace it once the cat is inside.

7. Practice closing the door and lifting the carrier, as well as getting it in and out of the car.

8. During car travel, secure the carrier by placing it on the floor or by using a seatbelt.

9. Place a towel over the carrier to prevent visual arousal during travel and on entrance to the veterinary clinic.

10. Provide palatable food treats to the cat continuously after the carrier door has been closed to maintain a positive association with being inside the carrier from the point of picking up the carrier to take it to the car, until the time of the examination. If the travel or wait time is prolonged, a small treat can be provided every 1 to 2 minutes.

Adapted from Rodan I, Sundahl E, Carney H, et al. AAFP and ISFM feline-friendly handling guidelines. J Feline Med Surg 2011;13:364–75.

- For cats that are calmed by this pressure, the shirt can be applied to the cat before entering the veterinary clinic and/or applied before the examination begins.
- Be careful that the suppression of mobility by the cat is caused by calming and not by fear (freezing) or inhibited mobility.
- Can be sprayed with feline facial pheromones before placement for added comfort.
- EZ Nabber (Campbell Pet Company, Brush Prairie, WA)
  - Mesh netting that is tightly secured to a metal enclosure that opens and closes manually to allow capture and restraint of cats (**Fig. 18**).

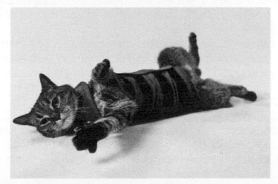

Fig. 17. Thundershirt for cats provides anxiety relief through firm, balanced pressure on the chest and torso. (*Courtesy of* ThunderWorks, Durham, NC; with permission.)

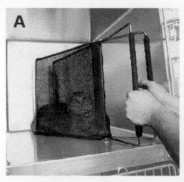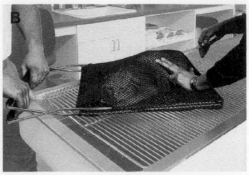

Fig. 18. EZ Nabber allows safe capture of fractious cats (*A*) and easy administration of chemical restraint (*B*). (*Courtesy of* Campbell Pet Company, Brush Prairie, WA; with permission.)

- o Especially helpful for feral or fractious cats that are fleeing or that are housed in a wall unit cage because it puts a 60-cm distance between a person's hands and the cat.
- o Used to administer chemical restraint intramuscularly because injections can easily be given through the mesh netting.
- o Cover the netting with a towel once the cat is captured to reduce visual exposure and stimuli that may exacerbate stress.

REFERENCES

1. The American Veterinary Medical Association's policy: veterinarians' oath. Available at: https://www.avma.org/KB/Policies/Pages/veterinarians-oath.aspx. Accessed August 1, 2013.
2. Jeyaretnam JH, Jones H, Phillips M. Disease and injury among veterinarians. Aust Vet J 2000;78:625–9.
3. Drobatz KJ, Smith G. Risk factors for bite wounds inflicted on caregivers by dogs and cats in a veterinary teaching hospital. J Am Vet Med Assoc 2003; 223:312–6.
4. August JR. Dog and cat bites. J Am Vet Med Assoc 1988;193:1394–8.
5. Volk JO, Felsted KE, Thomas JG, et al. Executive summary of the Bayer Veterinary Care Usage Study. J Am Vet Med Assoc 2011;238:1275–82.
6. Morgan KN, Tromborg CT. Sources of stress in captivity. Appl Anim Behav Sci 2007;102:262–302.
7. Mazur JE. Basic principle of classical conditioning. In: Learning and behavior. 6th edition. Upper Saddle River (NJ): Pearson Education; 2006. p. 76–81.
8. Yin S. Classical conditioning (aka associative learning). In: Low stress handling, restraint, and behavior modification of dogs and cats. Davis (CA): Cattle Dog Publishing; 2009. p. 83–4.
9. Veranic P, Jezernik K. Succession of events in desquamation of superficial urothelial cells as a response to stress induced by prolonged constant illumination. Tissue Cell 2001;33:280–5.
10. Pollard JC, Littlejohn RP. Behavioural effects of light conditions on red deer in a holding pen. Appl Anim Behav Sci 1994;41:127–34.
11. Gunter R. The absolute threshold for vision in the cat. J Physiol 1995;114:8–15.
12. Miller PE, Murphy CJ. Vision in dogs. J Am Vet Med Assoc 1995;207:1623–34.

13. Carlstead K, Brown JL, Strawn W. Behavioral and physiological correlates of stress in laboratory cats. Appl Anim Behav Sci 1993;38:143–58.
14. Kry K, Casey R. The effect of hiding enrichment on stress levels and behavior of domestic cats (*Felis sylvestris catus*) in a shelter setting and the implications for adoption potential. Anim Welf 2007;16:375–83.
15. Belew AM, Barlett T, Brown SA. Evaluation of the white-coat effect in cats. J Vet Intern Med 1999;13:134–42.
16. Crowell-Davis SL. White coat syndrome: prevention and treatment. Compend Contin Educ Vet 2007;29:163–5.
17. Anthony A, Ackerman E, Lloyd JA. Noise stress in laboratory rodents: I. Behavioral and endocrine responses of mice, rats, and guinea pigs. J Acoust Soc Am 1959;31:1437–40.
18. Herron ME, Shofer FS, Reisner IR. Survey of the use and outcome of confrontational and non-confrontational training methods in client-owned dogs showing undesired behaviors. Appl Anim Behav Sci 2009;117:47–54.
19. Wells DL, Graham L, Hepper PG. The influence of auditory stimulation on the behavior of dogs housed in a rescue shelter. Anim Welf 2002;11:385–93.
20. Kogan LR, Schoenfeld-Tacher R, Simon AA. Behavioral effects of auditory stimulation on kenneled dogs. J Vet Behav 2012;7:268–75.
21. Wells DL, Irwin RM. Auditory stimulation as enrichment for zoo-housed Asian elephants (*Elephas maximus*). Anim Welf 2008;17:335–40.
22. Davila SG, Campo JL, Gil MG, et al. Effects of auditory and physical enrichment on three measurements of fear and stress (tonic immobility duration, heterophil to lymphocyte ratio, and fluctuating asymmetry) in several breeds of layer chicks. Poult Sci 2011;90:2459–66.
23. Bear MF, Conners BW, Paradiso MA. The chemical senses. In: Neuroscience: exploring the brain. 3rd edition. Philadelphia: Lippincott Williams & Wilkins; 2007. p. 271–2.
24. MacDonald DW. The carnivores: order Carnivora. In: Brown RE, MacDonald DW, editors. Social odours in mammals. Oxford (United Kingdom): Clarendon Press; 1985. p. 619–722.
25. Bekoff M. Scent marking by free ranging domestic dogs: olfactory and visual components. Biol Behav 1979;4:123–39.
26. Stoddart DM. The ecology of vertebrate olfaction. London: Chapman and Hall; 1980.
27. Takahashi LK, Nakashima BR, Hong HC. The smell of danger: a behavioral and neural analysis of predator odor-induced fear. Neurosci Biobehav Rev 2005;29: 1157–67.
28. Kronen PW, Ludders JW, Erb HN, et al. A synthetic fraction of feline facial pheromones calm but does not reduce struggling in cats before venous catheterization. Vet Anaesth Analg 2006;33:258–65.
29. Kim YM, Lee JK, Abd el-aty AM, et al. Efficacy of dog-appeasing pheromone (DAP) for ameliorating separation-related behavioral signs in hospitalized dogs. Can Vet J 2010;1:380–4.
30. Siracusa C, Manteca X, Cuenca R, et al. Effect of a synthetic appeasing pheromone on behavioral, neuroendocrine, immune and acute-phase perioperative stress responses in dogs. J Am Vet Med Assoc 2010;237:673–81.
31. Mills DS, Ramos D, Estelles MG, et al. A triple blind placebo-controlled investigation into the assessment of the effect of dog appeasing pheromone (DAP) on anxiety related behaviour of problem dogs in the veterinary clinic. Appl Anim Behav Sci 2006;98:114–26.

32. Beata C. Appeasing pheromones in mammals. Vancouver (WA): World Congress; 2001.
33. Wells DL. Aromatherapy for travel-induced excitement in dogs. J Am Vet Med Assoc 2006;6:964–7.
34. Wells DL, Hepper PG. The influence of olfactory stimulation on the behaviour of dogs housed in a rescue shelter. Appl Anim Behav Sci 2005;91:143–53.
35. Crouse SJ, Atwill ER, Lagana M, et al. Soft surfaces: a factor in feline psychological well-being. Contemp Top Lab Anim Sci 1995;34:94–7.
36. Hawthorne AJ, Loveridge GG, Horrocks LJ. The behavior of domestic cats in response to a variety of surface textures. In: Holst B, editor. Proc. 2nd International Conference on Environmental Enrichment. Copenhagen (NY): 1995; p. 84–94.
37. Heath S. Aggression in cats. In: Horwitz D, Mills D, editors. BSAVA manual of canine and feline behavioural medicine. 2nd edition. Gloucester (MA): British Small Animal Veterinary Association; 2009. p. 233.
38. Waiblinger S, Menke C, Korff J, et al. Effects of different persons on the behaviour and heart rate of dairy cows during a veterinary procedure. Kuratorium für Technik und Bauwesen in der Landwirtschaft 2001;403:54–62.
39. Beerda B, Shilder MB, van Hooff JA, et al. Manifestations of chronic and acute stress in dogs. Appl Anim Behav Sci 1997;52:307–19.
40. Handelman B. Canine behavior: a photo illustrated handbook. Wenatchee (WA): Dogwise; 2008.
41. Aloff B. Canine body language: a photographic guide. Wenatchee (WA): Dogwise; 2005.
42. Milani MM. The body language and emotion of dogs: a practical guide to the physical and behavioral displays owners and dogs exchange and how to use them to create a lasting bond. New York: Quill William Morrow; 1997.
43. Keuster TD, Jung H. Aggression toward familiar people and animals. In: Horwitz D, Mills D, editors. BSAVA manual of canine and feline behavioural medicine. 2nd edition. Gloucester (MA): British Small Animal Veterinary Association; 2009. p. 182–210.
44. Bradshaw J, Cameron-Beaumont C. The signaling repertoire of the domestic cat and its undomesticated relatives. In: Turner DC, Bateson P, editors. The domestic cat. 2nd edition. Cambridge (United Kingdom): Cambridge University Press; 2000. p. 68–93.
45. Hemsworth PH. Human-animal interactions in livestock production. Appl Anim Behav Sci 2003;81:185–98.
46. Mills D. Training and learning protocols. In: Horwitz D, Mills D, editors. BSAVA manual of canine and feline behavioural medicine. 2nd edition. Gloucester (MA): British Small Animal Veterinary Association; 2009. p. 49–64.
47. Yin S. General handling principles. In: Horwitz D, Mills D, editors. Low stress handling, restraint, and behavior modification of dogs and cats. Davis (CA): Cattle Dog Publishing; 2009. p. 191–231.
48. Adaptil [package insert]. Lenexa, Kansas: Ceva Animal Health, LCC; 2013.
49. Pageat P, Gaultier E. Current research in canine and feline pheromones. Vet Clin North Am Small Anim Pract 2003;33:187–211.
50. Denenberg S, Landsberg GM. Effects of dog-appeasing pheromones on anxiety and fear in puppies during training and on long-term socialization. J Am Vet Med Assoc 2008;233:1874–82.
51. Sheppard G, Mills D. Evaluation of dog-appeasing pheromone as a potential treatment for dogs fearful of fireworks. Vet Rec 2003;152:432–6.

52. Tod E, Brander D, Waran N. Efficacy of dog appeasing pheromone in reducing stress and fear related behavior in shelter dogs. Appl Anim Behav Sci 2005;93: 295–308.
53. Grandin T. Calming effects of deep touch pressure in patients with autistic disorder, college students, and animals. J Child Adolesc Psychopharmacol 1992;2: 63–72.
54. Grandin T. A voluntary acceptance of restraint by sheep. Appl Anim Behav Sci 1989;23:257–61.
55. Cottam N, Dodman NH, Ha JC. The effectiveness of the Anxiety Wrap in the treatment of canine thunderstorm phobia: an open-label trial. J Vet Behav 2013;8:154–61.
56. Yin S. Restraint for standard positions in cats. In: Low stress handling, restraint, and behavior modification of dogs and cats. Davis (CA): Cattle Dog Publishing; 2009. p. 341–86.
57. Houpt KJ. Communication. In: Domestic animal behavior for veterinarians and animal scientists. 4th edition. Ames (IA): Blackwell Publishing; 2005. p. 3–35.
58. Griffith C, Steigerwals E, Buffington CA. Effects of a synthetic facial pheromone on the behavior of cats. J Am Vet Med Assoc 2000;217:1154–6.
59. Levine E. Fear and anxiety. Vet Clin North Am Small Anim Pract 2008;38: 1065–79.
60. Mills DS, White JC. Long-term follow up of the effect of a pheromone therapy on feline spraying behaviour. Vet Rec 2000;147:746–7.
61. Mills DS, Mills CB. Evaluation of a novel method for delivering a synthetic analogue of feline facial pheromone to control urine spraying by cats. Vet Rec 2001;149:197–9.
62. Ogata N, Takeuchi Y. Clinical trial with a feline pheromone analogue for feline urine marking. J Vet Med Sci 2001;63:157–61.
63. Frank D, Erb HN, Houpt KA. Urine spraying in cats: presence of concurrent disease and effects of pheromone treatment. Appl Anim Behav Sci 1999;61: 263–72.
64. Patel G, Heath S, Coyne K, et al. Pilot study to investigate whether a feline pheromone analogue reduces anxiety-related behavior during clinical examination of cats in a rescue shelter. J Vet Behav 2010;5:33.
65. Bonnafous L, Lafont C, Gaultier E, et al. Allomarking pheromone (F4) analog (Felifriend) during medical examination. In: Mills D, Levine E, Landsberg G, et al, editors. Current issues and research in veterinary behavioral medicine. West Lafayette (IN): Purdue University Press; 2005. p. 119–22.
66. Pozza ME, Stella JL, Chappuis-Gagnon AC, et al. Pinch-induced behavioral inhibition ('clipnosis') in domestic cats. J Feline Med Surg 2008;10:82–7.

Genetics and Behavior:
A Guide for Practitioners

Karen L. Overall, MA, VMD, PhD, CAAB[a,*], Katriina Tiira, PhD[b],
Desiree Broach, DVM[c], Deborah Bryant, DVM[d]

KEYWORDS

- Canine • Feline • Behavioral genetics • Temperament • Personality • Dog behavior
- Cat behavior

KEY POINTS

- Phenotyping behavior is difficult, partly because behavior is almost always influenced by the environment.
- Using objective terms/criteria to evaluate behaviors is always best; the more objective the assessment, the more likely any underlying genetic patterns will be identified.
- Behavioral pathologies, and highly desirable behavioral characteristics or traits, are likely to be complex, meaning that multiple genes are probably involved, and therefore simple genetic tests are less possible.
- Improvement in breeds can be accomplished using traditional quantitative genetic methods; unfortunately, this also creates the possibility of inadvertently selecting for covarying undesirable behaviors.
- Patterns of behaviors within families and breed lines still provide one of the best guidelines for genetic counseling in dogs.

INTRODUCTION: WHY SHOULD PRACTITIONERS CARE ABOUT BEHAVIORAL GENETICS?

Dogs have a relationship with humans unlike that of any other domestic animal. Dogs have been selected over time for true collaborative work with humans, and this selection has historically resulted in dog breeds and groupings based on the dog's ability to work with humans on certain tasks (eg, herding). As result, most of the emphasis on behavioral genetics in veterinary medicine has been on dogs, and that bias is reflected in this article.

[a] 10 County Lane, Glen Mills, PA 19342, USA; [b] Canine Genomics Research Group, Research Program's Unit, Molecular Neurology, Department of Veterinary Biosciences, The Folkhälsan Institute of Genetics, University of Helsinki, Helsinki, Finland; [c] JBSA-Lackland, 1219 Knight Street, San Antonio, TX 78236, USA; [d] PO Box 168, Sartell, MN 56377, USA
* Corresponding author.
E-mail address: overall.karen@gmail.com

Vet Clin Small Anim 44 (2014) 483–505
http://dx.doi.org/10.1016/j.cvsm.2014.01.006
0195-5616/14/$ – see front matter © 2014 Elsevier Inc. All rights reserved.

With respect to domestic dogs:

- Molecular data suggest that dogs separated from wolves 10,000 to 135,000 years ago.[1–7]
- Dogs have lived together with humans for 15,000 to 30,000 years,[8–10] as supported by anthropologic evidence.[11,12]
- Breed clusters of dogs of different shapes/sizes who engaged in different tasks have existed at least 3000 years.

Only in the past 150 years has selection/breeding emphasis largely shifted from what a dog could do to how society wanted that dog to look. Dog breeds represent pools of canalized genetic variation. Historically, they have been the result of many generations of selection for certain specific tasks, and therefore it is no accident that dogs bred for conformation may have more reliable looks than behaviors, and that those bred for work may have more reliable performance than looks. Understanding this pattern and how it shapes modern genetics is important for veterinarians who wish to provide the best information about genetic factors contributing to behavior.

GENOTYPE VERSUS PHENOTYPE

We are how we behave, and behavioral phenotypes are defined by the behaviors the dog exhibits under varied conditions. All phenotypes (what the behavior looks like) are influenced by the genetic, physical, and maternal (in utero and rearing) environments. The behavioral phenotype of any dog is also influenced by the interaction of the environment on the dog's neurochemistry, activity of various regions of the brain, and molecular responses to stimulation, within any given genotype. This fact is why even littermates from tightly tested and controlled breeding lines can be so variable (eg, one is terrified of storms and the other is not).

The genetic background (the genotype or genomic code) of the patient only tells what could happen in terms of behavior and personality, not what will happen. The genotype is a catalog of coded sequences of instructions, not all of which will be activated, used, or expressed. This concept is essential because it means that behavior is not deterministic. Even when diseases are heritable in a simple manner, their phenotypes and presentations can be altered through interaction with the environment. Nowhere is this truer than for behavior: it occurs when pharmacologic treatment and behavior modification are used for behavioral problems, and when problems are prevented simply because the patient is in a household that may not promote them. Unfortunately, misconceptions about determinism and the role of genetics have driven myths about breed-based behaviors and unfortunate breed-specific legislation. Given these limitations, on what should we focus with respect to behavioral genetics?

All behaviors are the result of the interaction of the genetic background with the physical and cognitive environments found in the individual patient. The concept of a response surface can help practitioners understand how patterns of behavior can individually vary with exposure to different environments depending on genetic background.

The response surface in **Fig. 1** represents a simple space created by behavioral traits, the environments in which they are displayed, and the genotype affecting them. In **Fig. 1**, dogs A and B seem to behave the same (they are the same color). Their responses to different environmental manipulations will expose how they are different. As dog A is exposed to a range of environments from right to left on the environmental axis, she remains unchanged; however, when dog B is similarly exposed, her behaviors alter dramatically (B1 in **Fig. 2**).

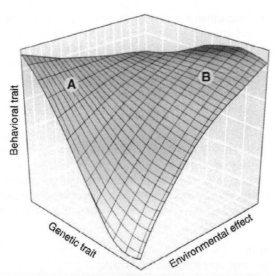

Fig. 1. A response surface for a series of expressions of a behavioral trait across different genetic and physical environments. A and B represent dogs whose behaviors seem the same (same color), but for whom the genetic and environmental contributions to their behaviors are vastly different. (*From* Overall KL. Proceedings of the Dogs Trust Meeting on Advances in Veterinary Behavioural Medicine London; 4th–7th November 2004. p. 65: Veterinary behavioural medicine: a roadmap for the 21st century. Vet J 2005;169:134; with permission.)

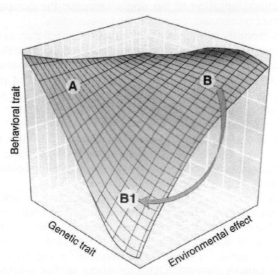

Fig. 2. Two dogs, A and B, who look alike in their behaviors. The underlying contribution of their genes to their behavior differs here, and when exposed to a series of environments, one of them alters her behavioral response surface considerably (patient B1) when compared with the other (patient A). This difference in response suggests that the underlying mechanisms (which are genetically determined in this example) for the 2 responses differ. A and B displayed the same behavioral phenotype in one environment, but they are not the same genetically and therefore do respond differently to different environments, such as tasks, training, and interventions. (*From* Overall KL. Manual of clinical behavioral medicine for dogs and cats. St Louis (MO): Elsevier; 2013. p. 66; with permission.)

Phenotyping behaviors is difficult, but phenotype is key to understanding genetic associations, complex mechanisms, or differential response to more specific treatments, particularly those involving medication. A diagnosis is almost never a phenotype, but it can help to develop the characterization of one. When done well, using rigorous criteria, behavioral diagnoses provide probabilistic associations among behaviors, pathology, and environment that can be represented using some kind of a decision tree reflecting possible outcomes. In behavior, diagnosis must rely on some objective representation of the behavior (eg, behavioral types, responses, transitions, and counts taken from video), evaluated over different contexts. Because many behaviors and behavioral sequences are nonspecific, they can only be interpreted within a context provided by the interaction of pattern (sequence of behaviors, duration, frequency, intensity), associated physiology, and species, breed, and ontogeny-typical behaviors. The more tightly these distinctions cluster, and the more diverse the measures of the clusters (eg, behavioral assay, plus physiologic assay, plus provocative test), the better the phenotype.

MEASURING BEHAVIOR
Temperament, Personality, and Behavioral Assays

Temperament can be broadly defined as the relatively stable individual characteristics of behavior that show some consistency over time and across situations,[13] and as differences in behavior between individuals that are relatively constant given similar evaluation situations.[14] Personality traits have been documented in several species. The concepts of temperament, personality,[15] and character[16] have been used to identify breeds or individuals suitable for specific behavioral tasks.[17] These terms provide only a summary characterization of the dog's behavior: the components used for assessment still must be defined, objective, and measurable.

Temperament/personality measures are often used to predict an association or correlation with a defined outcome, like succeeding as a working dog. Svartberg[18] found that the use of dogs as conformation show dogs (measured as the amount of merits of the breeding stock from dog shows) negatively correlated with 4 personality traits (playfulness, curiosity/fearlessness, sociability, aggressiveness) he had found to be stable in a standardized behavioral test that involved 13,097 Swedish dogs. However, using the dogs as working dogs in trials (measured as the amount of merits of the breeding stock from working dog trials) correlated positively with playfulness and aggressiveness in sires. These results were significant, regardless of breed. How the dog is used matters; breeding for different criteria (eg, for conformation vs field or other working trials) causes changes in the breed.

Certain personality traits may render humans vulnerable to psychiatric disorders, including anxiety disorders.[19] Anxiety disorders of genetic origin have been documented in dogs. One nervous strain of pointer dogs was more fearful than a stable strain from 2 months of age to maturity in dogs whose rearing environment and handling had been the same.[20,21] Overall and Dunham[22] noted that of dogs identified with obsessive-compulsive disorder (OCD) for whom familial information was available, multiple relatives were also affected. Breed task affected the form of the OCD for many breeds: German shepherds almost always spun and chased their tail. Breeding for different personality criteria may result in extremes of the selected behavior or unintended covariance with other undesired traits (ie, a focused working dog who also has OCD). A survey of the common behavior problems seen in military working dogs showed that aggression represented more than 30% of the behavioral complaints, with 25% involving repetitive behaviors.[23] Problems with object/reward release and overactivity were also significant.

A genetic association has been identified for Doberman pinschers exhibiting one form of OCD, flank sucking,[24] and an association has been suggested for Border collies and profound noise reactivity.[25] Overall and colleagues[26] assessed more than 1300 adult dogs of one breed at 12 to 18 months of age using an ethogram, and identified dogs who consistently withdrew when approached by humans. More than 800 offspring of these dogs were examined at 5 weeks of age, and the distribution of behaviors was similar to that in the adult populations; dogs who consistently withdrew from humans were readily identified, suggesting a heritable component to the fearful condition.

Hilliard and Burghardt[27] noted that the age at which they identified unsuccessful dogs differed from that at which they identified successful ones, and that these ages were not independent of breed. As a result, if dogs were sent to be raised by a foster family/puppy walker family, Belgian Malinois were returned to the colony for training at an earlier age (9 months) than were German shepherds (12 months).

Analyses of the records of training centers in England, the United States, and Australia have shown that dogs fail, not because of an inability to learn guide dog tasks, but because competing responses interfere with the dog's performance.[28–31] Reasons cited for failure were fearfulness, distractibility, and aggressive behaviors.

In one Japanese guide dog program, 80.6% of successful dogs had low scores for distractibility in a factor analysis, whereas 28.2% of failed dogs had high scores.[32] Distracted dogs performed less well in a sample of 33 Belgian military working dogs.[33] Distractibility was significantly related to failure in another program,[34] and showed a weak genetic relationship with the serotonin transporter protein haplotype, suggesting a potentially testable and measurable mechanism for some attribute of success. Some measure of distractibility/anxiety/uncertainty may ultimately allow performance to be assayed early. Heart rate combined with behavioral scores at 3 months help to identify distractible dogs.[32] Four behavioral responses associated with distractibility, restlessness, and anxiety predicted low suitability as a guide dog.[35] Earlier predictability of success in working dogs was found to be associated with 3 assessments: activity and vocalization (birth–7 weeks), fear of social and environmental stimuli (2 months), and absence of later fear of the environment (15 months).[17]

What Makes an Assessment "Good"?

Assessment of behavior must minimally meet 3 quality requirements[14,36,37]: standardization, reliability, and validity of selection procedures. These assessments represent a scientific standard that allows evaluation of how believable and consistent the data are, and whether similar data can be collected from other groups and compared in a meaningful way across groups.

- Tests must be standardized: when this criterion is met, the only source of variability is the animal being tested.
- The test must be reliable: if the same test is given to the same animal twice, the outcome should have a statistically significant and strong positive correlation. For this to happen, the test must also be sensitive so true behavioral differences can be assessed objectively, with only small variation in assessment among the assessors.
- A tests should be valid; it must measure what the evaluator is truly evaluating.

All of these requirements have been problematic, but the one that has been evaluated least often is validity.

Validity refers to how well a test measures and reports on the behaviors the test intends to measure. Validity assessment can be tricky for behavior, because what something is labeled may adversely affect its ability to be measured.[38,39] For example, not all fearful animals are fearful in the same way or for the same reason. In a comparison of specific behaviors exhibited by dogs subjected to an established temperament test, De Meester and colleagues[40] found that fearfulness on one subtest did not predict either the presence of fearfulness or how it appeared on another, related subtest. Contextually characteristic responses of the individual dogs were more important than was the subtest in determining the form of the fear.

Not all dogs that exhibit behaviors associated with an agonistic response are problematically aggressive: distinguishing normal agonistic/aggressive behavior from pathologic aggressive behavior requires a discrete assessment of context and excellent definitions of behaviors and conditions.[41] Studies that do not do this may not only label breeds or groups of dogs as aggressive[42–44] but also lose any phenotypic information that helps with further assessments of canine behavior or selection of breeding stock. The better subgroups of fear or problematic aggression can be characterized, the more likely genetic associations for undesirable traits within the breed or breeding program can be identified. Well-characterized trait subgroups may contain useful and easily recognizable phenotypes for identifying genetic regions associated with an enhanced risk of developing a problematic condition.[24]

Predictive ability (external validity) of behavioral tests for puppies varies greatly, and not just because of the test[37]; it depends on the complexity of the desired characteristics the test is intended to evaluate. If these desired behaviors are well defined and closely related to the test content, predictive ability can be as high as 91.7% for aptitude for police dogs.[45] If less of an association is present between the ultimate tasks that the test hopes to predict and the test battery, no predictive ability may be possible, as Rooney and Bradshaw[46] found for specialist search dogs. Predictive validity is enhanced when measures are specific and accurate.

Failure to identify specific behaviors that are well defined and closely related to the test content may be the single most worrisome aspect of most canine evaluations, especially if the concept of drive is involved.

The characteristics of drive involve:

- The definition from the craft of dog selection that is most often considered to be the propensity of a dog to exhibit a particular pattern of behaviors when faced with particular stimuli.
- That it is triggered by particular stimuli and expressed in a typical and predictable way associated with the particular stimulus.
- That it is enhanced or diminished through experience (eg, training, environment) but cannot be created or eliminated.

Assessments of drive are not quantified or standardized: one person's moderate-drive dog may be another's high-drive dog, and these tests usually lack an external referent that will assure the 3 aspects of validity are met: accuracy, specificity, and scientific validity. At best, tests assessing drive measure clusters or correlates of traits of interest, but they seldom measure any trait in a manner that would be useful to geneticists who require a useful phenotype.

When scores are used to assess behavior, the only way to assess whether dogs with lower scores perform worse than those with higher scores is to follow the dogs across time. Given that behaviors may change with development, tests hoping to identify behaviors that are valid and may be heritable should be evaluated for the sensitivity and specificity of the test. The *sensitivity* of a test is the probability that positive dogs test positively. The *specificity* of the test is the probability that negative dogs test negatively. The positive predictive value (PPV) of the test is the number of true positives, compared with the total number of positives; the negative predictive value (NPV) of the test is the number of true-negatives compared with the number identified as negative.

Van der Borg and colleagues[47] and De Meester and colleagues[40] used the Socially Acceptable Behavior (SAB) test to evaluate dogs for aggressive behavior to humans. The external referent is the actual bite to a human. The tests used were scored based on specific behaviors and their frequencies during timed intervals. Van der Borg and colleagues[47] found a sensitivity, specificity, and accuracy for the test of 0.33, 0.81, and 0.64, respectively, for 479 tests. The low sensitivity of the test was attributed to the decision to classify dogs as aggressive if they bit only once, coupled with the weak ability of the test to detect some types of aggression. The PPV of the test was approximately 0.30, but the NPV was approximately 0.85, meaning that aggression during the test did not predict aggression later, but lack of aggression during the test more often predicted lack of aggression later. De Meester and colleagues[40] compared subtests with the entire test and likewise found a low PPV (aggression by the dog during the test was not helpful for determining behavior later). When predictability and/or sensitivity fail, one aspect of test validity is missing. The small sample of studies using validity criteria seem to support convergent validity of behavioral assessments in adult dogs, but evidence for discriminant validity (when a measure does not correlate with other measures with which it should not be associated) is generally lacking.[48] This fact could be why so many tests of sheltered animals fail to identify types of behaviors that later appear,[49–52] and why investigators should focus on following dogs over time to assay the extent to which the evaluation procedures were truly valid and indicative of behaviors that may be worthy of future genetic study.

This discussion about measuring behavior shows why behaviors or phenotypes for accurate genetic assessment are so difficult to identify. The next section discusses the effect of these measures on heritability assessments.

IS BEHAVIOR HERITABLE?

When the question is asked whether behavior is heritable, 3 questions are really being asked: is this a behavior that contributes to the individual's fitness (for animals under natural selection); is this a behavior that could be enhanced or minimized through selective breeding within this group/breed (artificial selection and quantitative genetics); and is this a behavior that is transmitted by an identifiable region of the genomic code that in some way contributes to the mechanism of the behavior (molecular genetics)? This article focuses only on quantitative and molecular genetics. In fact, some of the changes in canine traits that were selected would be selected against if dogs would evolve merely under natural selection (eg, breeds that can only deliver puppies through Caesarian sections, behaviors such as severe compulsive behavior and extreme aggression or fearfulness).

Quantitative Approaches to Behavior

In quantitative genetics, heritability (h^2) is the proportion of the total phenotypic variance (V_P) that is attributable only to the additive genetic variance (V_A), and not to the variance from effects of dam or environment ($h^2 = V_A/V_P$).[53] V_A is available to be acted on by differential selection (eg, breeding for tighter hips or more milk fat). Heritability estimates pertain only to the population studied, not to the individual or any specific genetic region associated with any behavior or trait. Heritability estimates will not identify whether a certain dog has certain genes, and therefore cannot provide tests for genetic markers, but they can help change the frequency of a condition in a population of dogs. For example, through breeding only dogs with the tightest 20% of hips, hip laxity of a group of interbreeding Labrador retrievers could be greatly decreased over a decade without any knowledge of which genes are involved in sculpting hip dimensions. Behavior can be selected in the same manner, and most heritability focus on behavior has been on personality/temperament. Svartberg and Forkman[54–57] were the first to use the term *personality* in canine temperament studies when they identified 5 stable personality factors: playfulness, curiosity/fearlessness, sociability, aggressiveness, and chase-proneness, from a sample of 15,000 dogs of 164 breeds. Sociability, playfulness, curiosity/fearlessness, and chase-proneness were further found to correlate with each other: the more playful dogs were also more sociable, less fearful, and more interested in chasing.

Approximately 30% to 50% of the personality differences observed between humans are thought to be affected by genes.[58,59] Similar heritability estimates have been obtained for various personality traits in animals.[60–63] Because so much variation in behavior exists across breeds, dogs may provide one of the easiest routes to understanding the genetic component for behavior.[64]

Several studies have investigated the heritability of behavioral traits in dogs. Although heritability estimates calculated for any trait in one population (eg, boldness in Swedish Rottweilers) cannot be used as heritability estimates in another population (eg, Finnish golden retrievers), estimates for the same behavioral trait in different breeds should provide valuable information on the general heritability of particular traits, if the traits are evaluated in the same way.[65] This last condition is not usually met, and therefore caution is urged in overinterpreting breed and study comparisons.

Heritability values vary from 0 (no genetic variation) to 1 (all differences in a trait reflect genetic variation). Generally, heritability estimates larger than 0.40 are considered to be high, indicating that selective breeding can have a large effect on altering the proportion of the trait in the population. Heritability estimates of 0.20 to 0.40 are considered moderate, and estimates less than 0.20 are low and suggest that only a small proportion of the variation observed is of genetic origin in the population studied. In general, heritability estimates for behavior are usually lower than for morphologic traits,[66] and it should be considered that the extent to which this is true may be because of the failure to define clear, quantifiable behavioral measures, and therefore these estimates should be evaluated discretely within tests that can be validated. It is also important to remember that low h^2 values means that a small proportion of the observed differences in a particular population are caused by variation in genotypes, and not (necessarily) that the trait is not heritable.

Some heritability studies have evaluated personality traits important for working dogs, such as boldness, fear, general aggression, sociability, and reactivity to guns/sound sensitivity.[67–69] Heritabilities for boldness (or courage) in German shepherds have varied from low (0.05)[70] to moderate (0.27)[62] values. Fearfulness seems to have higher heritabilities in the breeds examined, with h^2 estimates from 0.46 and 0.58 in Labrador retrievers in training as guide dogs.[31,71] Similarly, reactivity to guns may have high h^2 estimates (0.56 in Labrador retrievers; 0.21 for German shepherds).[69]

Breeds and dogs within breeds vary in their reaction toward humans. Reactions can range from neutral to aggressive to extremely open/friendly. This sociability/amicability toward humans has a large h^2 in German shepherds (0.32) but an extremely low h^2 in Labrador retrievers (0.03),[69] suggesting that selection could change population norms in these shepherds but not in the retrievers. Is it possible that this retriever population is already the result of sustained selection (ie, all Labradors have a "friendly genotype," which results in no genetic variation for that trait)? Yes, but in the absence of continuous measures h^2 analysis, and discrete behavioral analyses, one should assume nothing.

Aggressiveness has been long known to have a strong genetic component, and aggressive and nonaggressive mouse strains have been bred for decades.[72] Similarly contrived dog breeds do not exist, but in a study investigating aggressiveness in golden retrievers, reactions to humans and dogs both had high heritabilities (0.77 toward humans; 0.81 toward dogs).[73] Aggressive responses to humans did not correlate with aggressive responses to dogs, suggesting that if the assessment was equally sensitive, these responses had different genetic backgrounds.[73] Heritability of dominance aggression (also called *impulse control aggression/conflict aggression*) in English cocker spaniels was calculated separately for dam (mother) and sire (father). Dam heritability was greater than that of the sire (0.46 vs 0.20),[74] but the higher heritability in dams includes both maternal genetic and maternal environmental factors in the calculation. Although diagnoses should not be considered phenotypes, they can identify patterns of behavior that can be quantified, and may help create subsequent assessments that can be validated.

Given the ongoing effort in selective breeding and the number of breeds involved, one would expect various aspects of hunting behavior to have high heritability. Liinamo and colleagues[75] found h^2 values of 0.06 to 0.13 for different hunting behaviors of the Finnish hound. Similarly, studies investigating heritability for different aspects of hunting behaviors (eg, speed, style, eagerness, cooperation, independence) have found low h^2 values (0.06–0.28 for German short-haired pointers, German wired-haired pointers, and Brittany spaniels; 0.18–0.29 for English setters[76]). However, in flat-coated retrievers in Sweden, Lindberg and colleagues[77] tested litters dogs of the same age, at the same time, and found high h^2 values for hunting excitement (0.48), willingness to retrieve (0.28), and independence (0.18). Heritability of herding behavior in Border collies was as high as 0.30 (average over 17 traits), indicating a strong genetic component for herding.[78,79] However, the h^2 estimates for the flat-coated retrievers and Border collies was based on actual behavioral testing, and not on questionnaires soliciting people's opinions (as was the case for the aggressive assessment in golden retrievers), and therefore may be the result of more repeatable and reliable behavioral measures. When questionnaires are used, they must be validated to ensure that the variance being studied is not that of human opinion or misperception; this is seldom done.

If behavior is clearly heritable, why do most studies of behavior find only very low heritabilities? Several possible explanations exist.

1. The test in which heritability is calculated may not measure the trait it is supposed to measure; instead, it may actually measure the owner's ability to train the dog (Courreau and Langlois[80] provide examples of heritability for heeling and jumping).
2. Hunting and working tests include a huge amount of noise in the data and do not test for interrater and intrarater reliability, which can be affected by factors such as opinion, bias, and lack of agreed terms. The use of several judges and testing places, and testing dogs at different times of year make measuring behaviors and estimating the genetic component more difficult.[75] Studies in which heritability values have been derived from properly standardized tests using only a few well-trained judges show much larger heritabilities for behavior.[67,68,78,79] The use of well-defined and/or objective criteria is a further improvement.[78,79]
3. The traits for which the heritability is calculated may have been split into pieces that are too numerous, and they correlate with each other. Reanalyzing existing data with some kind of factor analysis may reveal more reliable and independent personality components with larger heritabilities.[63,68,77]

4. Traits may be under strong genetic control, but the particular population studied may have no genetic variation; this also results in low heritability values.

To summarize, several behavioral traits in dogs seem to have a large genetic component because the behavior appears frequently in the pedigree (**Fig. 3**), but heritability studies may not identify these behaviors as having high heritability. This problem is largely because of the difficulty in capturing or evaluating the behavior's genetic component. Large heritability values observed for traits such as fear, activity, and noise sensitivity mean that most of the variation observed in these traits is caused by variation in the genotypes (ie, behavior is inherited in large degree from parent to offspring), and that selective breeding for these traits is possible in dogs. When these studies are used with molecular studies, problems with identifying and testing behaviors may be explained. For now, the primary use of heritability studies in canine behavior continues to be for purpose-bred dog groups (eg, service dogs) to make breeding decisions based on the direction in which breeders wish to encourage change in the population. Heritability studies are also useful for breeds or breeding groups if breeders decide that the dogs have a problem with a genetic basis and the breeders are going to use heritability to define the population that should be bred to minimize that problem (eg, the original example of hip laxity). These uses only work well when the assessments used are objective, repeatable, and reliable, and the data are recorded and used to make decisions. These constraints do not characterize the population of dogs from which average pets come, but should encourage the cooperation of breeders to realize that they have it in their power to improve the behavioral and welfare needs of pet dogs.

Molecular Approaches to Behavior

Methods to study genes behind complex traits

Molecular approaches in genetics seek to identify the genetic architecture of a trait or condition. Once a genetic basis/pattern has been established for a trait/condition, 2 types of methodologies can be used to map the putative genes: linkage and association studies. Gene association studies investigate whether statistically significant

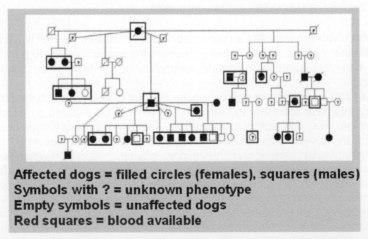

Affected dogs = filled circles (females), squares (males)
Symbols with ? = unknown phenotype
Empty symbols = unaffected dogs
Red squares = blood available

Fig. 3. Border collie pedigree for noise reactivity/phobia. (*From* Overall KL. Manual of clinical behavioral medicine for dogs and cats. St Louis (MO): Elsevier; 2013; with permission.)

differences in the allele frequencies exist between individuals with different pheno-types,[81] whereas linkage studies examine whether specific genetic markers cosegre-gate with trait/disease alleles.[82] Association studies are most likely more effective in complex traits (such as behavior) to which numerous genes are expected to contribute, each with a relatively small effect, whereas linkage analysis is effective in identifying rare and highly penetrant variants.[83,84] Association analysis can use both related and unrelated individuals, whereas linkage analysis is performed using a pedigree structure.

Candidate gene studies (a form of association study) mostly use a case-control study design, meaning that dogs are matched (and preferably unrelated, at least at the grandparental level) so that for every dog with the condition, one is without. Candi-date genes are chosen based on the function of the proteins for which the genes code, and therefore are hypothesis-driven. Candidate gene studies are cheap to perform, but they are vulnerable to population stratification—systematic ancestry differences between cases and controls—which is common in dog breeds. Underlying population structure may produce false-positive associations in candidate gene studies in which observed association is actually the result of different allele frequencies or cryptic relatedness, and not the result of a genetic disease effect.[85] To ensure this is a not a risk, candidate gene allele frequencies should be compared against the phenotype within one breed, and in some cases, within one breeding line, because breeds often have distinct conformation/show and working lines (eg, German shepherd, Border col-lies). Regardless, it is worth remembering that complex traits such as behavioral traits are most likely controlled by many loci, and by their interaction with each other and the environment. These considerations limit the usefulness of candidate gene studies in behavioral genetics.

Genome-wide association (GWA) studies have become increasingly popular, and the publication of the expanded canine genome (7.5x, Boxer) has made them possible.[4] GWA studies investigate the association between common genetic vari-ations and some phenotype. GWA studies are non–hypothesis-driven. These studies require a dense marker set that captures a substantial proportion of the common genetic variation across the genome. They also need a large sample size.[86] Single nucleotide polymorphisms (SNPs) are the most prevalent class of ge-netic variation used in human and canine GWA studies.[87] Copy number variations (deletions or multiple copies of sections of genome) are also frequently used as markers in association studies.[88,89] SNPs that are in proximity to each other are more often inherited together, which is referred as *linkage disequilibrium* (LD). In dogs, the average length of LD is 2 Mb, whereas in humans it is 0.28 Mb.[4,90,91] When combined with the large genetic homogeneity within breeds, this average LD means that many fewer individuals are needed in dog GWA studies than in hu-man GWA studies. But, because of the longer LD blocks, accuracy in dogs is typi-cally not as good as it is in humans. GWA studies investigating canine complex traits have successfully identified several affecting loci.[92] With sufficient sample size and detailed phenotyping, GWA studies should be able to find several loci that affect complex traits, such as behavior.

Whole-genome sequencing or next-generation sequencing (NGS) are now widely used in human genetics[93] and have also been used for dogs.[94,95] Whole-genome sequencing means simply sequencing the complete genome, whereas targeted NGS means sequencing certain area of interest. In the future, these methods will most likely increase the success of genetic studies in dogs, including those for behavior, because they provide the largest cover of genetic variants, which lowers costs.

GENETIC MARKERS AND CANINE STUDIES
Candidate Genes and Neurochemistry

Takeuchi and colleagues[96] used key word analysis of trainer observations in a factor analysis and found a significant association between the factor activity level and degree of polymorphism in genes associated with glutamate transporters and the catechol-O-methyltransferase (COMT) gene. COMT is important in dopamine metabolism, and glutamate has been implicated in impulsivity in aggression and neurocytotoxic events, such as stroke and seizures.

In a study of the dopamine D4 receptor (DRD4) in 96 unrelated German shepherds, Héjjas and colleagues[97] found significant associations between the exons ($P = 0.002$) and introns ($P = 0.003$) of the variable number of tandem repeats (VNTR) in the DRD4 gene and the social impulsivity phenotype of their Greeting Test. The phenotype was derived from a coded score that rated how a dog behaved during a staged human approach: 0 = the dog was not friendly; 1 = the dog was friendly but did not follow the person testing the dog; and 2 = the dog followed the person testing the dog when the person walked away. Higher scores were thought to indicate increased interest in novel social companions, which some authors characterize as social impulsivity. Although one could argue with this definition of impulsivity, this test was sufficient to characterize behavioral differences associated with the long (Q) and short form (P) polymorphisms of the DRD4 intron 2 VNTR and the DRD4 exon 3 VNTR. The scores for P/P (1.36 ± 0.58; $n = 50$), P/Q (0.84 ± 0.64; $n = 32$), and Q/Q genotypes (1.43 ± 0.51; $n = 14$) differed ($P = 0.006$), indicating that there was an association between the behaviors captured by the score and variability in gene expression. Similar patterns were shown for the DRD4 exon 3 VNTR. Whether these techniques will be valuable for screening or breeding pet and/or working dogs will depend on how variable the population of available dogs is and whether these behavioral assessments are representative of behavioral profiles useful for work or desired in pets. The population of German shepherds from which these dogs were sampled had the following genotype frequencies for the DRD4 intron 2 VNTR: 48.3% for P/P; 39.3% for P/Q; and 12.4% for Q/Q. Equivalent frequencies for Belgian Malinois, Belgian Tervuerens, Belgian Groenendael, and Siberian Huskies were, respectively, 30.0%, 14.9%, 29.5%, and 3.0% for P/P; 52.0%, 48.5%, 45.7%, and 5.1% for P/Q; and 18.0%, 36.6%, 24.8%, and 91.1% for Q/Q. Whether variation in genotype frequencies is functionally important for any dogs is unknown, but the question is especially relevant for working dogs.

Distractibility that was significantly related to failure[34] showed a weak genetic relationship with the serotonin transporter protein haplotype, suggesting a potentially testable and measurable mechanism for some attribute of success as a working dog. Whether these findings have any direct applicability for pet dogs, better characterization of any dog's behavior will provide clients with clearer expectations about their dog's behavioral style and needs, and may lead to more humane handling/training and better relationships.

The Special Case of Gene Mapping and Olfaction in Dogs

Olfactory receptors (ORs) are found on ciliated membranes of olfactory sensory neurons in the olfactory mucosa. Efficient odor discrimination requires that ORs bind with odorants and that this process trigger a signal transduction pathway that allows information to be processed and acted on via connections in the olfactory bulb and brain cortex. If dogs vary in odorant detection ability, are those who are more skilled more efficient in initiating the signal transduction cascade, or do they have different alleles encoding ORs with greater odorant affinity[96]? No simple answer to this question exists.

OR genes are members of the G protein–coupled receptor (GPCR) superfamily, which contains approximately 1300 genes in dogs[98] and is one of the largest gene families in mammals.[99,100] Intracellular and extracellular loops of GPCRs are polymorphic in all species studied, including dogs.[101] These polymorphisms are believed to play a large role in odor discrimination and, because of the large number of OR genes, the initial processing of information associated with the ability to discriminate odors has been thought to depend on the selective binding affinity of the ORs. However, ORs show only moderate affinity for scent molecules/odorants, and therefore binding affinity may also depend on the concentration of a particular odorant,[102] as has been confirmed for *Drosophila*, in which large concentration differences are treated like different odors.[103] Perception of odor relies on 3 stages of processing in the brain after OR binding: memory of odor quality, memory of odor intensity, and the range of intensities and qualities over which the odor is generalized.

Using 38 cloned OR genes belonging to the same canine OR gene family, Benbernou and colleagues[104] found considerable cross-receptor reactivity, suggesting that the number of combinations possible for the estimated 1000 receptors is sufficient to convey a portrait of the olfactory world to the dog in a manner that uniquely identifies the odors they encounter.

Assumptions made about breed superiority in olfactory skills have not been borne out by attempts to study the putative genes involved.[105–107] OR genes seem to be highly polymorphic across and within breeds.[101,102,107,108] Robin and colleagues[108] examined DNA sequences of 48 dogs from 6 breeds, of which 4 have been asserted to have strong olfactory detection skills (German shepherds, Belgian Malinois, English springer spaniel, Labrador retriever) and 2 have been asserted to have weak olfactory detection skills (greyhound, Pekinese). All sampled dogs were unrelated at least at the grandparental level, and every effort was made to sample dogs from diverse international sources. The number of SNPs differed among breeds, but their distribution did not. The number of OR genes without polymorphism differed markedly across breeds: German shepherds, greyhounds, and Labrador retrievers had, respectively, 24, 21, and 10 genes with no polymorphism. A total of 193 of 732 SNPs were restricted to a single breed, and their breed distribution varied significantly, with 10 private SNPs for German shepherds, 26 for Belgian Malinois, 47 for English springer spaniels, 18 for greyhounds, 8 for Labrador retrievers, and 84 for Pekinese. A total of 199 SNPs were common to all breeds, 79 were common to 3 breeds, and 50 were common to 2 breeds. These results suggest that the 199 SNPs that all breeds had in common likely arose before the separation of these 6 breeds, and that most of the private SNPs arose after these breeds developed. Comparison at the breed level found that the most polymorphic breed was the English springer spaniel (N value = 594), and the least polymorphic was the German shepherd (N value = 926), yet both of these breeds are favored as detection dogs.

These data strongly suggest that there has been no strong selection for more variable OR genes or proteins. Dogs with particularly acute olfactory detection capabilities may perform so well because they are particularly good at processing and acting on olfactory information, rather than at detecting it. If so, aspects of communication between the dog and handler may be more important for the success of detection dogs than has previously been believed.[109–112] Oddly, the modern view of relationships in the pet population is that good communication between dog and human is essential.

WHAT OTHER GENETIC ISSUES CAN AFFECT BEHAVIOR? EPIGENETICS IN BRIEF

Epigenetic changes are those changes in gene expression that are caused by mechanisms other than alterations in the underlying genetic sequence. Many epigenetic effects have been shown to be heritable. Some of the most common epigenetic effects involve methylation: tagging a CH_3 group onto a region of the DNA that affects how or whether it is transcribed.

For example, prenatal exposure to maternal stress causes epigenetic methylation of glucocorticoid receptor promoter regions, which leads to hyperreactivity in rodents and human beings.[113–115] Behavioral differences may not be present only in the first generation of offspring, they can also be apparent in the second generation, although none of these offspring experienced maternal stress themselves. In rodents, hippocampal expression of the glucocorticoid receptor gene and behavioral responses to stress are modulated by the amount of care mothers give their young in the first few days of life.[116] These processes also likely occur in dogs and cats and are known to affect task learning, which can be enhanced when stress and distress are mitigated. These effects may be responsible for the findings in one study that showed that canine puppies raised with their mothers and siblings through 56 days (8 weeks) developed fewer behavior problems and were less reactive than puppies adopted at 30 to 40 days, all other aspects being equal.[117] Similarly, early separation from the mother and lower-quality maternal care seems to be associated with frequent tail chasing in several breeds.[118] Raising puppies with their siblings and dam through at least 56 days, a time when most brain myelination is complete but when neuronal remodeling should be rapidly ongoing, may provide mitigation of potential epigenetic effects caused by acute neurodevelopmental stress.

Geneticists who study behavioral development have a strong sense that epigenetic effects may be extremely important for determining early genetic trajectories. Quick, inexpensive, and easy-to-use tools to test for these effects do not yet exist, but because so many of these effects are associated with prenatal, perinatal, and postnatal stress, the best advice veterinarians could give is to provide as excellent, stable, and enriched physical, nutritional, and behavioral environments as possible. The data to date also suggest that dogs and cats subject to stressors may be more at risk for becoming more reactive regardless, and should receive remedial intervention as soon as possible. These animals may include strays, shelter dogs/cats, feral dogs/cats, dogs/cats whose mothers were ill or malnourished or undernourished, puppies/kittens experiencing dystocia, or those experiencing less-than-optimal social and/or nutritional environments (puppy mills/farms, commercial catteries). Possible interventions may include diet, supplements, medication, and behavior modification that prompts learning of more appropriate responses.

FUTURE DIRECTIONS

Tables 1 and **2** contain lists of somatic conditions that can be confirmed/identified by genetic testing for cats and dogs, respectively (online resources in which updates can be found are listed in the Appendix). A quick look at these lists shows that genetic tests are restricted to conditions that are easily recognizable and that interfere in a clear, measurable way with physiologic or neurologic function. This characterization is a challenge in behavior, but progress can be made.

Gene discovery for behavioral traits in humans and other animal has not been as straightforward as for simple Mendelian traits. Although knowledge of the genetics of complex traits will increase hugely in a decade, the process to gain that

Table 1
Inherited diseases of cats that can be confirmed by genetic testing

Dermatologic conditions	Rex coat
	Alopecia
Ocular conditions	Retinal degeneration
Neurologic conditions	Deafness in white cats
	Cerebellar degeneration
	Feline hereditary neuroaxonal dystrophy
	Lysosomal storage diseases
Musculoskeletal conditions	Muscular dystrophy
	Dwarfism and chondrodystrophic disorders
	Polydactyly
	Split foot
	Short bent tail
	Curled ears
Cardiovascular conditions	Hypertrophic cardiomyopathy in Maine coon cats, only
Hematologic/immunologic conditions	Neonatal isoerythrolysis
	Inherited hyperchylomicronemia
	Bleeding disorders

Data from International Cat Care. Available at: http://www.icatcare.org/advice/cat breeds/inherited-disorders-cats. Accessed January 2, 2014.

knowledge may not get much simpler. The hope is that the roles of epigenetics, gene–gene interactions, and gene–environment interactions will become clearer, if the pattern in human psychiatric genetics is a model. After decades of work, efforts to understand the genetics of human anxiety are making progress, and one is reminded that genes do not follow diagnostic manuals. Several neuropsychiatric disorders seem to share predisposing loci,[119] and a similar result should be expected for canine behavioral genetics. A highly significant association between canine compulsive disorder and a neuronal adhesion protein, CDH2, on chromosome 7 has now been identified in Doberman pinschers.[24] This genetic locus was the first identified for any OCD in animals, but its role in the mechanism of the pathology remains unclear.

In the next decade, several novel loci associated with behavioral traits are likely to be discovered in dogs. However, potential gene discovery for conditions such as OCD, or noise phobia in one breed, does not necessarily mean that the puzzle is solved and a genetic test will be available for every breed. These conditions likely involve several genes, which may (at least partly) be breed-specific or breed group–specific (eg, herding dogs), as seems to be the case in heritable eye diseases and epilepsy in dogs.[120,121] In the future, potential gene tests may at most offer information on the risk for the allele carrier to develop, for example, noise phobia.

The challenge of behavioral genetics in all species is to characterize phenotypes sufficiently well that genetic studies illuminate both the risk of the condition and some of the mechanisms causing behavioral suffering. When this stage is reached, and it will be, therapies can be targeted that address specific malfunctions.

Until then, veterinarians are best advised to offer functional counseling about behavioral problems that involves advice to clients to understand normal, recognize any deviations from it, seek help from veterinarians and behavior specialists early, do not breed affected individuals, and, if the condition is common in the breed line (at least once every generation), seek genetic counseling and consider revision of all breeding

Table 2
Sample single-gene tests commercially available for specific disease conditions in dogs, among the more than 145 diseases listed as heritable

Genetic Trait	Disease Condition	Breeds Affected
GRM1 gene mutation	Neonatal ataxia	Coton de Tulear
CMR1 & CMR2: BEST1 gene mutations	Canine multifocal retinopathy	Australian shepherd, bull mastiff, bulldog, Cane Corso, Coton de Tulear, English bulldog, English mastiff
CNM gene: recessive trait	Centronuclear myopathy	Labrador retriever
CT gene: autosomal recessive gene	Copper toxicosis	Bedlington terrier
CN gene: autosomal recessive gene	Canine cyclic neutropenia (gray collie syndrome)	Collie
Cyst gene: autosomal recessive trait	Renal cysteine calculi	Newfoundlands
DCM: gene mutation	Dilated cardiomyopathy	Doberman pinscher
Factor VII deficiency: autosomal recessive	Mild to moderate hemorrhage	Alaskan Klee Kai, beagle, giant Schnauzer, Scottish deerhound
PN: autosomal recessive mutation	Greyhound polyneuropathy	Greyhound
Hem B: mutant X chromosome	Hemophilia B	Bull terrier, Lhasa Apso
HSF4 mutation	Hereditary cataract	Boston terrier, French bulldog, Staffordshire bull terrier
HN: X-linked dominant trait	Hereditary nephritis	Samoyed
HU: autosomal recessive trait	Hyperuricosuria	American Staffordshire, Australian shepherd Black Russian terrier, bulldog, Dalmatian, GSD giant Schnauzer, Parson Russell terrier, large Munsterlander, pit bull terrier, South African Boerboel, Weimaraner
L-2-hydroxyglutaric aciduria: recessive mutation	L-2-hydroxyglutaric aciduria	Staffordshire bull terrier

Abbreviations: BEST, bestrophin; CMR 1 and 2, canine multifocal retinopathy 1 and 2; GRM 1, metabotropic glutamate receptor 1.
Data from the CIDD Database. Available at: http://ic.upei.ca/cidd/disorder/overview. Accessed January 2, 2014.

decisions. For some breeds this will be difficult, because inbreeding has so greatly constrained the gene pool,[122] but if we are interested in the welfare of the animals who share our lives, we must invest in choosing to select for behaviors that do not cause animals suffering or distress, and in the tools that will help us identify these behaviors.

REFERENCES

1. Vilà C, Savolainen P, Maldonado JE, et al. Multiple and ancient origins of the domestic dog. Science 1997;276(5319):1687–9.
2. Savolainen P, Zhang YP, Luo J, et al. Genetic evidence for an East Asian origin of domestic dogs. Science 2002;298(5598):1610–3.
3. Sutter NB, Bustamante CD, Chase K, et al. A single IGF1 allele is a major determinant of small size in dogs. Science 2007;316(5821):112–5.
4. Lindblad-Toh K, Wade CM, Mikkelsen TS, et al. Genome sequence, comparative analysis and haplotype structure of the domestic dog. Nature 2005;438(7069): 803–19.
5. Cadieu E, Neff NW, Quignon P, et al. Coat variation in the domestic dog is governed by variants in three genes. Science 2009;326(5949):150–3.
6. von Holdt BM, Pollinger JP, Lohmueller KE, et al. Genome-wide SNP and haplotype analyses reveal a rich history underlying dog domestication. Nature 2010; 464:898–902.
7. Axelsson E, Ratnakumar A, Arendt ML, et al. The genomic signature of dog domestication reveals adaptation to a starch-rich diet. Nature 2013;495(7441): 360–4.
8. Boyko AR, Boyko RH, Boyko CM, et al. Complex population structure in African village dogs and its implication for inferring dog domestication history. Proc Natl Acad Sci U S A 2009;106(33):13903–8.
9. Pang JF, Kluetsch C, Zou XJ, et al. mtDNA data indicate a single origin for dogs south of Yangtze River, less than 16,300 years ago, from numerous wolves. Mol Biol Evol 2009;26(12):2849–64.
10. Castroviejo-Fisher S, Skoglund P, Valadez R, et al. Vanishing native American dog lineages. BMC Evol Biol 2011;11:73.
11. Germonpré MM, Lázničková-Galetová M, Sablin M. Paleolithic dog skulls at the Gravettian Předmostí site, the Czech Republic. J Archaeol Sci 2012;39(1): 184–202.
12. Wang G, Zhai W, Yang H, et al. The genomics of selection in dogs and the parallel evolution between dogs and humans. Nat Commun 2013;4: 1860.
13. Plomin R. Childhood temperament. In: Lahey BB, Kazdin AE, editors. Advances in clinical child psychology 6. New York: Plenum Press; 1983. p. 45–92.
14. Taylor KD, Mills DS. The development and assessment of temperament tests for adult companion dogs. J Vet Behav Clin Appl Res 2006;1(3):94–108.
15. Ledger RA, Baxter MR. The development of a validated test to assess the temperament of dogs in a rescue shelter. In: Mills DS, Heath SE, Harrington LJ, editors. Proceedings of the First International Conference on Veterinary Behavioral Medicine. Birmingham (United Kingdom): Universities Federation for Animal Welfare; 1997. p. 87–92.
16. Ruefenacht S, Gebhardt-Henrich S, Miyake T, et al. A behaviour test on German shepherd dogs: heritability of seven different traits. Appl Anim Behav Sci 2002; 79(2):113–32.
17. Diederich C, Giffroy JM. Temperament testing, from puppies to adulthood. J Vet Behav Clin Appl Res 2009;4(6):237–8.
18. Svartberg K. Breed-typical behaviour in dogs-historical remnants or recent constructs? Appl Anim Behav Sci 2006;96(3–4):293–313.
19. Deckersbach T, Dougherty DD, Rauch SL. Functional imaging of mood and anxiety disorders. J Neuroimaging 2006;16(1):1–10.

20. Murphree OD, Dykman RA. Litter patterns in the offspring of nervous and stable dogs. I: behavioral tests. J Nerv Ment Dis 1965;141:321–32.
21. Murphree OD. Inheritance of human aversion and inactivity in two strains of the pointer dog. Biol Psychiatry 1973;7:23–9.
22. Overall KL, Dunham AE. Clinical features and outcome in dogs and cats with obsessive-compulsive disorder: 126 cases (1989–2000). J Am Vet Med Assoc 2002;221(10):1445–52.
23. Burghardt WF Jr. Behavioral considerations in the management of military working dogs. Vet Clin North Am Small Anim Pract 2003;33(2):417–46.
24. Dodman NH, Karlsson EK, Moon-Fanelli A, et al. A canine chromosome 7 locus confers compulsive disorder susceptibility. Mol Psychiatry 2010;15:8–10.
25. Overall KL, Hamilton SP, Chang ML, et al. Noise reactivity in three breeds of herding dogs: what the crossroads of demography, ethology, and genetics can tell us. J Vet Behav Clin Appl Res 2009;4:70–1.
26. Overall KL, Dyer DJ, Dunham AE, et al. Update on the Canine Behavioral Genetics Project (CBGP): progress in understanding heritable fears and anxieties. J Vet Behav Clin Appl Res 2008;3(4):184–5.
27. Hilliard S, Burghardt WF Jr. Development and validation of behavioral testing instruments for longitudinal study of military working puppies. Presented at the International Working Dog Breeding Conference. San Antonio, September 10–12, 2001.
28. Baillie JR. The behavioural requirements necessary for Guide Dogs for the Blind in the United Kingdom. Br Vet J 1972;128:477.
29. Guide Dogs for the Blind. Annual report: the guide dogs for the Blind association. Windsor (Great Britain): Guide Dogs for the Blind; 1975.
30. Scott JP, Bielfelt SW. Analysis of the puppy testing program. In: Pfaffenberger CJ, Scott JP, Fuller JL, et al, editors. Guide dogs for the blind: their selection, development and training. Amsterdam: Elsevier; 1976. p. 39–75.
31. Goddard ME, Beilharz RG. Genetics of traits which determine the suitability of dogs as guide-dogs for the blind. Appl Anim Ethol 1983;9(3–4):299–315.
32. Arata S, Momozawa Y, Takeuchi Y, et al. Important behavioral traits for predicting guide dog qualification. J Vet Med Sci 2010;72(5):539–45.
33. Haverbeke A, Laporte B, Depiereux D, et al. Training methods of military dog handlers and their effects on the team's performances. Appl Anim Behav Sci 2008;113(1–3):110–22.
34. Maejima M, Inoue-Murayama M, Tonosaki K, et al. Traits and genotypes may predict the successful training of drug detection dogs. Appl Anim Behav Sci 2007;107(3–4):287–98.
35. Tomkins LM, Williams KA, Thomson PC, et al. Lateralization in the domestic dog (Canis familiaris): relationships between structural, motor, and sensory laterality. J Vet Behav Clin Appl Res 2012;7(2):70–9.
36. Martin P, Bateson P. Measuring behaviour: an introductory guide. 2nd edition. Cambridge (United kingdom): Cambridge University Press; 1993. p. 1–224.
37. Diederich C, Giffroy JM. Behavioural testing in dogs: a review of methodology in search for standardisation. Appl Anim Behav Sci 2006;97(1):51–72.
38. Overall KL. Proceedings of the Dogs Trust Meeting on Advances in Veterinary Behavioural Medicine London; 4th–7th November 2004: veterinary behavioural medicine: a roadmap for the 21st century. Vet J 2005;169:130–43.
39. Overall KL. Manual of clinical behavioral medicine for dogs and cats. St Louis (MO): Elsevier; 2013.

40. De Meester RH, Pluijmakers J, Vermeire S, et al. The use of the socially accept-
    able behavior test in the study of temperament of dogs. J Vet Behav Clin Appl
    Res 2011;6(4):211–24.
41. Haverbeke A, De Smet A, Depiereux E, et al. Assessing undesired aggression in
    military working dogs. Appl Anim Behav Sci 2009;117(1–2):55–62.
42. Duffy DL, Hsu Y, Serpell JA. Breed differences in canine aggression. Appl Anim
    Behav Sci 2008;114(3–4):441–60.
43. Serpell JA, Hsu Y. Development and validation of a novel method for evaluating
    behavior and temperament in guide dogs. Appl Anim Behav Sci 2001;72(4):
    347–64.
44. Hsu Y, Serpell JA. Development and validation of a questionnaire for measuring
    behavior and temperament traits in pet dogs. J Am Vet Med Assoc 2003;223(9):
    1293–300.
45. Slabbert JM, Odendaal JS. Early prediction of adult police dog efficiency—
    a longitudinal study. Appl Anim Behav Sci 1999;64:269–88.
46. Rooney NJ, Bradshaw JW. Breed and sex differences in the behavioural attri-
    butes of specialist search dogs—a questionnaire survey of trainers and han-
    dlers. Appl Anim Behav Sci 2004;86(1–2):123–35.
47. van der Borg JA, Beerda B, Ooms M, et al. Evaluation of behaviour testing for
    human directed aggression in dogs. Appl Anim Behav Sci 2010;128:78–90.
48. Jones AC, Gosling SD. Temperament and personality in dogs (Canis familiaris):
    a review and evaluation of past research. Appl Anim Behav Sci 2005;95(1–2):
    1–53.
49. Christensen E, Scarlett J, Campagna M, et al. Aggressive behavior in adopted
    dogs that passed a temperament test. Appl Anim Behav Sci 2007;106(1–3):
    85–95.
50. Bollen KS, Horowitz J. Behavioral evaluation and demographic information in the
    assessment of aggressiveness in shelter dogs. Appl Anim Behav Sci 2008;
    112(1–2):120–35.
51. Paroz C, Gebhardt-Henrich SG, Steiger A. Reliability and validity of behaviour
    tests in Hovawart dogs. Appl Anim Behav Sci 2008;115(1–2):67–81.
52. Segurson SA, Serpell JA, Hart BL. Evaluation of a behavioral assessment ques-
    tionnaire for use in the characterization of behavioral problems of dogs relin-
    quished to animal shelters. J Am Vet Med Assoc 2005;227(11):1755–61.
53. Falconer DS, Mackay TF. Introduction to quantitative genetics. 4th edition.
    Malaysia: Longman Publishing Group; 1996.
54. Svartberg K, Forkman B. Personality traits in the domestic dog (Canis familiaris).
    Appl Anim Behav Sci 2002;79(2):133–55.
55. Stamps J, Groothuis TG. The development of animal personality: relevance,
    concepts and perspectives. Biol Rev 2010;85(2):301–25.
56. König von Borstel U, Pasing S, Gauly M. Towards a more objective assessment
    of equine personality using behavioural and physiological observations from
    performance test training. Appl Anim Behav Sci 2011;135(4):277–85.
57. Gartner MC, Weiss A. Personality in felids: a review. Appl Anim Behav Sci 2013;
    144(1–2):1–13.
58. Jang KL, Livesley WJ, Vernon PA. Heritability of the big five personality dimen-
    sions and their facets: a twin study. J Pers 1996;64(3):577–91.
59. Bouchard TJ Jr, Loehlin JC. Genes, evolution, and personality. Behav Genet
    2001;31(3):243–73.
60. Dingemanse NJ. Repeatability and heritability of exploratory behaviour in great
    tits from the wild. Anim Behav 2002;64(6):929–38.

61. Drent PJ, van Oers K, van Noordwijk AJ. Realized heritability of personalities in the great tit (Parus major). Proc Biol Sci 2003;270(1510):45–51.
62. Strandberg E, Jacobsson J, Saetre P. Direct genetic, maternal and litter effects on behaviour in German shepherd dogs in Sweden. Livest Prod Sci 2005;93(1): 33–42.
63. Saetre P, Strandberg E, Sundgren P, et al. The genetic contribution to canine personality. Genes, Brain and Behav 2006;5(3):240–8.
64. Spady TC, Ostrander E. Canine behavioral genetics: pointing out the pheno-types and herding up the genes. Am J Hum Genet 2008;82(1):10–8.
65. Visscher PM. Sizing up human height variation. Nat Genet 2009;40:489–90.
66. Mousseau T, Roff D. Natural selection and the heritability of fitness components. Heredity 1987;59:181–97.
67. Wilsson E, Sundgren P. The use of a behaviour test for selection of dogs for ser-vice and breeding. II. Heritability for tested parameters and effect of selection based on service dog characteristics. Appl Anim Behav Sci 1997;54(2–3): 235–41.
68. Wilsson E, Sundgren P. Behaviour test for eight-week old puppies—heritabilities of tested behaviour traits and its correspondence to later behaviour. Appl Anim Behav Sci 1998;58(1–2):151–62.
69. van der Waaij EH, Wilsson E, Strandberg E. Genetic analysis of results of a Swedish behavior test on German shepherd dogs and Labrador retrievers. J Anim Sci 2008;86(11):2853–61.
70. Reuterwall C, Ryman N. An estimate of the magnitude of additive genetic vari-ation of some mental characters in Alsatian dogs. Hereditas 1973;73(2): 277–83.
71. Goddard ME, Beilharz RG. Genetic and environmental factors affecting the suit-ability of dogs as guide dogs for the blind. Theor Appl Genet 1982;62(2): 97–102.
72. Lagerspetz KM, Lagerspetz KY. Changes in the aggressiveness of mice result-ing from selective breeding, learning and social isolation. Scand J Psychol 1971;12(1):241–8.
73. Liinamo AE, van den Berg L, Leegwater PA, et al. Genetic variation in aggression-related traits in golden retriever dogs. Appl Anim Behav Sci 2007; 104(1–2):95–106.
74. Pérez-Guisado J, Lopez-Rodríguez R, Muñoz-Serrano A. Heritability of dominant-aggressive behaviour in English cocker spaniels. Appl Anim Behav Sci 2006;100:219–27.
75. Liinamo AE, Karjalainen L, Ojala M, et al. Estimates of genetic parameters and environmental effects for measures of hunting performance in Finnish hounds. J Anim Sci 1997;75:622–9.
76. Brenøe UT, Larsgard AG, Johannessen KR, et al. Estimates of genetic parame-ters for hunting performance traits in three breeds of gun hunting dogs in Nor-way. Appl Anim Behav Sci 2002;77(3):209–15.
77. Lindberg S, Strandberg E, Swenson L. Genetic analysis of hunting behav-iour in Swedish flatcoated retrievers. Appl Anim Behav Sci 2004;88(3–4): 289–98.
78. Arvelius P, Strandberg E. Genetic analysis of herding behavior in Swedish Border collie dogs. J Vet Behav Clin Appl Res 2009;4(6):237.
79. Arvelius P, Malm S, Svartberg K, et al. Measuring herding behavior in Border collie-effect of protocol structure on usefulness for selection. J Vet Behav Clin App Res 2013;8(1):9–18.

80. Courreau J, Langlois B. Genetic parameters and environmental effects which characterise the defence ability of the Belgian shepherd dog. Appl Anim Behav Sci 2005;91(3):233–45.
81. Cardon LR, Bell JI. Association study designs for complex diseases. Nat Rev Genet 2001;2(2):91–9.
82. Terwilliger JD. Handbook of human genetic linkage. Baltimore (MD): Johns Hopkins University Press; 1994.
83. Risch N, Merikangas K. The future of genetic studies of complex human diseases. Science 1996;273:1516–7.
84. Tabor HK, Risch NJ, Myers RM. Candidate-gene approaches for studying complex genetic traits: practical considerations. Nat Rev Genet 2002;3(5):391–7.
85. Voight BF, Pritchard JK. Confounding from cryptic relatedness in case-control association studies. PLoS Genet 2005;1:e32.
86. Frazer KA, Murray SS, Schork NJ, et al. Human genetic variation and its contribution to complex traits. Nat Rev Genet 2009;10(4):241–51.
87. Wheeler DA, Srinivasan M, Egholm M, et al. The complete genome of an individual by massively parallel DNA sequencing. Nature 2008;452:872–6.
88. Feuk L, Carson AR, Scherer SW. Structural variation in the human genome. Nat Rev Genet 2006;7:85–97.
89. Karyadi DM, Karlins E, Decker B, et al. A copy number variant at the KITLG locus likely confers risk for canine squamous cell carcinoma of the digit. PLoS Genet 2013;9(3):1–14.
90. Reich D, Cargill M, Bolk S, et al. Linkage disequilibrium in the human genome. Nature 2001;411(6834):199–204.
91. Sutter NB, Eberle MA, Parker HG, et al. Extensive and breed-specific linkage disequilibrium in Canis familiaris. Genome Res 2004;14:2388–96.
92. Wilbe M, Jokinen P, Hermanrud C, et al. MHC class II polymorphism is associated with a canine SLE-related disease complex. Immunogenetics 2009;61(8):557–64.
93. Davey JW, Hohenlohe PA, Etter PD, et al. Genome-wide genetic marker discovery and genotyping using next-generation sequencing. Nat Rev Genet 2011;12(7):499–510.
94. Hytönen MK, Arumilli M, Lappalainen AK, et al. A Novel GUSB mutation in Brazilian terriers with severe skeletal abnormalities defines the disease as mucopolysaccharidosis VII. PLoS One 2012;7(7):1–11.
95. Schoenebeck JJ, Hutchinson SA, Byers A, et al. Variation of BMP3 contributes to dog breed skull diversity. PLoS Genet 2012;8(8):1–11.
96. Takeuchi Y, Hashizume C, Arata S, et al. An approach to canine behavioural genetics employing guide dogs for the blind. Anim Genet 2009;40(2):217–24.
97. Héjjas K, Kubinyi E, Rónai Z, et al. Molecular and behavioral analysis of the intron 2 repeat polymorphism in the canine dopamine D4 receptor. Genes Brain Behav 2009;8(3):330–6.
98. Olender T, Fuchs T, Linhart C, et al. The canine olfactory subgenome. Genomics 2004;83(3):361–72.
99. Buck LB. The molecular architecture of odor and pheromone sensing in mammals. Cell 2000;100(6):611–8.
100. Buck LB. Olfactory receptors and odor coding in mammals. Nutr Rev 2004;62:184–8.
101. Tacher S, Quignon P, Rimbault M, et al. Olfactory receptor sequence polymorphism within and between breeds of dogs. J Hered 2005;96(7):812–6.

102. Lesniak A, Walczak M, Jezierski T, et al. Canine olfactory receptor gene poly-morphism and its relation to odor detection performance by sniffer dogs. J Hered 2008;99(5):518–27.
103. Masek P, Heisenberg M. Distinct memories of odor intensity and quality in Drosophila. Proc Natl Acad Sci U S A 2008;105(41):15985–90.
104. Benbernou N, Tacher S, Robin S, et al. Functional analysis of a subset of canine olfactory receptor genes. J Hered 2007;98(5):500–5.
105. Issel-Tarver L, Rine J. Organization and expression of canine olfactory receptor genes. Proc Natl Acad Sci U S A 1996;93(20):10897–902.
106. Quignon P, Kirkness E, Cadieu E, et al. Comparison of the canine and human olfactory receptor gene repertoires. Genome Biol 2003;4(12):R80.
107. Quignon P, Giraud M, Rimbault M, et al. The dog and rat olfactory receptor rep-ertoires. Genome Biol 2005;6(10):R83.
108. Robin S, Tacher S, Rimbault M, et al. Genetic diversity of canine olfactory recep-tors. BMC Genomics 2009;10:21.
109. Goodwin D, Bradshaw JW, Wickens SM. Paedomorphosis affects agonistic visual signals of domestic dogs. Anim Behav 1997;53:297–304.
110. Gazit I, Terkel J. Domination of olfaction over vision in explosives detection by dogs. Appl Anim Behav Sci 2003;82:65–73.
111. Szetei V, Miklósi Á, Topál J, et al. When dogs seem to lose their nose: an inves-tigation on the use of visual and olfactory cues in communicative context between dog and owner. Appl Anim Behav Sci 2003;83(2):141–52.
112. Lefebvre D, Diederich C, Delcourt M, et al. The quality of the relation between handler and military dogs influences efficiency and welfare of dogs. Appl Anim Behav Sci 2007;104(1–2):49–60.
113. Radtke KM, Ruf M, Gunter HM, et al. Transgenerational impact of intimate part-ner violence on methylation in the promoter of the glucocorticoid receptor. Transl Psychiatry 2011;1:e21.
114. Champagne FA. Epigenetic influence of social experiences across the lifespan. Dev Psychobiol 2010;52(4):299–311.
115. Morgan CP, Bale TL. Early prenatal stress epigenetically programs dysmasculi-nization in second-generation offspring via the paternal lineage. J Neurosci 2011;31(33):11748–55.
116. Weaver IC, Cervoni N, Champagne FA, et al. Epigenetic programming by maternal behavior. Nat Neurosci 2004;7:847–54.
117. Pierantoni L, Albertini M, Pirrone F. Prevalence of owner-reported behaviours in dogs separated from the litter at two different ages. Vet Rec 2011;169(18):468.
118. Tiira K, Hakosalo O, Kareinen L, et al. Environmental effects on compulsive tail chasing in dogs. PLoS One 2012;7(7):1–14.
119. Smoller JW, Craddock N, Kendler K, et al. Identification of risk loci with shared effects on five major psychiatric disorders: a genome-wide analysis. Lancet 2013;381(9875):1371–9.
120. Mellersh CS, Graves KT, McLaughlin B, et al. Mutation in HSF4 associated with early but not late-onset hereditary cataract in the Boston terrier. J Hered 2007;98(5):531–3.
121. Seppälä EH, Koskinen LL, Gullov CH, et al. Identification of a novel idiopathic epilepsy locus in Belgian shepherd dogs. PLoS One 2012;7(3):e33549.
122. Bateson P, Sargan DR. Analysis of the canine genome and canine health: a commentary. Vet J 2012;194(3):265–9.

APPENDIX: ONLINE RESOURCES

Canine Inherited Disorders Database	University of Prince Edward Island	http://ic.upei.ca/cidd/
Online Mendelian Inheritance in Animals	The University of Sydney	http://omia.angis.org.au/home
LIDA	The University of Sydney	www.sydney.edu.au/vetscience/lida
Inherited Diseases in Dogs	University of Cambridge	http://server.vet.cam.ac.uk
Orthopedic Foundation for Animals	Orthopedic Foundation for Animals	http://www.offa.org
American Kennel Club Canine Health Foundation	American Kennel Club Canine Health Foundation (AKC CHF)	http://www.akcchf.org
Fabcats	International Cat Care (formerly Feline Advisory Bureau)	http://www.fabcats.org/breeders/inherited_disorders

Data from Slutsky J, Raj K, Yuhnke S, et al. A web resource on DNA tests for canine and feline hereditary diseases. Vet J 2013;197(2):187.

Recognizing Behavioral Signs of Pain and Disease:

A Guide for Practitioners

Diane Frank, DVM

KEYWORDS

• Anxiety • Pain • Discomfort • Behavioral changes • Dog • Cat

KEY POINTS

- There is significant overlap in nonspecific signs of medical conditions, pain, and anxiety disorders.
- Lip licking, lip smacking, panting, pacing, trembling, aggression, agitation, hiding, withdrawal, and vocalizing can be seen in patients that are anxious, sick, or in pain.
- Sudden appearance of new behaviors (pica; aggression; anxious behaviors), especially in middle-aged or older animals, points to an underlying medical condition.
- Neuropathic pain is often worsened by stimuli that evoke a sympathetic response, such as the startle response and emotional arousal (stressful situations).
- Obtaining an accurate and complete history to collect all subtle signs and behavioral changes will help the veterinarian establish if the signs are more compatible with a medical condition, a behavioral disorder, or both.

INTRODUCTION

Disease is always associated with changes in behavior such as disappearance of normal behaviors or appearance of new behaviors. These changes are often considered abnormal behaviors, indicating illness and/or pain. Differentiating between normal and abnormal behaviors can be based on several aspects such as appropriateness of specific behaviors in a given context, appropriateness of the frequency, the severity or the duration of a behavior in a given context, and the behavioral sequence (normal or altered). The context in which the behavior occurs allows the clinician to distinguish between appropriate and inappropriate behaviors. Aggression, for example, can be an appropriate response in some contexts,[1] and serves different purposes depending on context. Aggression serves as normal communication in cats or dogs, signaling "stop," "leave me alone," or "stay away." Aggression in response to a threat as self-defense would also be considered normal. Behavior is generally

Department of Clinical Sciences, Centre Hospitalier Universitaire Vétérinaire, 1525, rue des Vétérinaires, Saint-Hyacinthe, Quebec J2S 7C6, Canada
E-mail address: diane.frank@umontreal.ca

Vet Clin Small Anim 44 (2014) 507–524
http://dx.doi.org/10.1016/j.cvsm.2014.01.002
0195-5616/14/$ – see front matter © 2014 Elsevier Inc. All rights reserved.

vetsmall.theclinics.com

a sequence of actions and reactions. A normal behavioral sequence of aggression in dogs would include (1) initiation, (2) pause, (3) response by the recipient, (4) end or further action, and (5) end of sequence. Initiation is the warning phase, such as a growl followed by a pause. The animal has communicated and is waiting for a response. If the recipient gives the desired response, the aggressive interaction may end at this early stage. The recipient may not always respond as desired by the instigator, in which case the instigator may proceed to bite (further action) and then release volitionally, signaling the end of the sequence. The bite may be single or multiple. In the context of communication, the aggressive behavior is generally controlled or inhibited (ie, one bite without teeth marks or injury). Inhibited aggression does not cause physical injury, and these aggressive behaviors would be considered normal given the context of communication. In the case of self-defense, the greater the fear, the more severe the injuries could potentially become. Behavior definitely becomes abnormal if some of the steps from the sequence are omitted or altered. A dog growling and biting simultaneously without any prior warning signal has an altered sequence because of the absence of clear initiation and pause. Such a sequence could not be considered normal, and thus becomes indicative of illness. Illness includes medical conditions and behavioral (mental) disorders. The aim of this article is to illustrate some examples of cases that might present as behavioral disorders but are in fact medical conditions.

ANXIETY DISORDERS
Dogs

Fear and anxiety result in a common stress response.[2] The range of responses to stressors seen in dogs can include avoidance, defensive aggression, panting, salivation, pacing, excessive activity, visual scanning, elimination, dilated pupils, vocalization, hiding, seeking out human contact, seeking out contact with other dogs or pets, attention-seeking behaviors such as pawing at a person, lowered body posture, flattened ear position, low tail position, anorexia, and digging. One study reported increased performance of tongue out, snout licking, paw lifting, and body shaking along with a lowered body posture[3] as well as increased heart rate and saliva cortisol in one dog subjected to noise (95 dB). The investigators concluded that these behaviors could indicate stress. In another study,[4] researchers found that dogs subjected to different types of stimuli (pushing the dog down by pressing on the neck and back, pulling the head of the dog down to the ground via a rope/bar system, opening an umbrella, dropping a bag filled with paper from the ceiling, noise, or an electric shock) performed more body shaking, crouching, oral behaviors (tongue out, tip of tongue briefly extended, snout licking, swallowing, smacking), yawning, and restlessness, and also presented a low posture. Dogs subjected to harsh training methods (physical corrections) exhibited mouth licking and front paw lifting, pulled their ears back, and had lowered standing or sitting postures[5]; they also vocalized, whereas dogs trained with rewards did not. A third study reported that dogs housed in the greatest degree of social isolation spent the most time moving, performed the greatest number of abnormal movements, and vocalized the most.[6] Many of these signs, though associated with various stressful stimuli, can also be associated with disease. Lip licking, repeated swallowing, and smacking can occur in animals that are nauseous.[7] Trembling can be seen in animals with fever (shivering) or neurologic disorders (tremors).[8,9] Restlessness, pacing, or increased activity can be seen in dogs with painful[10] or neurologic conditions.[11,12] Increased activity is associated with hyperthyroidism in

31% of cats.[13] In one retrospective study of 97 dogs diagnosed with brain tumors, circling was reported in 23% of cases, pacing in 10%, nonspecific behavioral changes or mentation changes in 7%, aggression in 5%, and wandering in 5%.[12] Vocalization can also be observed in some patients in pain.

The most common complaints in cases of canine separation anxiety are destructive behavior directed at the home, inappropriate elimination (defecation, urination), increased and repetitive motor activity (pacing, circling), and excessive vocalization (whining, barking, or howling) in the owner's absence.[14] Destructive behavior (chewing, digging, and scratching) can be directed at exit points such as doors, windows, and gates,[15] and specific objects in the home are scratched, chewed, or torn apart. Owners will not necessarily distinguish between destruction and pica. It is therefore crucial to question the owner specifically because in the author's opinion, pica is more likely a sign of gastrointestinal disorder than a behavioral disorder.

One study filming the behaviors of dogs diagnosed with separation anxiety when home alone[16] showed that dogs spent most of their time (22.95%) vocalizing (barking 11%, whining 10%, howling 1.95%), and a similar proportion of time (21%) remaining vigilant (expressed as oriented to the environment). Panting and destructive behavior were exhibited respectively for 14% and 6% (5% scratching at the cage, door, environment; 1% oral destruction of items or cage) of the time. Hourly average for lip licking and yawning was 27 and 3, respectively. None of these anxious dogs played during owner absence, 2 dogs trembled, and 3 dogs eliminated. Based on videotape records, panting tended to increase over time. Again, many of these nonspecific signs may also be seen in medical conditions. Panting can be associated with thermal regulation, fever, cardiovascular disease, metabolic disease, endocrine diseases such as hyperadrenocorticism,[17] hypertension, or painful conditions.[18] Anxiety will elicit behaviors that enable the animal to approach a source of perceived threat[19] by increasing attention and triggering risk assessment.[20,21] During risk assessment, nondefensive behaviors such as environmental exploration, self-grooming, feeding, and social interaction are inhibited,[22–24] and the degree of suppression of these behaviors may be used as an indirect index of defensiveness or anxiety.[24] Exploration can in fact be partially or completely inhibited by anxiety; therefore, reduced exploration might represent an indirect measure of anxiety.[21,25] In the previously reported study of dogs[16] with separation anxiety, self-grooming was never observed and exploratory behavior was observed only for short periods. These changes were compatible with a state of anxiety during owner absence. Similarly sick animals will generally not play, explore, self-groom, or interact socially.

Cats

The range of responses to stressors seen in cats can include avoidance, hiding, lowered body posture, defensive aggression, reduced activity, vocalization, elimination, flattened ear position, dilated pupils, pacing, seeking out human attention, visual scanning, anorexia, climbing, vigilance, spraying, and a reduction in maintenance behaviors such as sleeping, grooming, eating, and eliminating.[2] Lip licking and repeated swallowing can be seen in stressed cats during physical examination in the veterinary setting, and are observed during cat fights (chomping motion).[26] Again, several of these signs are also compatible with disease or pain. Lip licking and repeated swallowing are seen in nauseous cats.[27] Panting (increased respiratory rate), a sign of anxiety in the hospital environment[28] or during car rides, can also be a sign of acute pain[29] or hyperthyroidism.[13]

BEHAVIORAL SIGNS OF NEUROLOGIC DISEASE AND PAIN

Changes in behavior may occur with neurologic signs, but in some cases behavioral changes precede the other clinical signs by weeks or months.

Lysosomal storage diseases in cats and dogs are rare. In addition to neurologic signs animals may show behavioral changes, loss of learned behavior, or stereotypical behaviors.[30]

Sometimes dramatic hydrocephalus may be present, and owners will report few clinical signs other than slowness to learn.[31] Owners may report that a puppy is hard to house train or that the puppy was house trained but now is eliminating in the house again. Close attention to the animal's mentation and physical examination may reveal a neurologic disorder rather than a behavioral disorder.

Lissencephaly in dogs is rare. A case series[32] in Lhasa Apso dogs described that in one case, the owners had been unable to house train their 11-month-old female. Their dog was apprehensive of people, and on several occasions the dog was aggressive and failed to recognize its owner. The dog developed seizures at about 10 months of age. The other Lhasa Apso, a 1-year-old male, had a history, starting at 3 months of age, of sudden personality changes manifested as unprovoked attacks on the owner and other people.

Neuropathic pain is typically attributed to injury or disease that damages the axon or soma of sensory neurons or disrupts the myelin sheath of axons.[33] One of the most common causes of neuropathic pain is intervertebral disc herniation resulting in persistent or intermittent pain. Spinal cord injury (trauma, ischemia, hemorrhage, or extradural compression) can result in somatic or visceral neuropathic pain. Radicular (referred) pain is observed with impingement of nerve roots. Signs of central pain (secondary to central nervous system tumors or congenital/developmental lesions) highlight the importance of history taking with respect to changes in behavior (obvious and subtle). Behaviors such as scratching motion without touching the skin (Chiari-like malformation), continually biting or attacking an area on the body, frequently turning (looking) at the same area, or yelping for no reason should alert veterinarians to potential neuropathic pain. Cats that have undergone onychectomy may experience chronic neuropathic pain. Signs (within days to months after the surgery) can include obvious pain of the paw or paws as well as other nonspecific behavioral changes such as decreased activity, decreased appetite, or increased aggression. A multimodal perioperative analgesic plan is essential to prevent this type of chronic pain.[34] Some of the repetitive behaviors labeled as obsessive-compulsive disorders such as flank sucking, self-mutilation, and checking could in fact be secondary to somatic or visceral neuropathic pain. Anecdotally, the author has encountered a few cases of dogs with self-mutilation of the prepuce and penis that had back pain and improved significantly when treated with gabapentin.

Zulch and colleagues[35] reported the case of a 30-month-old Labrador retriever presented for acute tail biting leading to self-mutilation. On examination of the tail, an irregularity was noted midway on the dorsal surface. Radiographs of the tail showed soft-tissue swelling and presence of an ossicle between the midcaudal vertebrae. Analgesic treatment consisting of tramadol and paracetamol was implemented. Analgesia was discontinued after approximately 6 weeks.

In the case of aggression, it is important to always distinguish between appropriate, or normal, aggression and inappropriate, or abnormal, aggression. The latter will always be associated with a medical condition or behavioral disorder. Inappropriate aggression as a behavioral condition (mental disorder) is generally observed in young animals.[36] If inappropriate aggression appears as a new behavior in a middle-aged dog or cat, neurologic disease should be considered before a behavioral disorder.

Dogs

Clinical signs of tumors affecting the rostral cerebrum in 43 dogs,[37] ranging in age from 5 to 15 years (mean of 10 years), revealed that 5 dogs had recently reported abnormal behaviors (dementia, aggression, alterations in established habits) as a sole sign, 22 had seizures as their only initial sign, and 4 had seizures and behavioral changes. Thirty-one of these 43 dogs had normal neurologic examinations on initial presentation, but 25 eventually developed persistent neurologic deficits.

A published case of simultaneously occurring oligodendroglioma and meningioma in a 12-year-old neutered male Boxer reported a 3-week history of stumbling over objects, reluctance to climb stairs, standing in corners, and circling.[38] Three days before presentation, the dog became very agitated and started urinating inappropriately.

In a case report of clinical findings in 3 dogs with polycystic meningiomas,[39] an 8-year-old spayed female Labrador retriever was presented after a 1-month history of changes in behavior that included an initial increase in aggression toward people, a significant decrease in response to the owner, and increasing episodes of house soiling, panting, pacing, circling to the right, head pressing, and nightly vocalizations. A 9-year-old castrated Golden retriever was presented after a 3-week history of abnormal behavior and pacing and a 1-week history of right-sided circling and head pressing. In the third case, the dog had a 6-month history of seizures.

A case report[40] described progressive, abnormal signs observed before 9 months of age in a Dachshund diagnosed with ceroid lipofuscinosis. Changes in behavior included increased nervousness, decreased interactions with the other dogs in the household, a severe loss in the ability to recognize or respond to commands or his name, a loss of ability to recognize the owner or other people in the household, an increased sensitivity to loud noises, circling behavior, increasing inappropriate vocalization, loss of ability to climb stairs or other obstacles, tremors, loss of coordination, severe loss of vision, persistent head movements, and bumping into obstacles.

Dogs diagnosed with spinal meningiomas[11] have histories of clinical signs compatible with chronic discomfort. In one report, there was a prolonged delay between the onset of clinical signs and diagnosis (10 of 13 dogs), with an average 5.8 months for all dogs (range 3 days to 14 months). Owners reported signs such as restlessness, difficulty finding a comfortable sleeping position, and irritability. These signs preceded the appearance or recognition of limping or lameness by weeks or months.

One case report described a Boxer that had always growled and snarled[41] if owners disciplined the dog either verbally or physically, disturbed it when it was sleeping, tried to move it from furniture, or when petting the dog. However, the dog never bit in such circumstances. The aggression was appropriate for the contexts (the dog communicated that it did not want to be disturbed while resting, did not like physical contact, was feeling threatened when disciplined, and so forth). At 8 years of age, the dog was resting in a corner of the living room and suddenly entered the kitchen. He jumped at one of the adults and without warning bit her multiple times. The aggression was not triggered by any interaction on the part of the person. This aggressive behavior was novel, clearly inappropriate for the context, and the behavioral sequence was altered, thus pointing to an underlying medical condition. In addition, the dog had presented with seizures every 2 to 3 months during the 2 years before presentation. Following medical investigation and necropsy, the final diagnosis was a microcystic meningioma.[41]

A recent case report of abnormal behaviors[42] described a 5-year-old female spayed Cocker Spaniel presented with a history of intermittent episodes of vocalization and apparent fear since the age of 6 months. These episodes could happen at any time of day or night. Before the onset of vocalization (2–24 hours), the dog would appear fearful and quiet, and would hide under furniture, avoiding all interaction. Following these initial behavioral changes, the dog would start vocalizing and would exhibit a low head carriage. She would refuse to eat or drink. Occasionally she would also salivate excessively, swallow frequently, or vomit. Vocalization initially lasted 2 to 4 hours but progressed over time for to up to 3 days. The initial frequency was 1 to 2 episodes yearly progressing to 1 to 2 episodes monthly. After the episode of vocalization, she remained quiet for 1 to 2 days before returning to an apparently completely normal state. The owner of the dog was unable to identify any specific triggers. Physical, neurologic, and behavioral examinations were unremarkable. Blood analyses, bile acids, magnetic resonance imaging (MRI) of the brain, and cerebrospinal fluid analysis were all within normal limits. Thoracic radiographs and abdominal ultrasonography were normal. None of the initial pharmacologic treatments attempted were successful: opioids (morphine, methadone), diazepam, acepromazine, nonsteroidal anti-inflammatory drugs (carprofen, meloxicam), and phenobarbital. The dog was also presented during one episode that lasted over 2 days. She vocalized, and appeared photophobic and phonophobic. Physical and neurologic examinations were again unremarkable apart from a low head carriage with no detectable spinal pain. MRI of the entire spine was performed and was normal. Acetaminophen/codeine and pregabalin were prescribed but were unsuccessful at alleviating the signs. A migraine-like disorder was then suspected, and topiramate was prescribed. Clinical signs improved markedly. The dog continued to experience these episodes, but the duration was reduced to 1 to 3 hours. The intensity was also reduced as the dog would remain quiet, no longer vocalize, and be keen to go for walks, eat, and drink normally. The dog also no longer appeared to be photophobic and phonophobic. Eighteen months later she continued to respond well. The frequency of the episodes was reduced from 2 episodes monthly before the medication (topiramate) to 1 episode every 2 to 3 months.

Cats

A published case of intracranial meningioma in a 7.5-year-old cat[43] reported a 10-month history of visual impairment and altered behavior without specifying the changes. Following surgery, normal behavior was restored. A published case of extracranial expansion of a meningioma in a 13-year-old cat reported a 1-year history of behavioral changes with the first signs being reluctance to play and episodic lethargy, followed by episodes of aggressiveness.[44] The owner had noticed pain reactions when touching the head of her animal only 3 months before presentation. Behavioral changes thus preceded the signs of pain. Some geriatric cats diagnosed with meningioma are presented to their veterinarian as "just not being themselves."[45] Signs are typically present for 1 to 3 months in cats before diagnosis.

In one report of clinical features in 11 cats with *Cuterebra* myiasis of the central nervous system,[46] changes in behavior were reported in 2 of 11 cats but were not specified, other than aggression in 1 case. Depressed mentation was noted in 6 of 11 cats. The sequence of appearance of clinical signs was not specified.

A report on feline leukemia virus (FeLV)-associated myelopathy in 16 cats[47] indicated that clinical signs of some cats included abnormal vocalization (n = 1), fly biting (n = 1), undefined abnormal behavior (n = 1), catatonic behavior (n = 2), and pica (n = 1), along with other signs such as ataxia, hyperesthesia (n = 4), and paresis progressing to paralysis. Three cats presented with urinary incontinence and 1 cat had recurrent constipation. Signs generally progressed over the course of 1 year, but the article does not specify if the behavioral signs preceded the neurologic signs.

Lissencephaly with microencephaly in Korat cats has been reported, and is associated with signs of abnormal behavior and self-mutilation.[48]

BEHAVIORAL SIGNS OF UROGENITAL DISEASE AND PAIN
Cats

Numerous medical conditions (bacterial urinary tract infection, calculi, neoplasia) can result in urination outside the litter box[49] and urine spraying[49] in cats. One publication looked at urinalysis results in spraying and nonspraying cats, and found no difference.[50] However, the minimum data base should not only include urinalysis (with urinary specific gravity) but also abdominal radiographs if signs of lower urinary tract disease are present for more than 7 days.[49] A urine culture may be needed to rule out urinary tract infection in older cats. Urinary history should specify whether periuria (urinating outside the litter box) occurs on a vertical or horizontal surface, and a detailed environmental history should also be obtained.[49] In cats with recurrent episodes of lower urinary tract signs and in cats older than 10 years, serum thyroxine concentration in addition to serology for FeLV and feline immunodeficiency virus (FIV) should be performed because hyperthyroidism, FeLV, or FIV infection can result in abnormal urinary behavior.[49] Some cases will require ultrasonography to visualize uroliths larger than 2 mm in diameter, or contrast urethrocystography to evaluate the urethra and bladder.

Neuropathic pain is often worsened by stimuli that evoke a sympathetic response, such as the startle response and emotional arousal.[33] Feline interstitial cystitis (FIC) is associated with visceral neurogenic (neuropathic) pain. Treatment of FIC includes recommendations to decrease stress factors in the environment. One study reported that when looking at multicat households, cats with FIC were more likely than cats in the control population to be in conflict with a housemate.[51]

BEHAVIORAL SIGNS OF GASTROINTESTINAL DISEASE AND PAIN

Signs of esophageal disease include regurgitation, dysphagia, odynophagia, salivation, retching, gagging, and repeated swallowing.[52] Signs of gastric disease include nausea, salivation, vomiting, hematemesis, melena, unexplained breath changes, and anorexia. Clinical signs associated with large bowel diseases include, among others, dyschezia, tenesmus, and constipation. Signs of gastrointestinal foreign body include salivation, regurgitation, odynophagia, dysphagia, forceful retching, anorexia, and intermittent vomiting (free-floating gastric foreign body). Signs of gastric motility disorders in addition to gastric distension, food retention, and vomiting include belching and pica.[53]

Flatulence is excessive accumulation of gas in the gastrointestinal tract[54] and may be associated with eructation, borborygmus, or flatus. Eructation is the expulsion of gas from the stomach. Borborygmus is a rumbling noise caused by the propulsion of gas through the gastrointestinal tract, and flatus is the anal passage of gas. Flatulence and borborygmus are often considered normal for owners[54] but should not be dismissed too rapidly as insignificant,[7] as they can occasionally signal diseases of the intestine or pancreas.[54] Owners may report their dog having a tendency to bloat with or without belching, taking an arched stance (cramps?), and excessive expulsion of flatus. These behaviors may be associated with aerophagia (excitement; eating too rapidly), or eating foods that produce gas. However, in some cases a more serious disorder in dogs may be present, such as gastric hypomotility or gastric outflow obstruction. These dogs may experience intermittent to frequent signs of nausea.[7] Early in the course of the disease there may be minimal signs, but as the disorder progresses there may be significant discomfort. Dogs with inflammatory bowel disease (IBD) or irritable bowel syndrome may also experience abdominal discomfort caused by gas.[7] The symptom complex of bloating, fullness, and significant abdominal discomfort is recognized to occur in dogs but can be difficult to detect because of the nonspecific or subtle signs. In addition, restlessness (discomfort), changing position (discomfort), and lip licking (nausea) can all be confused with signs of anxiety.

IBD is frequently diagnosed in dogs and cats. Some anecdotal reports[33] of amitriptyline use in cats already adequately treated for their IBD, but still uncomfortable according to their owners, indicated improvement in behavior, thus suggesting a potential neuropathic component to IBD.

Flatulence is reported more commonly in dogs than in cats.[54] Borborygmi are rarely heard in cats.[7]

Anecdotal unpublished cases of IBD have been reported in both dogs and cats presenting with pica. Although more studies are needed, the author believes that in some species, conditions labeled as oral stereotypies or oral compulsive disorders are more likely signs of gastrointestinal disease than behavioral disorders. These repetitive behaviors in dogs include fly biting, excessive licking of surfaces, air licking, star gazing, flank sucking, and pica. IBD may in some cases be causing anal sac disease.[55] Therefore, checking behavior reported in Miniature Schnauzers should include gastrointestinal disease in the differential. These dogs may be experiencing pain and are therefore looking repeatedly at their hind end. Repetitive behaviors in cats, often labeled as obsessive-compulsive, include pica. In the author's opinion, pica in cats is more likely a gastrointestinal disease than a behavioral disorder, although further research is needed.

Dogs

One dog was referred to the behavior service for separation anxiety because of destruction during owner absence. However, when the dog was filmed home alone he showed no signs of anxiety. The dog also had a history of intermittent diarrhea, and the destruction was in fact associated with pica. The dog underwent medical investigation and was diagnosed with IBD. Both a change in diet and prednisone were required to treat the diarrhea and pica. When the prednisone dosage was decreased, the dog resumed pica. Gastrointestinal biopsies should always be taken when performing surgery for removal of a gastrointestinal foreign body in dogs or cats, especially in cases of repeat offenders.

In the author's opinion and based on preliminary studies,[56,57] gastrointestinal disease can manifest itself with unusual behavioral signs such as excessive licking of surfaces, fly biting, and star gazing. In general there are other subtle signs of gastrointestinal disease, such as presence of flatulence, borborygmus, belching, lip licking, swallowing, or drooling, though not always. Owners will not necessarily report these gastrointestinal signs unless asked specifically. It is therefore important to ask! In a study of 19 dogs licking surfaces excessively,[56] 14 dogs had gastrointestinal disorders including eosinophilic (n = 5) or lymphoplasmacytic infiltration (n = 3) of the gastrointestinal tract, delayed gastric emptying (n = 7), irritable bowel syndrome (n = 1), chronic pancreatitis (n = 1), giardiasis (n = 1), and gastric foreign body (n = 1). Mean duration of the behavior problem (ie, how long the dog had been licking surfaces) was 32 months (range 0.08–82 months). Sixteen of the 19 dogs exhibited daily licking of surfaces such as floors, walls, blankets and sofas. Following treatment of the underlying condition, complete resolution was achieved in 53% (9 of 17) after 90 days and in 59% (10 of 17) after 180 days.[56] Three additional dogs showed a decrease (more than 50%) in both duration and frequency of licking bouts at 180 days. Therefore, 76% of dogs (13 of 17) improved significantly clinically over the 6-month follow-up. Of the 5 dogs without gastrointestinal abnormalities and treated nonspecifically (hypoallergenic diet), 2 dogs stopped licking by day 90. One of the licking dogs was also "air licking", retching, and squinting. A painful facial expression in dogs can include ears back or down, eyes wide open with dilated pupils, or eyes partially closed.[10] Squinting with lowered head is also recognized as a sign of pain in cats.[58] This particular dog had a 12-inch piece of rope in his stomach for approximately 6 months before presentation. The owners were unaware that their dog had ingested the rope. Treatment included removal of the foreign body via endoscopy and a switch to a hypoallergenic diet. Air licking, surface licking, retching, and squinting all ceased once the foreign body was removed and the dietary change implemented.

A study on medical investigation of 7 fly-biting dogs[57] revealed that the age of the dogs at the onset of fly biting varied between 6 months and 10 years. Dogs had exhibited this behavior at the time of presentation from 6 days to 4 years. Frequency of bouts varied from once daily to once every hour. Duration of a single bout varied from seconds to 1 hour. At home, fly biting was more frequent following feeding in 3 dogs. The most significant finding in the fly-biting study was the occurrence of head raising and neck extension preceding jaw snapping in all dogs. In some cases, raising the head and extending the neck occurred more frequently than snapping (2 of 7). Underlying medical abnormalities included gastric and/or duodenal eosinophilic (n = 2) or lymphoplasmacytic infiltration (n = 4), and delayed gastric emptying (n = 2). Gastroesophageal reflux was observed on endoscopy in 2 dogs. One dog had no histologic abnormalities but presented a very flaccid and distended stomach on ultrasonographic and endoscopic examination. Medical treatment of the specific underlying gastrointestinal disease resulted in complete resolution of the fly biting in 5 of 6 dogs (within 30 days for 4 dogs, including 1 dog that had been fly biting for 2 years). Four dogs also presented behavioral changes compatible with anxiety (pacing, panting, hiding, increased attention-seeking) along with the fly-biting episodes. One dog paced continuously during the entire behavioral assessment. These signs disappeared once the underlying gastrointestinal disease was treated, and therefore were perhaps associated with pain or discomfort rather than strictly anxiety. Anxiety may also occur secondary to pain. One study[59] on postanesthetic esophagitis in dogs described clinical signs of esophageal pain that included extension of the neck during swallowing and abnormal posturing with the neck extended (possibly similar to the raised head and neck extension seen in fly-biting dogs).

Flank sucking in Doberman Pinschers is characterized by repetitive mouthing and sucking of the flank, resulting in consequences ranging from a dampened coat to alopecia and even raw open skin lesions. A study looking at blanket and flank sucking in 77 Doberman Pinschers[60] reported that 55 dogs only sucked blankets, 14 only sucked their flank, and 8 did both. Twenty-two of these dogs (18 blanket sucking and 4 flank sucking) exhibited pica as well, ingesting a wide variety of nonfood substances (fabrics; dirt; twigs and leaves; paper products; plastic, vinyl, and metal objects). Although more research is needed, the author hypothesizes that flank sucking and blanket sucking are more likely a sign of an underlying digestive problem (and possible neurogenic pain) than a strictly behavioral disorder.

In hindsight, when reading case reports of stereotypic motor behavior some of the abnormal behaviors described may have been associated with gastrointestinal discomfort. In one report,[61] a 4-year-old castrated male Rottweiler was evaluated for unusual behavior that was common at night, but could occur at any time during the day if someone scratched his back. At the start of his bouts, the dog would extend its neck and lick its lips (compatible with esophageal discomfort and nausea). The dog would swallow repeatedly and explore the room snuffling. During exploration, any objects encountered were ingested and could include plastic, pens, paper, paperclips, and toys. During bouts the dog would become excited, pace, circle, and ingest items. If restrained the dog would whine, become agitated, rock back and forth, and continue its ingestive movements (aerophagia). The dog had already had 2 gastrotomies within 18 months to remove foreign bodies. Biopsies were taken during the second gastrotomy, and a presumptive diagnosis of eosinophilic gastritis was made. No changes in behavior were seen with a change of diet. However, there is no mention of medication to treat the gastritis, and this dog may have also had gastric reflux. The report states that the drug clomipramine controlled the behavior, but does not specify if there was complete resolution of all the signs. Response to clomipramine in this case report may have been the result of neuropathic pain alleviation in a case of IBD. It is presumed that norepinephrine and serotonin reuptake inhibitors attenuate neuropathic pain. Blocking synaptic reuptake of norepinephrine and serotonin increases the postsynaptic levels of these neurotransmitters, which then sustain the activation of the descending pain inhibitory pathway. These actions result in alleviation of pain.[33]

Fecal incontinence can be divided into 2 main categories, reservoir incontinence and sphincter incontinence. In reservoir incontinence the colon and rectum are unable to retain feces.[62] The dogs will posture properly, but there is an urgency to defecate; they may therefore defecate excessively or in inappropriate areas. Diseases associated with reservoir incontinence include colitis and neoplasia.

Cats

Dyschezia is difficult or painful evacuation of feces from the rectum.[63] Tenesmus is ineffectual and painful straining at defecation or urination. Cats with tenesmus or dyschezia commonly vocalize or defecate outside the litter box.[63] It is therefore crucial in cases of defecation outside the litter box to question owners about the elimination behavioral sequence and all other associated behaviors prior to and during defecation. Tenesmus after defecation suggests irritation or inflammation. In the author's experience, cats with dyschezia or tenesmus often appear anxious or restless before defecation. If these cats use the litter box intermittently they will race out of the box after defecation, most likely because of pain or discomfort.

Pica in cats has been reported as a sign of FIV,[64,65] a sign of gastric motility disorder,[53] and to be associated with chronic anemia.[66] Cats may eat kitty litter or may lick concrete or ceramics. Compulsive licking at concrete, carpeting, or other cats was also reported in 3 of 16 cats with chronic feline infectious peritonitis (FIP).[65] Two were house soiling and one was incontinent (fecal and urinary).[65] Personality changes, although not specified, are also reported with FIP.[65]

BEHAVIORAL SIGNS OF DERMATOLOGIC DISEASE AND PAIN

Self-mutilation should always alert the veterinarian to pain, which can be local or neurogenic in origin.

Dogs

Infection is almost always present in acral lick dermatitis (ALD),[67] and antibiotics are one of the most important aspects in the treatment of ALD. These agents should be used systematically, and therapy may need to be as long as 4 to 6 months. Shumaker and colleagues[68] conclude that "lesions associated with ALD warrant tissue bacterial cultures as the majority of cases yielded positive growth of bacteria differing from superficial culture and often resistant to empirical drugs." Current text books and dermatology conference notes highlight that ALD should be considered as a primary disease that is complicated by perpetuating factors. Entrapped free hair shafts are very painful and most likely contribute in perpetuating the dog's licking behavior. Atopy, food allergy, and secondary deep pyoderma are among the most common differentials. In a case series,[69] 6 dogs presented with ALD-like lesions were diagnosed with various underlying causes, namely lymphoma, an orthopedic pin, deep pyoderma, mast cell tumor, leishmaniasis, and (presumptive) sporotrichosis. The author has personally not seen a single case of strictly anxiety-related ALD in 15 years of behavioral medicine practice. Other underlying causes have always been identified.

Cats

Feline symmetric alopecia (FSA) is a clinical reaction pattern whereby cats present with symmetric alopecia over the thorax, flanks, ventral abdomen, or pelvic regions.[70] Initially it is important to determine if the overgrooming is associated with pain or a medical condition. Excessive grooming of the ventral abdomen may indicate abdominal pain, particularly of the bladder. Radiographs may reveal arthritic changes in older cats, particularly intervertebral arthritis. Resolution of the overgrooming and regrowth of the hair following the treatment of pain provide compelling evidence that pain can be a trigger for overgrooming.[70] True behavioral causes of overgrooming are rare. A case series of 21 cats with presumptive psychogenic alopecia[71] showed medical causes of pruritus in 16 cats. Three cats had a combination of psychogenic alopecia and a medical condition, and 2 were found to have psychogenic alopecia.

BEHAVIORAL SIGNS OF ENDOCRINE DISEASE
Dogs

Behavioral manifestations have been attributed to hypothyroidism, but there is no strong evidence of a causal association.[72] A study comparing thyroid analytes in 31 dogs aggressive to familiar people and in 31 nonaggressive dogs found no significant differences in the complete blood cell (CBC) count, serum chemistry panel, total thyroxine, free thyroxine by equilibrium dialysis, total triiodothyronine, free triiodothyronine, triiodothyronine autoantibodies, thyroid-stimulating hormone, and thyroglobulin autoantibodies.[73] Significant differences were found only with thyroxine autoantibodies. Levels were increased in the aggressive dogs but were still within normal reference range.

Cats

Hyperthyroid cats may be restless, vocal, and anxious looking. Night yowling can be associated with hyperthyroidism, hypertension, both hyperthyroidism and hypertension, and cognitive dysfunction.[13]

A 14-year-old spayed female cat was presented for a 1-year history of aggression toward other cats and urine spraying.[74] The cat's urine had recently developed a strong "tom cat" smell. The cat was diagnosed with hyperadrenocorticism, resulting in oversecretion of sex steroid hormones. In a similar case,[75] a 13-year-old neutered male domestic shorthair was evaluated for urine spraying that had a strong odor and aggressive behavior. The cat had been spraying urine and was aggressive for approximately 2 years before presentation. The owner had also noticed that the cat's face appeared larger. A mass associated with the right adrenal gland was found, and the adrenal gland and mass were removed during laparotomy. Final diagnosis was an adrenocortical adenoma. Eight weeks after surgery, the cat was no longer spraying urine and the strong odor had resolved.

A 15-year-old spayed female domestic shorthair cat was evaluated[76] for cyclic intermittent estrous behavior of 1 year's duration. Clinical signs reported were posturing, licking the vulva, vocalizing, rolling on the ground, and head rubbing. These behaviors occurred every 2 weeks and were similar to estrus behaviors exhibited by this cat at 6 months of age. The cat was diagnosed with an adrenocortical carcinoma.

A 12-year-old castrated male domestic longhair cat with a 2-year history of urine spraying was diagnosed with a functional ectopic interstitial cell tumor.[77] In addition to the spraying behavior, the cat had a round and full head with a general muscular body condition, similar to the appearance of a sexually intact male.

A 1-year-old female spayed Birman cat was presented to the referring veterinarian for inappropriate urination and defecation 1 month before presentation at a referral center.[78] Initially urinalysis revealed high levels of whole red blood cells (sediment and dipstick) and the CBC count revealed thrombocytopenia. One week later the cat became lethargic, had a decreased appetite, and was "more clingy" than usual. Following medical investigation, a diagnosis of atypical hypoadrenocorticism was made.

Diabetic neuropathy is a well-recognized cause of neuropathic pain in people.[33] Many cats with diabetes exhibit an aversion to being petted and cuddled. Owners refer to them as "cranky and aloof." Many of these cats also do not like to have their paws touched. Amitriptyline may help alleviate these pain-associated behaviors.

BEHAVIORAL SIGNS OF DENTAL DISEASE OR PAIN

In cases of dental disease or pain the animal is hesitant to pick up, chew, or swallow food. The animal may drop food, toys, or training articles from the mouth. Quivering of the jaw or chattering of the teeth may be reported. Oral pain can also cause pawing, tilting, bobbing, shaking, and sliding of the head and mouth along the floor. Chronic ptyalism or drooling may be seen and is most commonly caused by an inability or reluctance to swallow.[79]

Feline orofacial pain syndrome (FOPS) is considered to be an episodic neuropathic pain disorder, caused by a dysfunction of central or ganglion processing of sensory trigeminal information.[80] Affected cats usually exhibit exaggerated licking, unusual chewing movements, and pawing at the mouth. Mutilation of the tongue, lips, and labial and buccal mucosa may also be noted. Sensitization of trigeminal nerve endings from tooth eruption or oral disease and environmental stress are most likely important contributing factors in the etiology of the disease. Social incompatibility, if present in a multicat household, should be addressed as part of the treatment plan of this syndrome. In a retrospective study of 113 cases of FOPS,[81] the investigators stated that external factors could influence the disease. One or more FOPS events were directly linked to anxiety in 24 cats. In 14 cases, social incompatibility in a multicat household was listed as a source of stress. In 8 of these cats, stressful events included stay at a cattery, builders in the environment, death of the primary carer and moving house.

BEHAVIORAL SIGNS OF OSTEOARTHRITIS OR PAIN
Dogs

The most common sign of osteoarthritis in dogs is lameness.[82] Owners will report loss of normal performance (early signs) but will only seek veterinary care once their dog is lame. Stiffness after rest is a cardinal sign of joint disease, and is often present before onset of overt lameness. Stiffness will last only a few minutes. Anecdotally, dogs in constant joint discomfort can also exhibit increased nervousness, aggression, depression, and loss of appetite.[82] Muscle atrophy in some or all muscle groups of the legs can be a sign that the dog has stopped bearing weight evenly and/or is not exercising its limbs as it normally would. This type of muscle loss may occur slowly and develop before any overt lameness.

Cats

Changes in lifestyle and behavior are the main clinical features of osteoarthritis in cats. One study[83] used a questionnaire to identify lifestyle or behavioral changes noticed by owners that could be associated with chronic pain in 23 cats aged 9.4 to 19 years (mean 13.4 years). The changes were scored on a scale of 1 (minor) to 10 (severe). Owners rated the behaviors observed before and after analgesic therapy (meloxicam). Behaviors were grouped as mobility, activity, grooming, and temperament changes. The mobility category included jumping, height of jump, gracefulness, and changes in elimination behaviors (reluctance to go outside or use the litter pan; difficulties using the pan; missing the pan; and so forth). Activity included sleeping habits, playing, and hunting. Temperament addressed tolerance to owner or other animals and general attitude. There was a statistically significant reduction in owner scores in all categories, with the greatest reduction in the activity category. An earlier prospective study of 28 cats with osteoarthritis had already reported[84] that alterations in the ability to jump (20 of 28 cats or 71%) and height of jump (19 of 28 cats or 67%) were the most frequent signs of the disease. Data on demeanor, lameness, food intake, behavior, lifestyle, and other orthopedic parameters before and after analgesic administration (meloxicam) were recorded. Behavioral characteristics such as seeking seclusion, resentment, vocalization or aggression when handled, abnormal elimination habits, and lifestyle alterations such as unwillingness to jump and/or reduced height of jump and abnormal gait were all recorded. There were statistically significant improvements in willingness to jump, height of jump, stiff gait, activity level, and lameness. There were no significant changes in behaviors such as seeking seclusion, vocalization, resentment, or aggression when handled. The latter signs were present in a small number of cats (n = 6–10); the lack of improvement following analgesic treatment may simply indicate that the cat did not like being handled, and seeking seclusion may have been normal for that given individual. Lameness is rarely a sign of osteoarthritis in cats, and was absent in 15 of the 28 cats.[84] Stiffness after resting was reported in 8 of 50 cats in a study of owner-perceived signs of feline osteoarthritis.[85] Five owners reported a change in posture for claw sharpening (ie, the cat scratched a horizontal instead of a vertical surface).[85] Changes in how cats performed jumping included hesitation, stumbling or falling, or doing small jumps at a time. Stair use was described as climbing a few stairs at a time instead of the entire flight. This study also reported more specifically on changes in litter-box use. According to owners, 11 cats were eliminating outside the litter box because of either an inability to reach the box in time (urgency to urinate) or reluctance to climb stairs. Nine of these cats were thought to have difficulty maneuvering in the litter box.[85] No study to date has clearly shown house soiling as a consequence of osteoarthritis. Other medical conditions seen in older cats could also account for changes in litter-box use.

SUMMARY

Observing and collecting complete histories of obvious and subtle changes in behavior will help veterinarians identify and define more precisely all of the signs associated with medical and painful conditions as well as those associated with behavioral disorders. Pain identification remains a challenge in veterinary medicine, and should always be considered in the list of differential diagnoses when patients are presented with behavioral changes.

REFERENCES

1. Overall KL. Appendix B. In: Duncan LL, editor. Clinical behavioral medicine for small animals. St Louis (MO): Mosby; 1997. p. 461.
2. Casey R. Fear and stress in companion animals. In: Horwitz D, Mills D, Heath S, editors. British Small Animal Veterinary Association (BSAVA) manual of canine and feline behavioral medicine. Gloucester (United Kingdom): Br Small Anim Vet Assoc; 2002. p. 144–53.
3. Beerda B, Schilder MB, Van Hooff JA, et al. Manifestations of chronic and acute stress in dogs. Appl Anim Behav Sci 1997;52:307–19.
4. Beerda B, Schilder MB, Van Hooff JA, et al. Behavioral, saliva cortisol and heart rate responses to different types of stimuli in dogs. Appl Anim Behav Sci 1998; 58:365–81.
5. Schwizgebel D. Zusammenhänge zwischen dem Verhalten des Tierlehrers und dem Verhalten des Deutschen Schäferhundes im Hinblick auf tiergerechte Ausbildung. Aktuelle Arbeiten zur artgemassen Tierhaltung 1982;138–48.
6. Hetts S, Clark JD, Arnold CE, et al. Influence of housing conditions on beagles behavior. Appl Anim Behav Sci 1992;34:137–55.
7. Tams TR. Gastrointestinal symptoms. In: Tams TR, editor. Handbook of small animal gastroenterology. 2nd edition. St Louis (MO): Saunders; 2003. p. 1–50.
8. Miller JB. Hyperthermia and fever of unknown origin. In: Ettinger SJ, Feldman EC, editors. Textbook of veterinary internal medicine. Diseases of the dog and cat. 7th edition. St Louis (MO): Saunders Elsevier; 2010. p. 41–5.
9. Thomas WB. Movement disorders. In: Ettinger SJ, Feldman EC, editors. Textbook of veterinary internal medicine. Diseases of the dog and cat. 7th edition. St Louis (MO): Saunders Elsevier; 2010. p. 216–9.
10. Mich PM, Hellyer PW. Clinical pain identification assessment and management. In: Ettinger SJ, Feldman EC, editors. Textbook of veterinary internal medicine. Diseases of the dog and cat. 7th edition. St Louis (MO): Saunders Elsevier; 2010. p. 48–63.
11. Fingeroth JM, Prata RG, Patnaik AK. Spinal meningiomas in dogs: 13 cases (1972-1987). J Am Vet Med Assoc 1987;191:720–6.
12. Bagley RS, Gavin PR, Moore MP, et al. Clinical signs associated with brain tumors in dogs: 97 cases (1992-1997). J Am Vet Med Assoc 1999;215:818–9.
13. Baral RM, Peterson ME. Hyperthyroidism. In: Little S, editor. The cat: clinical medicine and management. St Louis (MO): Elsevier Saunders; 2012. p. 571–84.
14. King JN, Simpson KL, Overall KL, et al. Treatment of separation anxiety in dogs with clomipramine: results from a prospective, randomized, double-blind, placebo controlled, parallel group, multicentre clinical trial. Appl Anim Behav Sci 2000;67:255–75.
15. McCrave EA. Diagnostic criteria for separation anxiety in the dog. Vet Clin North Am Small Anim Pract 1991;21:247–55.
16. Palestrini C, Minero M, Cannas S, et al. Video analysis of dogs with separation-related behaviors. Appl Anim Behav Sci 2010;124:61–7.
17. Melian C, Pérez-Alenza MD, Peterson M. Hyperadrenocorticism in dogs. In: Ettinger SJ, Feldman EC, editors. Textbook of veterinary internal medicine.

Diseases of the dog and cat. 7th edition. St Louis (MO): Saunders Elsevier; 2010. p. 1816–40.

18. Forney S. Dyspnea and tachypnea. In: Ettinger SJ, Feldman EC, editors. Textbook of veterinary internal medicine. Diseases of the dog and cat. 7th edition. St Louis (MO): Saunders Elsevier; 2010. p. 253–5.

19. McNaughton N, Corr PJ. A two-dimensional neuropsychology of defence: fear/anxiety and defensive distance. Neurosci Biobehav Rev 2004;28: 285–305.

20. Lang PJ, Davis M, Ohman A. Fear and anxiety: animal models and human cognitive psychophysiology. J Affect Disord 2000;61:137–59.

21. Ohl F, Arndt SS, Van Der Staay FJ. Pathological anxiety in animals. Vet J 2008; 175:18–26.

22. Blanchard RJ, Hebert MA, Ferrari P, et al. Defensive behaviours in wild and laboratory (Swiss) mice: the mouse defense test battery. Physiol Behav 1998;65: 561–9.

23. Mastripieri D, Martel FL, Nevison CM, et al. Anxiety in rhesus monkey infants in relation to interactions with their mother and other social companions. Dev Psychobiol 1992;24:571–81.

24. Shuhama R, Del-Ben CM, Loureiro SR, et al. Animal defense strategies and anxiety disorders. An Acad Bras Cienc 2007;79:97–109.

25. Crawley J, Goodwin FK. Preliminary report of a simple animal behavior model for the anxiolytic effects of benzodiazepines. Pharmacol Biochem Behav 1980;13: 167–70.

26. Dards JL. The behaviour of dockyard cats: interaction of adult males. Appl Anim Ethol 1983;10:133–53.

27. Baral RM. Approach to the vomiting cat. In: Little S, editor. The cat: clinical medicine and management. St Louis (MO): Elsevier Saunders; 2012. p. 428–31.

28. Quimby JM, Smith ML, Lunn KF. Evaluation of the effects of hospital visit stress on physiologic parameters in the cat. J Feline Med Surg 2003;13:733–7.

29. McKune C, Robertson S. Analgesia. In: Little S, editor. The cat: clinical medicine and management. St Louis (MO): Elsevier Saunders; 2012. p. 90–111.

30. Skelly BJ, Franklin RJ. Recognition and diagnosis of lysosomal storage diseases in the cat and dog. J Vet Intern Med 2002;16:133–41.

31. O'Brien D, Coates JR. Brain disease. In: Ettinger SJ, Feldman EC, editors. Textbook of veterinary internal medicine. Diseases of the dog and cat. 7th edition. St Louis (MO): Saunders Elsevier; 2010. p. 1413–46.

32. Greene CE, Vandevelde M, Braund K. Lissencephaly in two Lhasa Apso dogs. J Am Vet Med Assoc 1976;169:405–10.

33. Mathews KA. Neuropathic pain in dogs and cats: if only they could tell us if they hurt. Vet Clin North Am Small Anim Pract 2008;38:1365–414.

34. Gaynor JS. Chronic pain syndrome of feline onychectomy. NAVC Clinician's Brief 2005;11–3.

35. Zulch HE, Mills DS, Lambert R, et al. The use of tramadol in a Labrador retriever presenting with self-mutilation of the tail. J Vet Behav 2012;7:252–8.

36. Horwitz DF, Neilson JC. Aggression/canine: classification and overview. In: Horwitz DF, Neilson JC, editors. Canine and feline behavior, Blackwell's five-minute veterinary consult. Ames (IA): Blackwell Publishing; 2007. p. 10–7.

37. Foster ES, Carrillo JM, Patnaik AK. Clinical signs of tumors affecting the rostral cerebrum in 43 dogs. J Vet Intern Med 1988;2:71–4.

38. Stacy BA, Stevenson TL, Lipsitz D, et al. Simultaneously occurring oligodendroglioma and meningioma in a dog. J Vet Intern Med 2003;17:357–9.

39. James FM, da Costa RC, Fauber A, et al. Clinical and MRI findings in three dogs with polycystic meningiomas. J Am Anim Hosp Assoc 2012;48:331–8.

40. Sanders DN, Farias FH, Johnson GS, et al. A mutation in canine *PPT1* causes early onset of neuronal ceroid lipofuscinosis in a Dachshund. Mol Genet Metab 2010;100:349–56.

41. Fatjo J, Martin S, Manteca X, et al. Animal behavior case of the month. J Am Vet Med Assoc 1999;215:1254–6.

42. Plessas IN, Volk HA, Kenny PJ. Migraine-like episodic pain behavior in a dog: can dogs suffer from migraines? J Vet Intern Med 2013;27:1034–40.

43. Goulle F, Meige F, Durieux F, et al. Intracranial meningioma causing partial amaurosis in a cat. Vet Ophthalmol 2011;14(Suppl 1):93–8.

44. Karli P, Gorgas D, Oevermann A, et al. Extracranial expansion of a feline meningioma. J Feline Med Surg 2013;15:749–53.

45. Sessums K, Mariani C. Intracranial meningioma in dogs and cats: a comparative review. Compend Contin Educ Vet 2009;31:330–9.

46. Glass EN, Cornetta AM, deLahunta A, et al. Clinical and clinicopathologic features in 11 cats with *Cuterebra* larvae myiasis of the central nervous system. J Vet Intern Med 1998;12:365–8.

47. Carmichael KP, Bienzle D, McDonnell JJ. Feline leukemia virus-associated myelopathy in cats. Vet Pathol 2002;39:536–45.

48. Barone G. Neurology. In: Little S, editor. The cat: clinical medicine and management. St Louis (MO): Elsevier Saunders; 2012. p. 734–67.

49. Chew DJ. Non obstructive idiopathic or interstitial cystitis in cats. In: Chew DJ, Dibartola SP, editors. Canine and feline nephrology and urology. 2nd edition. St Louis (MO): Elsevier Saunders; 2011. p. 306–40.

50. Tynes VV, Hart BL, Pryor PA, et al. Evaluation of the role of lower urinary tract disease in cats with urine-marking behavior. J Am Vet Med Assoc 2003;223:457–61.

51. Cameron ME, Casey RA, Bradshaw JW, et al. A study of environmental and behavioural factors that may be associated with feline idiopathic cystitis. J Small Anim Pract 2004;45:144–7.

52. Sherding RG. Diagnostic evaluation of the esophagus. In: Washabau RJ, Day MJ, editors. Canine and feline gastroenterology. St Louis (MO): Elsevier Saunders; 2012. p. 570–80.

53. Washabau RJ, Hall JA. Dysmotility. In: Washabau RJ, Day MJ, editors. Canine and feline gastroenterology. St Louis (MO): Elsevier Saunders; 2012. p. 630–4.

54. Matz ME. Flatulence. In: Ettinger SJ, Feldman EC, editors. Textbook of veterinary internal medicine. Diseases of the dog and cat. 7th edition. St Louis (MO): Saunders Elsevier; 2010. p. 210–2.

55. Zoran DL. Infection. In: Washabau RJ, Day MJ, editors. Canine and feline gastroenterology. St Louis (MO): Elsevier Saunders; 2012. p. 784–5.

56. Bécuwe-Bonnet V, Bélanger MC, Frank D, et al. Gastrointestinal disorders in dogs with excessive licking of surfaces. J Vet Behav 2012;7:194–204.

57. Frank D, Bélanger MC, Bécuwe-Bonnet V, et al. Prospective medical evaluation of 7 dogs presented with fly biting. Can Vet J 2012;53:1279–84.

58. Brondani JT, Luna SP, Padovani CR. Refinement and initial validation of a multidimensional composite scale for use in assessing acute postoperative pain in cats. Am J Vet Res 2011;72:174–83.

59. Wilson DV, Walshaw R. Postanesthetic esophageal dysfunction in 13 dogs. J Am Anim Hosp Assoc 2004;40:455–60.

60. Moon-Fanelli AA, Dodman NH, Cottam N. Blanket and flank sucking in Doberman Pinschers. J Am Vet Med Assoc 2007;231:907–12.

61. Overall KL. Use of clomipramine to treat ritualistic stereotypic motor behavior in three dogs. J Am Vet Med Assoc 1994;205:1733–41.
62. Chen AV, Bagley RS, West CL, et al. Fecal incontinence and spinal cord abnormalities in seven dogs. J Am Vet Med Assoc 2005;227:1945–51.
63. Foley P. Constipation, tenesmus, dyschezia and fecal incontinence. In: Ettinger SJ, Feldman EC, editors. Textbook of veterinary internal medicine. Diseases of the dog and cat. 7th edition. St Louis (MO): Saunders Elsevier; 2010. p. 206–9.
64. Diaz JV, Poma R. Diagnosis and clinical signs of feline infectious peritonitis in the central nervous system. Can Vet J 2009;50:1091–3.
65. Foley JE, Lapointe JM, Koblik P, et al. Diagnostic features of clinical neurologic feline infectious peritonitis. J Vet Intern Med 1998;12:415–23.
66. Abrams-Ogg A. Nonregenerative anemia. In: Ettinger SJ, Feldman EC, editors. Textbook of veterinary internal medicine. Diseases of the dog and cat. 7th edition. St Louis (MO): Saunders Elsevier; 2010. p. 788–97.
67. MacDonald JM, Bradley DM. Acral lick dermatitis. In: Bonagura JD, editor. Kirk's current veterinary therapy XIV. St Louis (MO): Saunders Elsevier; 2009. p. 468–73.
68. Shumaker AK, Angus JC, Coyner KS, et al. Microbiological and histopathological features of canine acral lick dermatitis. Vet Dermatol 2008;19:288–98.
69. Denerolle P, White SD, Taylor TS, et al. Organic diseases mimicking acral lick dermatitis in six dogs. J Am Anim Hosp Assoc 2007;43:215–20.
70. Moriello KA. Dermatology. In: Little S, editor. The cat: clinical medicine and management. St Louis (MO): Elsevier Saunders; 2012. p. 371–424.
71. Waisglass SE, Landsberg GM, Yager JA, et al. Underlying medical conditions in cats with presumptive psychogenic alopecia. J Am Vet Med Assoc 2006;228: 1705–9.
72. Scott-Moncrieff JC. Clinical signs and concurrent diseases of hypothyroidism in dogs and cats. Vet Clin North Am Small Anim Pract 2007;37:709–22.
73. Radosta LA, Shofer FS, Reisner IR. Comparison of thyroid analytes in dogs aggressive to familiar people in non-aggressive dogs. Vet J 2012;192:472–5.
74. Boag AK, Neiger R, Church DB. Trilostane treatment of bilateral adrenal enlargement and excessive sex steroid hormone production in a cat. J Small Anim Pract 2004;45:263–6.
75. Millard RP, Pickens EH, Wells KL. Excessive production of sex hormones with an adrenocortical tumor. J Am Vet Med Assoc 2009;234:505–8.
76. Meler EN, Scott-Mongrief JC, Peter AT, et al. Cyclic estrous-like behavior in a spayed cat associated with excessive sex-hormone production by an adrenocortical carcinoma. J Feline Med Surg 2011;13:473–8.
77. Rosen DK, Carpenter JL. Functional ectopic interstitial cell tumor in a castrated male cat. J Am Vet Med Assoc 1993;202:1865–6.
78. Hock CE. Atypical hypoadrenocorticism in a Birman cat. Can Vet J 2011;52: 893–6.
79. Wiggs RB, Lobprise HB. Oral examination and diagnosis. In: Wiggs RB, Lobprise HB, editors. Veterinary dentistry principle and practice. Philadelphia: Lippincott-Raven; 1997. p. 87–103.
80. Reiter AM. Dental and oral diseases. In: Little S, editor. The cat: clinical medicine and management. St Louis (MO): Elsevier Saunders; 2012. p. 329–70.
81. Rusbridge C, Heath S, Gunn-Moore DA, et al. Feline orofacial pain syndrome (FOPS): a retrospective study of 113 cases. J Feline Med Surg 2010;12: 498–508.

82. Bennett D. Canine and feline osteoarthritis. In: Ettinger SJ, Feldman EC, editors. Textbook of veterinary internal medicine. Diseases of the dog and cat. 7th edition. St Louis (MO): Saunders Elsevier; 2010. p. 750–61.

83. Bennett D, Morton C. A study of owner observed behavioural and lifestyle changes in cats with musculoskeletal disease before and after analgesic therapy. J Feline Med Surg 2009;11:997–1004.

84. Clarke SP, Bennett D. Feline osteoarthritis: a prospective study of 28 cases. J Small Anim Pract 2006;47:439–45.

85. Klinck MP, Frank D, Guillot M, et al. Owner-perceived signs and veterinary diagnosis in 50 cases of feline osteoarthritis. Can Vet J 2012;53:1181–6.

Stress—Its Effects on Health and Behavior: A Guide for Practitioners

Daniel Mills, BVSc, PhD, CBiol, FSBiol, FHEA, CCAB, MRCVS *,
Christos Karagiannis, DVM, MSc, MRCVS,
Helen Zulch, BVSc (Hons), MRCVS

KEYWORDS

- Stress • Health • Behavior • Arousal • Emotions • Stress audit

KEY POINTS

- Stress may affect the physical, mental, and social health of an animal.
- The effect of stressors is individual to the animal concerned and results from the appraisal of the stressor by the animal.
- Emotional states are not mutually exclusive and emotional conflict can also have serious behavioral consequences.
- Treatment of animals presenting with problems deemed to be stress-related should focus on the amelioration of background stress as well as specific stress-related triggers.
- Providing animals with certain coping mechanisms as well as teaching them some key life skills may be beneficial for the prevention of stress-related problems.

INTRODUCTION

The impact of stress on human health is widely recognized but recognition in the veterinary literature seems more limited. Health has physical, mental, and social dimensions,[1] and the growth of veterinary behavioral medicine has led to the development of paradigms for assessing the impact of stress on each of these. All of these health dimensions impact on the well-being of the patient, albeit in different ways, and perceived problems in any dimension are often a cause for concern by owners. It is therefore important not only that practitioners recognize the relationship between stress and these problems but also that they are prepared to manage them. Achieving this requires a clear understanding of the nature of the risk factors, which increase the likelihood of a stress response (stressors) and how this response may be manifest in the physical, mental, and social health of the individual. Only then can sound preventive advice and intervention be offered with confidence.

The stress response consists of the physiologic, behavioral, and psychological changes that occur in the face of a challenge to an individual's state of well-being.[2]

Animal Behaviour, Cognition and Welfare Group, School of Life Sciences, University of Lincoln, Brayford, Lincoln LN6 7TS, UK
* Corresponding author.
E-mail address: dmills@lincoln.ac.uk

Vet Clin Small Anim 44 (2014) 525–541
http://dx.doi.org/10.1016/j.cvsm.2014.01.005
0195-5616/14/$ – see front matter © 2014 Elsevier Inc. All rights reserved.

Many approaches are used to infer an animal's level of stress, but there is no single valid way of doing this, nor is there ever likely to be, because, contrary to the initial theories regarding the stress response (eg, general adaptation syndrome[3]), responses are in fact determined by the nature of the stressor. Appreciation of this fact should lead to clinical recognition that different types of stressors require different interventions to manage them according to the fundamental quality of the stressor involved. As discussed in this article, this quality is defined by the emotional processes that the stressor arouses within the individual.

ASSESSING SPECIFIC STRESS RESPONSES

Cortisol has historically been used as a biomarker of stress, but raised cortisol level is really just a physiologic reaction to environmental changes that increase arousal, whether that is in a positive or negative way. To assess emotional distress, it is necessary to systematically triangulate a range of measures to make an inference with the necessary objectivity for this process to be considered scientific. For example, for the evaluation of the effect of a potential auditory stressor on a dog (eg, a loud noise), all available indicators of physiologic (eg, tachypnea, tachycardia, drooling, pupil dilation) and behavioral change (eg, dog runs up to its owner or runs away, dog shows hypervigilance or increased tendency to startle) need to be considered to evaluate the psychological quality of this stimulus *to this dog, in this situation*. This statement is particularly important, but potentially challenging, when trying to differentiate an active emotional response to aversion from a conditioned response (learned habit) that gains the owner's attention.

In addition, it must be noted that stressors may differ not only in type (qualitative aspect) but also quantitatively (in intensity), and that different behavioral and physiologic signatures may be associated with these differences or a change in the stressor's quality and/or quantity. Continuing the previous example, this might involve a shift from freezing to flight behavior in the case of a more intense (louder) or less predictable sound, which may also indicate the need for different interventions, although still focused on the same broad type of emotional response (fear).

To infer that a given event evokes an emotional response, 4 lines of evidence should be used[4]:

1. The event is of personal importance to the individual and the response is associated with its anticipated or actual arrival or removal. From an affective neuroscientific perspective, it has been argued (Mills and colleagues[5] adapted and developed from Panksepp[6]) that the stimuli associated with these events (emotionally competent stimuli) can be broadly classified into
   a. Desirables (resources the animal wants)
   b. Frustrations (the denial or absence of things that the animal wants)
   c. Fears (threats to the animal)
   d. Pains (bodily damage)
   e. Those with whom an affectionate bond is shared (social play and similar positive interactions)
   f. Attachment figures and objects (sources of safety and security)
   g. Offspring (parental activity)
   h. Potential sexual partners (courtship and reproductive activity), to which a ninth category is now added:
   i. Undesirables (avoidance, including aggressive responses focused on stimuli which do not pose an actual or perceived physical threat)

2. The response reflects a change in arousal (increase or decrease depending on the emotional state involved), which provides underlying physiologic support for the action to be taken in association with the triggering event
3. The response is associated with general changes in behavioral tendency (eg, the tendency to escape), which may vary with the options available to the animal (ie, the form of escape used varies with the circumstances). A relatively invariate response may imply either an extreme reaction or the development of a conditioned habit
4. The event produces changes in behavior associated with communication of the animal's internal state (eg, certain facial expressions)

Emotional responses are not mutually exclusive and more than one may occur at any given time within an individual. For example, a dog that does not appear comfortable around other dogs may be reacting for many reasons, but to take just 2 of these possibilities: he may be afraid of other dogs or he wants to approach but is frustrated by being on the leash (2 concurrent emotions). In both scenarios, the dog may appear superficially to express similar responses (eg, lunging behavior and barking), but fear will typically include well-established elements of body posture, such as the ears drawn backwards, gaze aversion, tail tucking, and a lowered body stance before any aggressive response.[7] By contrast, an animal that is frustrated from interacting with another will show signs of positive approach and engagement before any aggressive behavior, with ambivalent, displacement, or redirected behaviors, like walking on the spot, circling, yawning, leg cocking, when he is excited.[5] It is worth emphasizing, that, in this example, the different emotional responses are associated with different emotionally competent stimuli, even though the general circumstances are the same — in the first, it is the arrival of the dog, and in the second, it is the combined stimuli of the presence of the dog and the presence of the leash. These circumstances may be partly differentiable because of the evidence provided by the animal's behavior when off leash. Also, if the frustrated dog is punished by its owner for this display, a change in (or addition of) emotion may occur with fear displayed that has the owner as its focus (**Fig. 1**). If this situation of the dog reacting to dogs occurs regularly with either a specific dog (or dogs in general), the other dog (or dogs in general) may become an undesirable stimulus so that a pre-emptive aggressive display is made to prevent contact, before any signs of fear or frustration. The subtleties of the distinguishable ethological elements associated with this latter response are the subject of ongoing research by the authors' research group.

Another important consideration when assessing the stress response in any given individual revolves around the neurochemistry of the underlying behavior. In behavioral medicine it has been noted that not all patients with the same broad behavioral diagnosis respond in the same manner to the same intervention and this may reflect different underlying mechanisms, giving rise to a common end point. Different neurotransmitters may be implicated in the presentation of the same superficial behavior. For example, Pageat and colleagues,[8] described a positive correlation between anxious behaviors and prolactinemia and that prolactinemia may be useful in guiding the choice of medication; thus, animals with behavioral manifestations of anxiety and lower levels of prolactinemia tend to improve after fluoxetine (a selective serotonin reuptake inhibitor) administration, whereas dogs with increased prolactinemia improved more after administration of selegiline (a monoamine oxidase inhibitor). As with individualized medicine in humans, looking beyond superficial diagnostic categories allows one to be more specific with interventions,[9] especially in the case of an acute response. This intervention eases treatment for clients (which makes

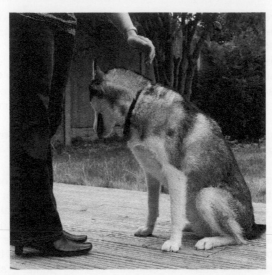

Fig. 1. It is important for clients to recognize the subtle signs of discomfort, such as a head turn, rather than force the animal into stressful situations that may provoke a more overt response. (*Courtesy of* P. Baumber, Lincoln, United Kingdom.)

compliance more likely), because redundant measures can be identified and excluded more effectively. If left untreated or treated inappropriately, the chronic arousal associated with long-term stress can also have serious physical health impacts, once again emphasizing the importance of accurate assessment and appropriate interventions (**Box 1**).

THE IMPACT OF STRESS ON PHYSICAL HEALTH

Stress has been shown to directly shorten an animal's lifespan,[10] but it is also associated with various detrimental changes in physical health (eg, through its impact on the immune system, gastrointestinal function, and the urogenital system), which affect the animal's quality of life. Several well-documented associations in the companion animal veterinary literature are reviewed briefly below in this section, but it should be noted that associations do not necessarily indicate causality and indeed the 2 will interact, because disease is by definition stressful (it is a state of changed or "dis" ease). In some situations the relationship may be unclear. For example, hyperthyroidism in cats is more common in cats kept indoors (increasing the odds by

---

Box 1
Assessing the specific stress response

- A single measure of stress such as cortisol is inadequate when assessing a patient because these general measures may simply indicate a level of arousal with no regard to the underlying emotional state of the individual.

- Assessing emotion through triangulation of features is critical for the implementation of a plan to manage or treat stress.

- Emotional states are not mutually exclusive and the emotion(s) elicited in a specific situation can undergo alteration over time.

a factor of 4 to 11.2)[11] and although this might be associated with increased stress, recent data suggest the coincident increased exposure to fire retardants, which are widely used to treat home furnishings and have been shown to affect thyroid function, may be very important in this increased risk.[12]

Urinary System

An increased risk of interstitial cystitis in cats is associated with a range of stressors (eg, moving to a new home, dogs or other cats in the house, and especially, conflict between cats and difficulty accessing a litter tray).[13,14] Three different studies have also shown an increased risk for cystitis correlated with the time that cats spent indoors.[15–17] In addition, this condition is associated with increased plasma norepinephrine.[18] A possible pathophysiological mechanism for these associations might relate to a change in bladder permeability associated with stress.[19]

A recent study found that behaviorally normal and problematic cats from households including a urine sprayer had elevated fecal glucocorticoids (an indicator of chronic arousal), compared with individuals from homes with a cat that was failing to use the litter tray,[20] suggesting that urine spraying is a more common behavioral outcome of chronic stress than failure to use the litter tray. It is worth noting that in this study, 7/18 (39%) of the spraying cats who seemed otherwise physically normal to their owners had signs of physical disease on clinical examination. By comparison, 11/23 (48%) of the toileting cats were subsequently found to have physical problems, suggesting that failure to use the litter tray often has medical complications, but these do not seem to be associated with ongoing chronic stress.

This finding demonstrates the importance of careful evaluation of health and behavioral indicators when a sign such as house soiling is presented because there is no simple means of determining the influence of stress on the presenting signs.

Reproductive System

In dogs, decreased sperm quality, azoospermia, has been associated with an anxious temperament.[21] Fear and anxiety may also inhibit complete erection and ejaculation in the dog[22] and reduce proceptive and receptive behaviors. On the other hand, environmental stress in bitches may result in a failure to breed.[23] In young bitches, stress may play a role in the development of "split cycles," an estrous cycle that begins with normal follicular development and estrogen secretion but fails to progress to ovulation or can be a contributory factor for delayed puberty.[23]

Immune System

Although small bouts of stress can enhance the immune response toward a pathogen, chronic stress can dampen immune responses to invasive pathogens.[24] In humans, chronic stress seems to result in suppression of the immune response[25] and 2 studies in shelter dogs support a similar association.[26,27] In catteries, it has been found that cats exhibiting high levels of stress are about 5 times more likely to develop upper respiratory tract infection compared with cats exhibiting lower levels.[28] Stress during pregnancy in both human and nonhuman animals can also reduce immunocompetence in the offspring.[29,30]

Gastrointestinal System

Stress has been associated with various gastrointestinal diseases in humans, including functional bowel disorders, inflammatory bowel disease, peptic ulcers, and gastroesophageal reflux.[31] In both cats and dogs it has been associated with intermittent diarrhea, vomiting, or decreased appetite, especially when the stressor is associated with isolation or confinement.[32,33] Cats faced with unexpected changes to their management may decrease appetite and water intake, avoid elimination for 24 hours (potentially increasing the risk of constipation), and defecate outside the litter tray.[34] In general, food intake and stress seem to be negatively correlated in cats,[28] whereas in dogs, associations have been made between increased stress and coprophagia[35] and inflammatory bowel disease.[36]

The Integument

The skin and nervous system are both derived from embryonic ectoderm[37] and so it is not surprising that they share functional relationships through a substantial number of common hormones, neuropeptides, and receptors.[38] Thus, under stressful conditions, these common factors might play a role in the pathogenesis of dermatoses, such as atopic dermatitis,[39] or lead to the expression of pruritus.[40] The management of identifiable environmental stressors or concurrent behavioral problems in dogs with recurrent pyoderma can be an important part of the long-term treatment of these conditions.[41] An increased severity and frequency of dermatologic conditions has been reported among dogs with fears and anxieties,[10] and the importance of multimodal treatment addressing concurrent psychological conditions in dogs with pruritus, such as anxiety, fearfulness, or aggressive behavior, is increasingly being recognized.[42] Indeed it has been suggested that behavioral therapy in combination with psychopharmacology can be important in achieving an improvement of 50% or more in dermatologic expressions of repetitive behaviors in cats and dogs.[43]

In cats, self-grooming and scratching are often immediate responses to conflict without any pathologic impact.[44] However, within repeatedly stressful situations over which the cat has very limited control, maladaptive over-grooming may develop.[45] Although a range of environmental and social stressors have been associated with this disorder,[43] others suggest that psychogenic alopecia is overdiagnosed and that in most cases the cause is primarily an underlying medical factor.[46] In reality, attention should be given to both physical and psychological elements because the former probably increases the risk of the latter even if they are not specifically causal (**Fig. 2**).

THE IMPACT OF STRESS ON MENTAL HEALTH

Not only is anxiety a mental health problem in its own right and a risk factor for the development of a range of physical health problems as described in the previous

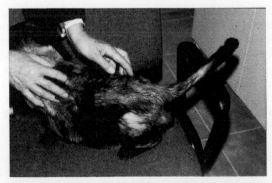

Fig. 2. Stress may not only trigger bouts of over-grooming but also play an important role in maintaining chronic dermatopathies. Multimodal management of such cases is essential. (*Courtesy of* S. Stariha Pipan, Lincoln, United Kingdom.)

section, it can also increase the risk of other psychological problems. In humans, it has been reported that generalized anxiety increases the risk of separation anxiety in children, social phobias in adults, and more generally, the risk of obsessive-compulsive behavior and posttraumatic stress disorders, all of which may have companion animal analogues.[43]

Unavoidable and unpredictable fear-eliciting stressors may result in more general disturbances to mental health if the animal is unable to find an appropriate way to cope. For example, a dog with a sound aversion may become more generally anxious during fireworks season, necessitating the use of combination psychopharmacological therapy to control both the emotional response to specific noises (benzodiazepines) and the more general change in mood (specific or nonspecific serotonergic agents).

Chronic frustration may similarly evoke more general behavioral changes, especially when the animal is faced with an insoluble problem.[5] Depending on the individual and the circumstances, the pet might respond passively with depressed behavior, or actively with a state of heightened arousal and possibly chronic displacement behaviors that may ultimately become stereotypic (eg, tail chasing).[47] Genetic factors inevitably play a role in the expression of specific displacement activities, for example, flank-sucking is often associated with Dobermans,[48] tail chasing and spinning with German shepherds and bull terriers,[49] and wool sucking with Oriental cat breeds.[50] However, it important to note that although genetic factors constitute a heightened risk for the development of the behavior, a stressor still needs to be present to trigger its expression.

Mental health problems may arise not only from the prolonged effects of specific emotions but also from the emotional consequences of motivational conflict. For example, a dog that is inconsistently treated by a member of the family may suffer from such conflict anxiety. This conflict anxiety is distinguished from the anxiety that arises from the anticipation of an aversive event, because it is associated with uncertainty about the current state, rather than a concern about the future and may be evident from a greater prevalence of ambivalent behaviors such as approach-avoidance and hesitancy. Treatment of such a problem needs to focus on resolving the conflict; accordingly desensitization regimes are of less value than respondent counterconditioning of the emotion, for example, with powerful rewards to encourage approach.

Finally, it is worth noting again that the increased arousal associated with stress is normally mediated through the endogenous glucocorticoid system. In addition to mobilizing energy reserves, these chemicals seem to have significant effects on cognitive processing, resulting in greater sensitivity to aversive events, which may be of mental health significance, in both normal animals and those already suffering some degree of dementia. Stress responses may increase cerebral metabolic demand and so have the potential to increase the rate of cognitive decline in animals with cognitive dysfunction. Concern over the deleterious psychological effects of raised levels of glucocorticoids has also caused some[51] to recently recommend using caution in the chronic administration of related chemicals for therapeutic reasons. An initial survey by these authors indicated that around 30% of dogs treated with glucocorticoids showed increased sensitivity to aversive events (eg, nervousness and/or restlessness, increased startle responses, food guarding, increased avoidance responses including irritable aggression, and increased barking).[51] Obviously these drugs have many beneficial effects, but, given the precautionary principle, these data suggest a cost-benefit analysis should be performed before they are prescribed, noting the potential increased risk of behavior problems related to an increased sensitivity to aversive stimuli and also the significance of possible negative psychological effects on welfare.

THE IMPACT OF STRESS ON SOCIAL HEALTH

Social health includes a wide range of interactions with others, both con-specifics and hetero-specifics. Perhaps the most widely recognized problems in this domain include the "social phobias,"[39] but conditions like agoraphobia also impact on normal social interactions, albeit indirectly. In a study of 1040 dogs with aggressive behavior problems, more than a third of them involved family members and around 12% involved dogs living in the same household,[52] indicating poor social relationships likely to result in stress with an associated risk to health (**Box 2**). Fear and frustration are commonly cited as the most common reason for these problems[53] and this may result from chronically inconsistent interactions that give rise to stress. Thus it can be seen that where relationship problems occur, stress can be a cause and/or a consequence (**Table 1**).

Behavior problems (and especially aggressive behavior) are among the most common reasons given for the relinquishment of dogs and cats,[54] and this abandonment may also be considered another social health cost associated with chronic stress. Accordingly, as the veterinary profession increasingly takes on a responsibility for the total health care of pets, it is essential that techniques aimed at managing and preventing these problems are embraced. These interventions form the focus of the second part of this article.

PRINCIPLES OF STRESS AUDITING AND INTERVENTION MANAGEMENT

Behavior problems arise as a result of the accumulation of risk factors of varying importance and are rarely entirely related to a single cause. Accordingly, management should focus on addressing relevant factors based on both their significance and also the ease with which they can be addressed. Although many behavior problems may have a clear trigger that may be considered a stressor, these are not the focus of this article, because this embraces much of veterinary behavioral medicine. Instead, the focus here is on the management of factors that increase the risk of a problem, which may provide the tipping point for the expression of a problematic behavior or exacerbate its intensity to an unacceptable level. In some situations focusing on these may resolve the problem and be easier for clients to address.

Box 2
The impact of stress on health

- Several organ systems have been shown to be susceptible to developing pathologic abnormality as a result of stress, for example, the urinary, gastrointestinal, reproductive, and immune systems as well as the integument.

- For these reasons, where the underlying cause of a disease process is unclear and especially in the case of recurrent problems, stress should be investigated as a contributory cause.

- There is now evidence that corticosteroids may give rise to changes in behavior; therefore, their use needs to be even more carefully scrutinized, especially their long-term use or use in patients already at risk of developing certain behavior problems related to negative affect.

- Stress can lead to alterations in behavior that impact on relationships between individuals and vice versa.

Table 1		
Stress' impact on dogs' and cats' health		
	Species	**Impact**
Physical health		
General	Dog	Shortened lifespan
Urinary system	Cat	Increased risk of interstitial cystitis
		Increased risk for cystitis
		Association between spraying and medical complications
Reproductive system	Dog	Decreased sperm quality (azoospermia)
		Inhibit complete erection and ejaculation
		Failure to breed in bitches
		"Split cycles"
		Delayed puberty in female animals
Immune system	Dog	Suppression of the immune system
	Cat	Increased risk to develop upper respiratory tract infection
Gastrointestinal system	Dog, cat	Intermittent diarrhea, vomiting, or decreased appetite
	Cat	Decreased appetite and water intake, avoiding elimination for 24 h, defecation out of the litter tray
	Dog	Coprophagia
		Inflammatory bowel disease
Integument	Dog	Pyoderma
		Pruritus
		Increased severity and frequency of dermatologic conditions
	Dog, cat	Repetitive behaviors
	Cat	Repetitive behaviors, eg, over-grooming
Mental health	Dog, cat	Chronic frustration
	Dog	Deleterious psychological effects of raised levels of glucocorticoids
		Nervousness and/or restlessness, increased startle responses, food guarding, increased avoidance responses including irritable aggression, and increased barking
		Tail chasing
		Flank sucking in Dobermans
		Tail chasing and spinning in German shepherds and bull terriers
	Cat	Wool sucking in Oriental cat breeds
Social health	Dog, cat	"Social phobias"
	Dog	Aggressive behavior toward family members or toward dogs living in the same household

Data from Refs.[5,10–18,20–23,26–28,32–36,39–45,47–53]

As with specific stress responses, this background stress may have a predominant quality, which alters the likelihood of an overt emotional reaction in a given circumstance. For example, if the home is relaxed, the animal may be less likely to show a specific fear response, but if there is an undercurrent of anxiety, these responses may be more likely to occur. In clinical practice, increased levels of background stress in the home have been found to be one of the most pervasive risk factors for aggression by cats toward humans.[55] To address this issue, it is essential to first recognize the background context of the problem. A framework for this systematic evaluation of circumstances requiring intervention is provided by the stress audit process, which aims to identify these nonovert risk factors.[5] Each of a series of contexts is systematically evaluated for the predominant affective responses (as detailed above) with which they are associated. These stresses are listed in **Box 3**, together with indicators

534

Box 3
Stress audit

- Husbandry
  - Daily management
  - Rules and regulations
    - Training given to enable the pet to understand them
    - Consistency of enforcement by all spending time with the pet
  - Level of routine
  - General environment quality both physical and social
- Expectations placed on the animal by its owner
  - Animal's role and whether it is the same for all family members
  - Clarity and consistency of expectations by all family members
  - Provision of resources needed by the animal to achieve these expectations
- Ongoing change
  - Amount and type of change
  - Predictability within changing situations
  - Preparation for change and communication of ability to cope
  - Availability of coping strategies
- Specific stressors in the home affecting the client's family
  - Changes in behavior or circumstance that might impact on the animal
    - Associated changes in expectations of animal's behavior (see specific stressors affecting the pet, below)
    - Associated changes in animal's management
- Specific stressors in the home affecting the pet
  - Physical characteristics of the stressor
    - Affective quality
    - Intensity
    - Magnitude
    - Duration
    - Predictability
  - Expectation of animal's behavior in relation to this stressor
    - Preparation given to enable coping
    - Appropriateness of response to the pet's behavior including variants of it
  - Opportunities for control over the stressor by the pet
  - Supportive or conflicting social relationships in the home (see also support for the pet, below)
- Support for the pet
  - Communication
    - Clarity: instruction provided or animal expected to initiate appropriate behavior
    - Provision made for the animal to succeed in the above
  - Feedback
  - Consistency

of some more specific characteristics to be explored. Elements are then discussed further in the following sections. With practice, the assessment of these in the clinical setting can be made from questions framed into a conversation of just a few minutes, alongside a written history.

Demands and Expectations

The first goal of the stress audit process is to examine the demands being made of the animal in terms of its daily management, including its level of routine (predictability), the quality of the general environment, and the support given to the animal to ensure it is able to adapt to these expectations. For example, a dog that is home alone for an extended period of time may be more prone to certain forms of separation-related problems if it has not been trained to cope with either the frustration of being confined or separation from an attachment figure. By way of further example, if a family expects a dog not to jump on the sofa, but he has never been consistently taught this, there is likely to be frustration as the animal is sometimes punished for jumping on the sofa but is at other times allowed up (without it being clearly cued that this is acceptable) when members of the family want company (**Fig. 3**).

Second, the stress audit considers the physical characterization of specific demands and the preparation and available resources given to the animal to help it cope (**Box 4**). An animal may be able to cope with stressors individually, but together, especially if the stressors are of the same emotional quality, these events may overwhelm the individual. In this regard, predictability and control may be particularly important considerations. If an animal is able to cope, predictability may reduce the impact of the stressor, but if not, both predictable and unpredictable stressors will lead to a significant stress response—in predictable situations anxiety may develop from the time the animal can predict the triggering event; however, in the case of unpredictable stressors, the animal may generalize its state of anxiety to many extraneous stimuli.

Control implies that the animal has acceptable choices available to it that it can use to reduce the impact of the stressor for itself; for example, a dog that is not at ease with unfamiliar people and does not have anywhere to retreat to when visitors arrive has no

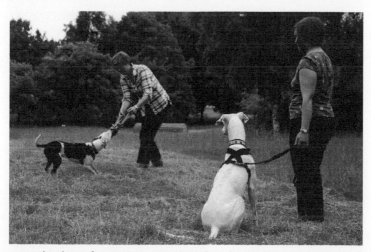

Fig. 3. Dogs need to learn frustration control, so they do not get over-aroused when denied the opportunity to engage in a pleasurable activity. (*Courtesy of* P. Baumber, Lincoln, United Kingdom.)

Box 4
The stress audit

- Stressors are cumulative and therefore all aspects of an animal's life need to be assessed when planning an intervention to manage stress.

- Both the physical and the social environment, as well as changes in both, need to be assessed as part of the stress audit.

- Control and predictability are important for stress reduction.

- Owners who offer support (rather than consolation) to help their pet's coping ability in the face of the pet reacting to stressors can reduce their pet's stress, whereas a punitive owner response will exacerbate this.

---

control over the situation and may respond aggressively as a consequence. The provision of an area of safe and secure retreat, however, puts it in control (**Fig. 4**). Provision of such a safe haven is extremely important in the effective and safe management of a dog and is described further in **Box 5**.

When an animal faces a demand, it will cope best if those around it are supportive rather than indifferent or in conflict with it. Often, owners feel the urge to punish their pets when they do not behave as they would like (**Fig. 5**). Punishment not only potentially exacerbates an animal's anxiety and/or frustration, but also impacts on the dog's perception of the individual as a consistent source of security (secure base; see below, **Box 5**), affecting its wider coping capacity. It is therefore not surprising that physical punishment is significantly associated with all forms of dog-related aggression (ie, toward owner, unfamiliar people, and other dogs).[56]

INTERVENTION MEASURES FOR MANAGING STRESS

As already mentioned, specific problems may require specific interventions, but this falls outside the scope of this article and the reader is referred to other texts for advice

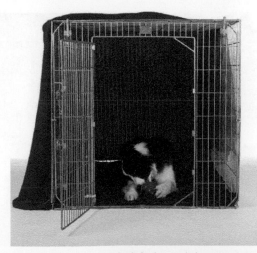

Fig. 4. A safe haven is not the same as a bolt hole, and the association with safety, security, and control needs to be made, away from stressful situations. (*Courtesy of* P. Baumber, Lincoln, United Kingdom.)

> **Box 5**
> **A note on safe havens and secure bases**
>
> A safe haven is an area where the animal is in control and which has become a conditioned place of safety outside of times when there are significant stressors. Consequently, when the animal is faced with potential stressors, it can retreat to this place and feel relatively safe. This safe place is not the same as a "bolt hole," which is a place to which the animal goes hoping that the aversive event will pass (ie, the animal is not confident of a desirable outcome). When establishing a safe haven, it is important that training takes place when the animal is calm and not anxious and that the philosophy of this area is respected by all family members (ie, the animal should not be forced to come out of the safe haven); no one forces their attention on the animal when it is in its safe haven, and there are only ever positive associations with the place (eg, tasty treats or toys can be placed when the animal is not there for it to find). Pheromonatherapy may provide unconditioned chemical safety signals to help enable the creation of this area, especially in an otherwise chaotic home environment.[5]
>
> A secure base is a place or individual that allows an animal to explore uncertainty with confidence. Accordingly, a safe base cannot be associated with aversives and in the case of the person there may be an expectation that the individual will recognize and intervene to abort situations in which the animal is expressing discomfort.[62]

on these matters (eg, Refs.[5,39]). Nonetheless, it should be remembered that support measures need to be tailored to the individual patient, their family, and circumstances, because there is no point overwhelming a client with tasks beyond their competence or resources.[5] Therefore, simple management and environmental changes, such as avoidance of exacerbating stressful circumstances and the use of pheromonatherapy where relevant, are often preferable as initial interventions, although specific behavioral intervention may be required.[5] Where possible, training and learning exercises should be framed within the context of normal daily interactions, because time is often the most limited resource for many clients, impacting on their compliance with training.[57]

Interventions to manage stress will always be important, but minimizing the stress response in the first place would be ideal. To this end, early life experiences can be manipulated to help pets cope with stimuli that may put them at risk for arousal and negative emotion. A review of the literature of puppy and kitten development is outside the scope of this article, but there is extensive evidence of correlations between certain early life events and the expression of problem behavior later in life.[58,59] Although

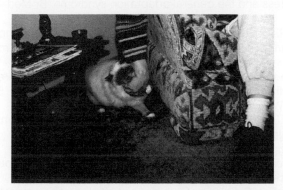

Fig. 5. Encouraging inappropriate play can not only lead to problematic behaviors like biting, but also become part of a stressful cycle as the owners try to punish what they see as inappropriate behavior by the cat. (*Courtesy of* Daniel Mills, Lincoln, United Kingdom.)

causal relationships are often difficult to prove and scientific assessment of early life interventions is scant (see Seksel and colleagues[60] as an example of such a study), appropriate puppy training, habituation, and socialization are generally advised. More specific to developing coping strategies for stressors, Zulch and Mills[61] postulate that owners should take a more proactive role in creating resilience through educating puppies in life skills. Examples of the type of skills that puppies can learn to assist them in coping with everyday life include an ability to experience novelty with confidence, not immediately take fright at startling stimuli, tolerate frustration, and understand the boundaries. Hand in hand with this go owner skills of responding appropriately to the communicative behavior of their pets so that they can serve as a secure base.[62]

SUMMARY

Stressors impact on all areas of a pet's life, potentially to the detriment of their well-being. In addition, should this lead to behavior change, it is likely to cause strain in the owner-pet relationship with an increased risk of relinquishment. Understanding why events may be perceived as stressful to a given individual is essential in remedying their effect. Clinicians need to be skilled in recognizing and categorizing potential stressors as well as auditing the background stress in the animal's environment as only once this has been accomplished can measures be implemented to reduce the effects of specific stimuli. In addition, a thorough understanding of both the features of a stimulus that elicit a stress response and the cumulative effect of stressors allows the clinician to structure interventions that are tailored to the individual. An individualized approach is likely to be more effective of itself and because it will reduce the resource commitment and skill set required by owners, which through increased compliance is beneficial to the overall outcome of sometimes challenging behavior problems.

REFERENCES

1. World Health Organization. Preamble to the Constitution of the World Health Organization as adopted by the International Health Conference. New York, June 19–22, 1946; signed on 22 July 1946 by the representatives of 61 states and entered into force on 7 April 1948. (Official Records of the World Health Organization, no. 2. p. 100).
2. Carlstead K, Brown JL, Strawn W. Behavioral and physiological correlates of stress in laboratory cats. Appl Anim Behav Sci 1993;38(2):143–58.
3. Selye H. Stress and the general adaptation syndrome. Br Med J 1950;1(4667): 1384–92.
4. Scherer KR. On the nature and function of emotion: a component process approach. In: Scherer KR, Ekman P, editors. Approaches to emotion. Hillsdale (NJ): Erlbaum; 1984. p. 293–317.
5. Mills D, Braem Dube M, Zulch H. Principles of pheromonatherapy. Stress and pheromonatherapy in small animal clinical behaviour. Wes Sussex (United Kingdom): Wiley-Blackwell; 2013. p. 127–45.
6. Panksepp J. Affective neuroscience: the foundations of human and animal emotions. New York: Oxford University Press; 1998.
7. Bain M. Aggression towards unfamiliar people and animals. In: Horwitz D, Mills DM, Heath S, editors. BSAVA manual of canine and feline behavioural medicine. Gloucester (United Kingdom): BSAVA Publications; 2009. p. 154–63.
8. Pageat P, LaFont C, Falawee C, et al. An evaluation of serum prolactin in anxious dogs and response to treatment with selegiline or fluoxetine. Appl Anim Behav Sci 2007;105(4):342–50.

9. Savard J. Personalised medicine: a critique on the future of health care. J Bioeth Inq 2013;10(2):197–203.
10. Dreschel NA. The effects of fear and anxiety on health and lifespan in pet dogs. Appl Anim Behav Sci 2010;125(3–4):157–62.
11. Scarlett JM, Moise NS, Rayl J. Feline hyperthyroidism: A descriptive and case-control study. Prev Vet Med 1998;6(4):295–309.
12. Dye JA, Venier M, Zhu L, et al. Elevated PBDE levels in pet cats: sentinels for humans? Environ Sci Technol 2007;41(18):6350–6.
13. Cameron ME, Casey RA, Bradshaw JW, et al. A study of environmental and behavioural factors that may be associated with feline idiopathic cystitis. J Small Anim Pract 2004;45:144–7.
14. Pryor PA, Hart BL, Bain MJ, et al. Causes of urine marking in cats and effects of environmental management on frequency of marking. J Am Vet Med Assoc 2001;219(12):1709–13.
15. Reif JS, Bovee KC, Gaskell CJ, et al. Feline urethral obstruction: a case-control study. J Am Vet Med Assoc 1977;170:1320–4.
16. Walker AD, Weaver AD, Anderson RS, et al. An epidemiological survey of the feline urological syndrome. J Small Anim Pract 1977;18:282–301.
17. Willeberg P. Epidemiology of naturally-occurring feline urologic syndrome. Vet Clin North Am Small Anim Pract 1984;14:455–69.
18. Buffington CT, Pacak K. Increased plasma norepinephrine concentration in cats with interstitial cystitis. J Urol 2001;165(6):2051–4.
19. Westropp JL, Kass PH, Buffington CA. Evaluation of the effects of stress in cats with idiopathic cystitis. Am J Vet Res 2006;67(4):731–6.
20. Ramos D, Reche-Junior A, Mills D, et al. Are cats with housesoiling problems stressed? A case-controlled comparison of faecal glucocorticoid levels in urine spraying and toileting cats. In: Mills, Da Graca Pereira, Jacinto, editors. Proceedings of the Ninth International Veterinary Behavioural Meeting Conference. Lisbon, Portugal; 26–28, September 2013. p. 113–4.
21. Memon MA. Common causes of male dog infertility. Theriogenology 2007;68(3): 322–8.
22. Kutzler MA. Canine semen collection and management of male infertility. Fifth Congreso Latinoamericano de Emergencias y Cuidados Intensivos, 2012, Mexico. Available online from http://www.congreso.laveccs.org/res2012/m2012.php.
23. Grundy SA, Feldman E, Davidson A. Evaluation of infertility in the bitch. Clin Tech Small Anim Pract 2002;17(3):108–15.
24. Radek KA. Antimicrobial anxiety: the impact of stress on antimicrobial immunity. J Leukoc Biol 2010;88(2):263–77.
25. Maddock C, Pariante CM. How does stress affect you? An overview of stress, immunity, depression and disease. Epidemiol Psichiatr Soc 2001;10:153–62.
26. Beerda B, Schilder MB, van Hooff, et al. Behavioural, saliva cortisol and heart rate responses to different types of stimuli in dogs. Appl Anim Behav Sci 1998;58(3):365–81.
27. Hennessy MB, Williams T, M, et al. Influence of male and female petters on plasma cortisol and behaviour: can human interaction reduce the stress of dogs in a public animal shelter? Appl Anim Behav Sci 1998;61(1):63–77.
28. Tanaka A, Wagner DC, Kass PH, et al. Associations among weight loss, stress, and upper respiratory tract infection in shelter cats. J Am Vet Med Assoc 2012; 240(5):570–6.
29. Kinney DK, Hintz K, Shearer EM, et al. A unifying hypothesis of schizophrenia: abnormal immune system development may help explain roles of prenatal

hazards, post-pubertal onset, stress, genes, climate, infections, and brain dysfunction. Med Hypotheses 2010;74(3):555–63.

30. O'Connor TG, Winter MA, Hunn J, et al. Prenatal maternal anxiety predicts reduced adaptive immunity in infants. Brain Behav Immun 2013;32:21–8.

31. Bhatia V, Tandon RK. Stress and the gastrointestinal tract. J Gastroenterol Hepatol 2005;20(3):332–9.

32. Schwartz S. Separation anxiety syndrome in cats: 136 cases (1991-2000). J Am Vet Med Assoc 2002;220(7):1028–33.

33. Sherman BL, Mills DS. Canine anxieties and phobias: an update on separation anxiety and noise aversions. Vet Clin North Am Small Anim Pract 2008;38(5):1081–106.

34. Stella JL, Lord LK, Buffington T. Sickness behaviours in response to unusual environmental events in healthy cats and cats with FIC. J Am Vet Med Assoc 2011;1:67–73.

35. Hart BL, Tran AA, Bain M. Canine conspecific coprophagia: who, when and why dogs eat stools. In: Proceedings Behavior Symposium of American College of Veterinary Behaviorists/American Veterinary Society of Animal Behavior, 8, 3 August 2012, San Francisco, California, US.

36. Monte F, Basse C, Lynch A. Stress as a factor in inflammatory bowel disease; pilot study to investigate whether affected dogs differ from unaffected controls in their response to novel stimuli. In: Proceedings of the European Veterinary Behavioral Meeting, 46–49, 24–26 September 2010, Hamburg, Germany.

37. Fuchs E. Scratching the surface of skin development. Nature 2007;445(7130):834–42.

38. Panconesi E, Hautmann G. Psychophysiology of stress in dermatology: the psychobiologic pattern of psychosomatics. Dermatol Clin 1996;14(3):399–422.

39. Landsberg G, Hunthausen W, Ackerman L. Behavioural problems of the dog and cat. 3rd edition. Edinburgh, UK: Saunders Limited; 2013. p. 76–112.

40. Nagata M, Shibata K, Irimajiri M, et al. Importance of psychogenic dermatoses in dogs. J Am Vet Med Assoc 2008;233:1105–11.

41. Nagata M, Shibata K, Irimajiri M, et al. Importance of psychogenic dermatoses in dogs with pruritic behavior. Veterinary Dermatology 2002;13(4):211–29.

42. Klinck MP, Shofer FS, Reisner IR. Association of pruritus with anxiety or aggression in dogs. J Am Vet Med Assoc 2008;233(7):1105–11.

43. Overall K. Self-injurious behavior and obsessive-compulsive disorder in domestic animals. In: Dodman NH, Shuster L, editors. Psychopharmacology of animal behavior disorders. Malden (MA): Blackwell Science; 1998. p. 222–52.

44. van den Bos R. Post-conflict stress-response in confined group-living cats (Felis silvestris catus). Appl Anim Behav Sci 1998;59(4):323–30.

45. Willemse T, Mudde M, Josephy M, et al. The effect of haloperidol and naloxone on excessive grooming behavior of cats. Eur Neuropsychopharmacol 1994;4(1):39–45.

46. Waisglass SE, Landsberg GM, Yager JA, et al. Underlying medical conditions in cats with presumptive psychogenic alopecia. J Am Vet Med Assoc 2006;228(11):1705–9.

47. Mills D, Luescher A. Veterinary and pharmacological approaches to abnormal behaviour. In: Mason G, Rushen J, editors. Stereotypic animal behaviour: fundamentals and applications to welfare. Wallingford, Oxon, UK: CABI; 2008. p. 286–324.

48. Dodman NH, Karlsson EK, Moon-Fanelli A, et al. A canine chromosome 7 locus confers compulsive disorder susceptibility. Mol Psychiatry 2010;15(1):8–10.

49. Moon-Fanelli AA, Dodman NH. Description and development of compulsive tail chasing in terriers and response to clomipramine treatment. J Am Vet Med Assoc 1998;212(8):1252.
50. Bradshaw JW, Neville PF, Sawyer D. Factors affecting pica in the domestic cat. Appl Anim Behav Sci 1997;52(3):373–9.
51. Notari L, Mills D. Possible behavioral effects of exogenous corticosteroids on dog behavior: a preliminary investigation. J Vet Behav 2011;6(6):321–7.
52. Fatjo J, Amat M, Mariotti VM, et al. Analysis of 1040 cases of canine aggression in a referral practice in Spain. J Vet Behav 2007;2(5):158–65.
53. Beaver BV. Clinical classification of canine aggression. Appl Anim Ethol 1983; 10(1):35–43.
54. Salman MD, Hutchison J, Ruch-Gallie R, et al. Behavioral reasons for relinquishment of dogs and cats to 12 shelters. J Appl Anim Welf Sci 2000;3(2):93–106.
55. Ramos D, Mills DS. Human directed aggression in Brazilian domestic cats: owner reported prevalence, contexts and risk factors. J Feline Med Surg 2009;11(10):835–41.
56. Hsu Y, Sun L. Factors associated with aggressive responses in pet dogs. Appl Anim Behav Sci 2010;123(3):108–23.
57. Corridan CL, Mills DS, Pfeffer K. Comparison of factors limiting acquisition versus retention of companion dogs. In: Heath SE, editor. Proceedings of the 7th International Veterinary Behaviour Meeting, 197, 28–31 October 2009 Edinburgh, UK.
58. Appleby DL, Bradshaw JW, Casey RA. Relationship between aggressive and avoidance behaviour by dogs and their experience in the first six months of life. Vet Rec 2002;150:434–8.
59. Jagoe JA, Serpell J. Early experience and the development of behaviour. In: Serpell J, editor. The domestic dog: its evolution, behaviour and interactions with people. Cambridge (United Kingdom): Cambridge University Press; 1996. p. 79–103.
60. Seksel K, Mazurski EJ, Taylor A. Puppy socialisation programs: short and long term behavioural effects. Appl Anim Behav Sci 1999;62:335–49.
61. Zulch HE, Mills DS. Life skills for puppies: laying the foundation for a loving lasting relationship. Dorchester (United Kingdom): Hubble and Hattie; 2012.
62. Gácsi M, Maros K, Sernkvist S, et al. Human analogue safe haven effect of the owner: behavioural and heart rate response to stressful social stimuli in dogs. PLoS One 2013;8(3):e58475.

Abnormal Repetitive Behaviors in Dogs and Cats: A Guide for Practitioners

Valarie V. Tynes, DVM[a],*, Leslie Sinn, DVM, CPDT-KA[b,c]

KEYWORDS

- Repetitive behaviors • OCD • Obsessions • Compulsive disorders • Stereotypies
- Frustration • Conflict • Self-injurious

KEY POINTS

- Stereotypies and compulsive/impulsive disorders represent 2 different forms of repetitive behaviors. Although they share similarities and possibly overlapping neurophysiology, they are not the same thing.
- Stereotypy and compulsive disorder (CD) are not diagnoses to be made carelessly; too little is currently known about their underlying pathophysiology, and no clear diagnostic criteria exist.
- Many medical conditions can result in or contribute to repetitive disorders, so treatment of concurrent or underlying conditions are a critical part of the overall treatment plan.
- Abnormal repetitive behaviors (ARBs) that are not caused by medical conditions, pain, paresthesia, or dysesthesia are likely a result of anxiety due to feelings of conflict or frustration.
- Complete resolution of an ARB is uncommon, but a variety of treatments, both pharmacologic and nonpharmacologic, may be used to decrease the frequency of the behavior and thus improve the quality of life for the patient.

INTRODUCTION

The ARBs represent a highly heterogeneous group of behaviors the neurobiology of which is poorly understood. These behaviors have been observed in a large variety of captive wild and domestic species, are commonly associated with certain husbandry practices, and are generally believed to be reflective of poor welfare. The ARBs have historically been referred to as stereotypies, obsessive-compulsive disorders (OCDs), and compulsive disorders (CDs) by various investigators. Although the veterinary literature regularly uses the term stereotypies and obsessive-compulsive or compulsive disorders interchangeably, evidence continues to grow that these are 2 distinctly different, yet complexly related, behaviors, about which there is much to

a Premier Veterinary Behavior Consulting, PO Box 1413, Sweetwater, TX 79556, USA;
b Northern Virginia Community College, Veterinary Technology Program, 21200 Campus Drive, Sterling, VA, 20164, USA; c Behavior Solutions, PO Box 116, Hamilton, VA 20159, USA
* Corresponding author.
E-mail address: pigvet@hughes.net

Vet Clin Small Anim 44 (2014) 543–564
http://dx.doi.org/10.1016/j.cvsm.2014.01.011
0195-5616/14/$ – see front matter © 2014 Elsevier Inc. All rights reserved.
vetsmall.theclinics.com

learn. Prematurely attempting to assign these different labels to companion animal behavior problems may have led to confusion in our thinking.[1] In addition, the careless application of labels may prevent prompt and appropriate treatment of animals afflicted with these behaviors. **Box 1** lists some useful definitions of the current terminology. For the purpose of this article, the term abnormal repetitive behaviors is used to include all the aforementioned behaviors. Although the use of the term abnormal

---

Box 1
Some useful definitions

Perseveration

The inappropriate repetition of behaviors elicited in an experimental or diagnostic context. There are 3 recognized forms of perseveration, and they each reflect brain dysfunction at a different level of executive processing.

Stereotypic behaviors

A descriptive term referring to any behavior that is repetitive or stereotypic in form and whose mechanism is either not known or not of concern. Some stereotypic behaviors are normal, such as grooming sequences or ritualized courtship behaviors.

Stereotypies

The repetitive, unvarying behavior patterns with no apparent goal or function, commonly displayed by captive animals.[15]

Frustration

Occurs when an individual is motivated to perform particular behavior but is somehow prevented from doing so.

Conflict

Occurs when an individual is motivated to perform 2 opposing behaviors at the same time.

Displacement behaviors

Normal behaviors shown at an inappropriate time or out of context for the situation. Grooming behaviors are commonly seen as displacement behaviors in a variety of species.

Redirected Behaviors

Behaviors that are redirected away from the target stimulus and toward a different target that did not trigger the original behavior. Many animals redirect aggression toward a more convenient target when they are prevented from reaching the target that triggered their aggressive response.

Vacuum activities

The performance of a behavior in the absence of the normal substrate required for the performance of the behavior. One example is vacuum chewing in sows, where they perform the motor patterns associated with chewing in the absence of any food.

Obsessive-compulsive disorders

OCDs are characterized by obsessions, recurrent thoughts, urges or images, and compulsions, the repetitive mental acts or behaviors that an individual feels driven to perform in response to the obsessions.

Obsessive-compulsive spectrum disorders

This term is used to cover conditions that are included in the Diagnostic and Statistical Manual of Mental Disorders, Fifth Edition, under OCDs but recognized to have important differences and similarities. Examples include conditions such as trichotillomania and pathologic gambling, conditions that are also often referred to as impulse control disorders.

could be debated, in the context of this article it is used to signify the likely maladaptive nature of these behaviors, as well as the possibility that they may represent an underlying pathologic condition. Whether that pathologic condition is a result of an inappropriate environment or something inherent in the affected individual (or more likely a complex interaction between the two) is also yet to be determined.

Many have posited that anxiety, associated with conflict, frustration, or other stressors, contributes to the development of repetitive behaviors. In addition, a genetic predisposition has been well documented in several species[2,3] and in certain dog and cat breeds,[4-7] and autoimmune mechanisms have been identified in the development of some forms of OCD in humans.[8,9] Different neurotransmitter systems have also been implicated in these problems and have included the opioid-mediated, dopaminergic, serotonergic, and glutamatergic systems. Continuing to recognize and attempting to differentiate between the differing forms of ARBs are critical to better understand them and improve the ability to treat them successfully or even prevent them.

NATURE OF THE PROBLEM

ARBs are often looked upon by pet owners as a source of amusement[10] and thus are not always presenting complaints to the veterinarian. In many cases, the pet owner does not perceive the behavior as a problem until it either results in self-harm or the animal spends an inordinate amount of time performing the behavior, thus interfering with their ability to function optimally in the environment with the pet owner or other pets.

Repetitive behaviors documented in dogs and cats have included spinning and tail chasing, hind end checking, staring, light and shadow chasing, fly snapping, wool sucking, flank and blanket sucking, and even some self-injurious behavior (SIB), such as acral lick dermatitis (ALD). Such enormous variation exists between these different behaviors, as well as in the same behavior in different individuals, that at this time, one cannot even state that all these conditions are indeed homologous or share similar neurophysiologic underpinnings. To further complicate matters, as diagnostic capabilities continue to improve, new evidence is arising that suggests that many of these problems may arise from underlying medical conditions.[11,12]

Although stereotypic behavior may be a component of obsessive-compulsive behaviors, the 2 terms are not interchangeable. Within psychiatry, a diagnosis of OCD is distinct from a diagnosis of stereotypy and other body-focused repetitive disorders such as trichotillomania. These conditions are all recognized to be related and possibly overlapping but may result from completely different underlying mechanisms. Some investigators suggest that the term stereotypy should be restricted to a specific subset of stereotypic behaviors, those manifested by recurrent or continuous perseveration associated with basal ganglia dysfunction.[13] Stereotypies in humans are seen most often in a range of neurodevelopmental syndromes or disorders, such as certain forms of mental retardation or autism. Similar to animals, these patients are often nonverbal and therefore their stereotypies are defined based entirely on behavioral signs, which is in contrast to OCDs in humans whereby the patient's cognitive experiences are a requisite part of the definition of the behavior.[14]

STEREOTYPIES

The stereotypic behaviors of farm animals and captive wild animals have been recognized and studied for more than 50 years. The most fascinating feature of these behaviors is the diverse array of stereotypies shown by different species and even the variations seen within species. Common stereotypic behaviors in rodents include bar chewing, jumping, back flipping, digging, and circling. Stereotypic behaviors seen in ungulates are more likely to be oral in form and include crib biting in horses, sham chewing in sows, and tongue rolling in cattle and giraffe. Captive carnivores typically perform locomotor stereotypies such as pacing, circling, or weaving. This clear distribution of different forms of stereotypic behaviors among different taxons is striking and should raise the question, is a pacing bear suffering from the same condition as a back flipping mouse or a tail chasing Bull Terrier?

The variation among these different types of behavior has actually made it challenging to even answer the question, "What is a stereotypy?", but most agree that a stereotypy is a behavior performed in an invariant and repetitive manner, which has no apparent function. (**Box 2** lists features shared by all stereotypies.) However, these repetitive behaviors are not seen in animals in the wild, leading to the theory that stereotypies are caused by developing and/or living in an environment that is barren or somehow inappropriate. Efforts to enrich environments as a treatment of stereotypic behaviors succeed in some cases but fail to completely resolve the problem in many. In addition, the question that remains is, Why do some animals in a particular environment develop stereotypies, whereas others of the same species in the same environment do not?

A variety of different factors have been suggested as the basis for stereotypy development, including a heightened sensitivity to stress, a general disinhibition of behavioral control mechanisms, or a lack of opportunity to perform a normal array of species-typical behaviors.[15] The result is that animals repeat the same behavior patterns to the point that other behaviors are performed less often, and the one behavior pattern, the stereotypy, is repeated, to the detriment of other behaviors. With repetition, behaviors become less variable.

It has also been proposed that the brain contains a set of executive systems that filter, integrate, and translate stimuli into expressed behavior. Disruptions to this system have been shown to interfere with an individual's ability to shift tasks or motor patterns, resulting in perseveration or an inappropriate repetition of behaviors.[17] The possibility that stereotypies reflect acquired brain pathology due to poor housing conditions has yet to be determined. It is also possible that normal individual variation in brain function results in the tendency to perform stereotypies.

Possible Functions of Stereotypies

Although it may seem strange to attempt to understand the function of something that is defined as being functionless, the definition of stereotypies as being functionless is simply an indication of how little is known about these behaviors.[16]

Box 2
Features of stereotypies

- They develop from motor patterns typical for the species, which have been referred to as source behaviors.[15]

- Most agree that one feature common to all situations in which stereotypies develop is the presence of frustration.[16]

- They develop slowly, becoming more fixed and invariant with repetition.

- Eventually, stereotypies continue to be performed even in the absence of the original eliciting stimulus. They are then referred to as emancipated.

- Stereotypies have been hypothesized to help animals cope with an environment that is somehow inappropriate or inadequate. This theory was based on the suggestion that repetitive behavior led to increased release of endogenous opioids and that stereotyping animals were self-narcotizing.[15]
- The coping hypothesis was at first partially supported by the fact that stereotypies were often stopped by administering narcotic antagonists.[15]
- However, when treated successfully with narcotic antagonists, stereotypies were usually stopped immediately. This result is inconsistent with the theory that the behavior is intrinsically rewarding. If that were the case, the behaviors would be more likely to increase before stopping (an extinction burst).
- Overall, there is no good evidence that all stereotypies help animals to cope, although some may have beneficial effects. Whether coping effects cause stereotypies or are simply beneficial side effects remains to be elucidated.[16]

Another more popular theory behind the development of stereotypies is that they are reflective of the thwarting of highly motivated behaviors.[16] Although most captive animals' needs for food, water, and shelter are met (consummatory needs), the species-typical behaviors normally associated with the acquisition of those needs (appetitive needs) are not, in most cases. This situation may leave these animals in a highly motivated state to perform particular motor behaviors for which hundreds or thousands of years of evolution have prepared them. Thus, the pacing of carnivores may represent the appetitive search phase of the hunt[18] and the cribbing of horses the unfulfilled feeding motivation that results when eating high-concentrate, low-fiber diets.[19] The possibility that certain stereotypic behaviors of dogs (such as light chasing by herding breeds) may represent the frustrated drive to perform behaviors for which they have been bred, but too often are unable to perform in the typical pet household, needs to be explored.

Neurobiology of Stereotypies

Psychomotor stimulant drugs, such as amphetamines and apomorphine, can induce stereotypies, it is thought, by their activation of the dopaminergic systems in the basal ganglia. Increasing doses of these drugs leads to increased rigidity and intensity of the behaviors.[20] Captive animals experiencing high levels of stress also experience massive release of endogenous opioids that modulate dopaminergic pathways. It has been hypothesized that rather than simply having an affect due to their rewarding properties, these opioids are sensitizing the dopaminergic pathways in the basal ganglia.[21]

OBSESSIVE-COMPULSIVE DISORDERS

OCDs have been well documented in people, yet many questions remain unanswered about their cause, development, and treatment. OCD in humans is a severe, disabling, chronic condition that affects 2% to 3% of the US population.[22] People with OCD experience intrusive and unwanted thoughts or images. Compulsions are the mental acts or behaviors that the person feels driven to perform to deal with the obsessions. Many patients describe that feelings of anxiety are associated with the obsessions and that the performance of the compulsive behaviors relieve these feelings of anxiety.[14]

OCD has been noted to develop in one subset of the population early, before puberty, and in another subset, later in adulthood, leading some to suggest that 2 different subtypes of OCD should be recognized because they may have different neurobiological underpinnings.[23] For example, early-onset OCD is more prevalent in males, whereas adult-onset OCD is more prevalent in females and is more sensitive to treatment.[23] OCDs seem to be familial, but their genetics are poorly understood.

The neurobiology of OCDs has been the subject of much research in the last 20 years, and modern neuroimaging techniques have led to greater understanding of many neuropsychiatric conditions in people. OCD and the OCD spectrum disorders may best be viewed as a group of multiple overlapping syndromes rather than a single entity. It is currently proposed that abnormal metabolic activity in the orbitofrontal cortex, anterior cingulate/caudal medial prefrontal cortex, and the caudate nucleus is associated with OCD and OC spectrum disorders.[24] Numerous corticostriatal loops are involved in the sequencing of goals, behaviors, and movements. It is generally believed that there is an indirect pathway and a direct pathway, with the indirect pathway decreasing stimulation of the thalamus and the direct pathway increasing activity of neurons in the thalamus. The direct pathway functions in the initiation and continuation of behaviors and the indirect pathway is important for the inhibition of and switching between behaviors.[25] These pathways are modulated by opiates, dopamine, serotonin, and several other neurotransmitters.[26] The complex way in which these pathways and neurotransmitters interrelate contributes to the challenge of medicating patients with OCDs and related disorders. No single neurotransmitter causes the problem, and few drugs effect only a single neurotransmitter.

OCD in people can be refractory to treatment, and medication, as well as cognitive therapy and other nonpharmacologic therapies, is often required to achieve satisfactory treatment results. Serotonin reuptake inhibitors are the first line of treatment of human OCDs, and it is serotonin's inhibitory role on dopamine that is thought to contribute to their efficacy. Dopamine plays a dual role on the balance between the direct and indirect frontal striatal pathways.[25] However, other drugs, such as the atypical antipsychotics, clomipramine, buspirone, and clonazepam, have also been used as augmenting agents,[27] because there remains a population of people who do not respond to treatment with serotonergic drugs. Deep brain stimulation has recently been shown to have beneficial effects in treating some patients with OCD.[28]

STEREOTYPY VERSUS COMPULSIVE DISORDERS

The term stereotypy has traditionally been used as a descriptive term that gives no information about underlying neurobiology or possible pathophysiology. In fact, the stereotypies commonly seen in captive animals are so numerous and varied that it is unlikely that they are homogenous in regards to cause, development, physiology, or function.[1]

OCD is a psychiatric diagnosis and a disease in humans that shares similarities between some repetitive behaviors in animals, but the research suggesting that certain repetitive behaviors in dogs or cats can serve as models for human OCDs are rife with weaknesses. The more common conditions in dogs and cats that have been referred to as CDs are covered in more detail later. **Table 1** lists some of the behaviors often labeled as CDs and the breeds thought to be more commonly affected.

An investigation into the differences and similarities between stereotypies and OCDs, using a systems approach to the problem, has led to the hypothesis that stereotypies arise from disruption of basal ganglia systems. OCDs and related impulse control disorders arise from disruptions in the prefrontal cortex and the numerous pathways between the prefrontal cortex and the rest of the brain.[17] Research on humans with brain damage or dysfunction show different neurologic signs depending on which part of the brain is affected and support the concept that the difference between stereotypies and between impulsive/compulsive disorders lies in *what* is

Table 1
A compilation of multiple studies and case reports that suggest an increase in incidence of particular ARBs in specific breeds

Breed	Behavior	Reference
Dobermans	Flank sucking	6,29–33
Bull Terriers, German Shepherd dogs, Australian Cattle dogs	Tail chasing	5,29,30,32–41
Schnauzers	Hind checking	30,41
Cavalier King Charles Spaniels, Border Collies, Terriers	Light (shadow) chasing	30,33,40,42,43
Siamese cats	Fabric sucking and ingestion	40,41
Bengals	Overgrooming	40

Data from Refs.[5,6,29–43]

repeated. In impulsive/compulsive disorders, an inappropriate goal is repeated (such as the plucking of hair by a person with trichotillomania), and in stereotypies, a particular motor pattern is repeated.[17] Although this still does not answer the question as to whether behaviors in animals labeled as compulsive are homologous in any way to those in humans, or not, it does support the concept that stereotypies and CDs are 2 distinctly different conditions that need further study both in humans and animals in order for one to be able to use these labels in dogs and cats with any accuracy (**Fig. 1**).

COMPULSIVE DISORDERS IN ANIMALS

The term compulsive disorders was initially coined when certain repetitive behaviors of dogs and cats were hypothesized to be similar to OCDs in humans. It was suggested that because one could not ascertain whether or not animals obsessed it was best to refer to these as CDs.

CDs in dogs and cats have been categorized as locomotor, hallucinatory, self-injurious or self-directed, and oral.[44] Several of these categories seem to overlap,

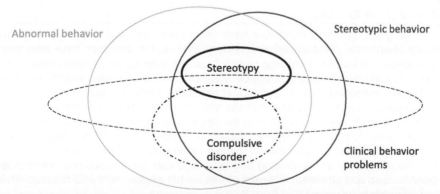

Fig. 1. Relationship between stereotypies, compulsive disorders, and stereotypic behaviors as they may occur within the range of abnormal behaviors and clinical behavior problems. (*Adapted from* Mills DS, Luescher AU. Veterinary and pharmacological approaches to abnormal behaviour. In: Mason G, Rushen J, editors. Stereotypic animal behaviour: fundamentals and applications to welfare. 2nd edition. Wallingford (WA): CABI; 2006. p. 293; with permission.)

and some repetitive behaviors seem to lie on a continuum between the categories. For example, tail chasing or spinning has been described as a locomotor CD, but if the tail is also attacked and mutilated, the behavior would be considered a self-injurious one. Staring at lights and shadows could seem to be a hallucinatory CD, but if the animal also chases lights and shadows, then the behavior would be considered a locomotor CD.

Oral CDs such as pica and surface licking can easily be a result of an underlying medical condition, and it is far too easy to label them as a CD simply because a medical condition was not identified. However, recent research supports the likelihood that in many cases, gastrointestinal disease leads to behaviors such as surface licking and fly snapping or air biting.[11,12]

A working definition of CDs in animals was proposed by Hewson and Luescher[45] in 1996 and reads as follows:

"Behaviors that are usually brought on by conflict, but that are subsequently shown outside of the original context. The behaviors might share a similar pathophysiology (eg, Changes in serotonin, dopamine and beta endorphin systems). Compulsive behaviors seem abnormal because they are displayed out of context and are often repetitive, exaggerated or sustained."

This definition is strikingly similar to the definition and features of stereotypies, so it does little to clarify attempts to diagnose and treat a repetitive behavior in a dog or cat.

Overall defines the behaviors in this way: "OCDs are characterized as behaviors that are not only stereotypic and ritualistic but those in which the urge to engage in them or the process of engaging in them severely interferes with normal functioning."[46]

This definition is similarly problematic in that many repetitive behaviors in dogs and cats that are commonly referred to as CDs are not described as interfering with the animals' normal functioning according to their owners.[6]

Few controlled studies have been performed on CDs in dogs and cats. The studies that have examined treatment efficacy have included such a variety of different behaviors referred to as compulsive behaviors that the usefulness of the results is questionable. The studies that have examined specific repetitive behaviors in pets are discussed in more detail later.

Tail Chasing and Spinning

Tail chasing and spinning behaviors have often been reported in Bull Terriers and German Shepherds, although other breeds displaying this behavior have also been documented. Although tail chasing seems to run in families, its genetic basis is unknown. A study that included pedigree analysis of 44 tail chasing and/or spinning Bull Terriers proposed that an autosomal recessive mode of inheritance exists for the condition.[47] Tail chasing can include slow to rapid spinning in both directions and often, although not always, leads to the dog actually grasping and eventually mutilating its tail tip. Some dogs begin by focusing on their tail and then slowly begin to spin, whereas others simply spin in circles without particularly focusing on their tail.[39] The affect seen in tail chasing dogs can also vary greatly; some of these dogs appear frenzied and stressed, whereas others simply appear calm and focused while being completely disassociated from their environments.

Most studies of tail chasing behavior report that the median age of onset of tail chasing behavior is before sexual maturity in the dog (or at least within the first year of life), which is consistent with the development of most OCDs in humans.[5,38] However, staring, trancelike behavior, fly snapping, and episodic aggression have also been documented in many dogs with tail chasing behavior.[38] Epileptiform activity has been identified on electroencephalographs of some tail chasing Bull Terriers and combined with the other commonly seen clinical signs further supports the possibility that the behavior may represent focal seizure activity in some cases.[48] One study of tail chasing dogs found structural abnormalities in some, including hydrocephalus,[5] but another more recent study found no abnormalities on magnetic resonance imaging (MRI) or histologic examination of a subset of the affected dogs.[47]

Studies that have included observations of the dogs' temperament have found tail chasing dogs to be more active and excitable in some cases and shyer and more fearful in others,[39] and phobias have been found to have a high incidence of comorbidity with tail chasing behavior.[38] These data suggest that temperament differences may predispose some dogs to tail chasing behavior. One study reported that 31% of triggers for tail chasing involved situations that increased the dog's level of arousal or frustration.[38] Unpredictable or restricting environments and a lack of physical or mental stimulation made up a large percentage of the documented triggers. Only 10% of owners reported no discernible triggers for the dog's behavior.[38] These data lead further support to the theory that tail chasing is a displacement behavior performed by many dogs in response to conflict or frustration. However, the investigators suggest that due to the cluster of clinical signs found in the tail chasing Bull Terriers of this study, the syndrome may have features in common with autism in humans.[38] Attention-seeking behavior, middle ear infection, and play have all also been suggested as potential causes of tail chasing behavior, in addition to the possible diagnosis of stereotypy or CD.[13]

It is important for the clinician to keep in mind that numerous medical conditions can potentially lead to tail chasing behavior, and one documented case of tail mutilation responded to a combination of tramadol and a nonsteroidal antiinflammatory.[49] Self-mutilation is not always a component of tail chasing or spinning and in some cases may be considered a secondary problem to tail chasing. Conversely, self-mutilation is not always presented as a repetitive behavior. Anecdotally, however, pain within the tail, lower back, or around the region of the tail has been identified in cases of tail chasing, and these cases often responded to appropriate treatment of the medical conditions. In at least 2 cases, MRI and computed tomographic scans have documented lumbosacral disease in tail chasing dogs (Marsha Reich, personal communication, DVM, DACVB) that responded well to treatment with varying combinations of surgery and antiinflammatories. Because advanced imaging of this type is not within the budget of many clients, underlying medical conditions can easily be overlooked in these cases and treatment with antiinflammatories or analgesics is often indicated to rule out pain-related conditions.

Acral Lick Dermatitis

ALD or lick granuloma is a dermatologic disease that is a result of self-trauma directed at the leg. Repetitive licking of the limb eventually results in a well-circumscribed, alopecic, firm, red raised, ulcerated plaque. Lesions are seen most commonly on the cranial carpus or metatarsus, but they have also been seen, although less commonly, on the cranial radius, metatarsus, and tibia. The condition is seen more often in large breed dogs but other breeds with the condition have also been documented.[50,51]

Lick granulomas have long been suspected of being psychogenic in origin, and some have labeled it a canine CD.[50,51] Other behavioral causes that have been proposed include stress, anxiety, phobias, attention seeking and inadequate exercise, mental stimulation, or social interaction. However, the cause of acral lick is most likely multifactorial. A variety of causes, in addition to behavioral causes, have been proposed. These have included pruritus due to allergies (food sensitivity or atopy), trauma, and joint disease. Research has confirmed that a variety of less common medical conditions can also result in ALD or similar-appearing lesions. These conditions include lymphoma, the presence of an orthopedic pin, deep pyoderma, and a mast cell tumor.[52] In addition, one study found deep bacterial infection present in 95% of ALD lesions that were biopsied. To further complicate matters, this study found a poor association between bacterial isolates cultured from the surface compared with those cultured from deep tissue. More than half of the cultures were resistant to the antibiotics used most commonly to treat skin infections.[53] Deep bacterial infection and the ruptured hair follicles and free keratin in the dermis that occur secondary to the self-trauma are important contributing factors. These lead to intense pruritus and the perpetuation of the itch-scratch cycle.

Although grooming has been noted to be a common displacement behavior, most dogs respond to a lesion present on their skin by licking it. Dogs presented with ALD should have a thorough medical workup and a behavioral history collected. The behavioral history should be used to identify possible signs of anxiety or stress due to frustration or conflict that contribute to the licking behavior. Other anxiety-based conditions, such as noise phobias, or separation anxiety are also likely if the ALD has developed primarily because of stress or anxiety. In the authors' experience, it is highly unusual for ALD to be the only behavioral disorder in a patient. Even if other signs of behavior problems are present, ALD is not resolved without complete resolution first of the pyoderma. The lesion should be cultured if initial empiric treatment is not effective, and a biopsy of deep tissues should be included. Antibiotic therapy should be continued until at least 2 weeks after complete resolution of the lesion. Other treatment aimed at breaking the itch-scratch cycle may include symptomatic allergy medication, such as antihistamines or glucocorticoid (possibly both oral and topical). Physically preventing the dog from continuing to lick may be a critical component of the treatment, so e-collars, bandages, socks, leggings, or body suits may be tried depending on the patient. Any comorbid behavioral conditions should also be addressed separately.

Support for ALD as a model of human OCD is poor at this time. The use of clomipramine, desmipramine, fluoxetine, and naltrexone in the treatment of ALD has all been documented.[50,51,54,55] However, most studies strictly measured licking behavior, and few clearly documented whether or not lesions were completely resolved during the trial.[50,51,55] Some decrease in licking behavior but rarely a total cessation of licking behavior was documented. Any mention of treatment with antibiotics was also missing in some of these studies, which could be why complete healing of lesions was uncommon.[50,51] The antihistaminic effects of drugs such as clomipramine could be responsible for the cessation of licking behavior. Finally, the average age of onset of ALD in all studies that included that information was greater than 1 year of age, which is inconsistent with the age of development of OCDs in humans.

Other Self-Injurious Behaviors

No other peer-reviewed publications have been published on SIBs in pets. However, this problem has been studied extensively in humans and nonhuman primates. In humans, SIB has been postulated to help an individual to gain control over an overwhelming emotional state, the so-called affect regulation model.[56] SIB in nonhuman primates is considered to be phenomenologically similar to SIB in humans and is believed to be a maladaptive coping mechanism. Rearing in a suboptimal environment is a common feature linking most cases of SIB in nonhuman primates, with social isolation being an important risk factor.[56] As with many ARBs, all animals reared in inappropriate environments or in social isolation do not develop SIBs, so other yet-to-be-determined factors, such as a genetic predisposition, are likely present as well.

Nevertheless, it must also be kept in mind that self-injury has often been documented in cases in which pain, paresthesia, or dysesthesia was suspected,[56–58] so a thorough physical examination and diagnostics are critical when faced with a case of SIB in a dog or cat. Empiric treatment with analgesics or antiinflammatories may be necessary before determining that SIB is occurring as a primary behavioral disorder.

Blanket and Flank Sucking in Doberman Pinschers

Blanket and flank sucking are unique repetitive behaviors that have been documented primarily in Doberman Pinschers and occur with a remarkably high frequency in North America.[7] Because of its presence primarily in one breed, a genetic predisposition has been suspected. Recent research has identified a locus on chromosome 7 (within the CDH2 region) where the particular allele occurs significantly more often in Dobermans exhibiting these behaviors than in unaffected controls.[31] Blanket sucking behavior involves the dog taking a blanket into its mouth and mouthing or sucking on it. Flank sucking behavior is characterized by a repetitive mouthing and sucking of the dogs own flank region. Both behaviors are a type of nonnutritive suckling and may be seen immediately before the animal falls asleep, similar to a suckling neonate. Nonnutritive suckling has been considered to be a displacement behavior performed as a result of anxiety due to conflict and thus may serve a self-comforting purpose.[59] Some have deemed blanket and flank sucking a form of CD.[40,41]

One study examining a convenience sample of 77 Doberman Pinschers with blanket sucking, flank sucking, or both found the age of onset of blanket sucking to be significantly earlier than that for flank sucking, although the median age of development for both behaviors occurred before 1 year of age.[6] There was no significant difference between the 2 behaviors in frequency, duration, triggers, or interruptability. Sex distribution between the 2 behaviors was similar. The most common triggers reported by owners of flank and blanket sucking dogs were inactivity and increased arousal. Owners defined inactivity as bedtime, when bored or crated, when relaxing, and so on.[6] Examples of situations of increased arousal described by owners in this study included kenneling, separation from owners, new or uncertain situations, or loud noises. All these triggers also represent situations potentially leading to conflict or frustration, emotional states that can readily lead to anxiety and thus the expression of displacement behaviors.

In this study, only 17% of dogs with blanket sucking and 32% of dogs with flank sucking sustained any injuries or illness associated with the behavior.[6] In addition, most owners claimed that the behaviors did not interfere with their relationship with the dog nor the dog's quality of life. Many owners provided their dog with its own blanket to suck. Because some dogs only began sucking on their flanks when a blanket or fabric was not available, this may have been considered by many owners to be the better, safer option for the dog. Although a small number of dogs that suck fabric also ingested it and developed obstructions requiring surgery, most of these dogs do not ingest fabric. The physical signs reported by some owners of flank sucking dogs included hair loss and skin lesions or ulcerations. These results are actually in contrast to at least one definition of canine CD that states the behavior should "interfere with normal daily activities and functioning."[46] Although recent research has identified brain structural abnormalities in Dobermans with blanket and flank sucking behaviors, these abnormalities are similar to those in humans with anxiety disorders but not specific to those seen in human OCD,[31] a reminder that there is much to learn before assuming that canine repetitive behaviors are in fact homologous to human OCDs. Because many Dobermans owners do not perceive this condition as problematic, little has been documented on the actual treatment of blanket or flank sucking behavior, so there is no way to know if the condition shares face validity with human OCD.

It has been suggested that blanket and flank sucking may be a variation of pica.[6] Pica, the persistent consumption of nonfood items,[4] is commonly associated with a variety of medical conditions but has been considered by some to represent an oral compulsive behavior.[41] It is worth noting that significantly higher number of blanket and flank sucking dogs (29% of affected dogs) in this study also exhibited pica, when compared with unaffected control dogs,[6] suggesting that all these behaviors may lie on a continuum and pointing to the necessity of ruling out underlying medical conditions that may promote the development of these behaviors.

Wool Sucking and Pica in Cats

The oral repetitive behaviors common to cats include pica (the consumption of unusual or nonfood items) and wool sucking (also sometimes referred to as fabric chewing). However, despite its common name, many cats exhibiting this behavior target several different materials such as plastic, rubber, or leather in addition to a variety of fabrics, including cotton and synthetic.[60] No controlled studies have been performed on this condition, and as is the case with much of the literature about repetitive behaviors in dogs and cats, much of the published research did not discriminate between consuming unusual objects and simply sucking on them. This difference may prove to be critical between differing behavioral diagnoses.

Pica and wool sucking or fabric chewing has been reported to occur more commonly in Siamese cats than other breeds,[61] with one study finding that Siamese cats were evaluated more frequently than expected for behavior problems related to aggression and ingestive problems such as pica.[62] However, pica is also a sign of a diverse number of different medical conditions associated with gastrointestinal problems and nutrient imbalances. Studies have documented pica associated with pyruvate kinase deficiencies, feline infectious peritonitis, and anemia in cats.[63–65] Damage to particular areas of the brain has been demonstrated to lead to pica,[66] once again suggesting that labeling it a CD is often premature and may put the patient at risk of delayed or inappropriate treatment.

RECOGNIZING/DIAGNOSING THE PROBLEM

Nonpharmacologic management of ARBs does not so much require determining which diagnostic label to assign to the problem, as it does attempting to identify the underlying affective state or motivation for performance of the behavior. The welfare of the animal is placed in jeopardy if any pain, discomfort, or altered sensation that may be causing or contributing to the repetitive behavior is not carefully ruled out. The role that stress and anxiety may play in the development of certain medical conditions, such as gastrointestinal disease, skin disease, and urinary tract disease, must not be overlooked either. See the chapters by Mills et al and Frank elsewhere in this issue for a review of these conditions.

Once medical conditions are identified and treated, the next goal of the clinician may best be focused on identifying other sources of anxiety that contribute to the performance of the repetitive behaviors. Environments that are unpredictable or understimulating can lead to feelings of conflict, frustration, and anxiety. When routines are disrupted or animals experience chronic, recurring situations that cause fear or anxiety, then displacement, vacuum activities, or redirected behaviors may develop and become repetitive over time. Inappropriate use of punishment is a common mistake made by pet owners that often leads to fear and anxiety in pets.

The ability to interrupt a repetitive behavior is not necessarily diagnostic for CD or stereotypy. Dogs experiencing seizure activity are difficult if not impossible to stop and may or may not demonstrate the appearance of being disassociated with the environment. The author has witnessed dogs with severe pruritus being equally difficult to interrupt. Many animals, if interrupted often enough, simply learn to move to another area, away from their owners so that they can continue to perform the behavior. Video of the animal alone can be useful in ruling out attention seeking as the cause of repetitive behaviors.

Ruling out focal seizures is challenging because they can be associated with twitching of facial musculature or whole body trembling, as well as unusual behaviors such as frantic running and colliding with objects, piloerection, dilated pupils, and unilateral limb motions with no loss of consciousness. Repeated presentations of this type of seizure activity might be easily confused with an ARB.

There are no clear diagnostic criteria for identifying a CD. It is a diagnosis of exclusion.

MANAGEMENT OF REPETITIVE BEHAVIORS
Pharmacologic Strategies

The challenge of pharmacologic therapy for repetitive behaviors, in addition to not knowing if all repetitive behaviors truly share the same underlying neurophysiology or neuropathology, lies in the fact that it is not known exactly which neurotransmitter systems need to be affected by therapy. Existing information suggests that stereotypies are sensitive to opioid and dopaminergic antagonists early on in their development and once established are only sensitive to dopaminergic control.[15,67] However, to date, antipsychotic drugs that block dopamine receptors have not been proved to be effective in the treatment of ARBs in animals.

As is the case with many behavioral problems in animals, pharmacotherapy, although not always necessary, can play a useful role in treatment. Pharmacotherapy has been used in a variety of cases of repetitive disorders in pets and has been shown to be helpful in many. The use of several different families of drugs has been documented, and the ones found to be most effective are the serotonin reuptake inhibitors. Beta-endorphin antagonists such as naloxone, naltrexone, and nalmefene have been used to treat repetitive behaviors, but few studies of their use in animals have been published.[34,54,67] These drugs are, however, expensive and their effects short lived.

- Serotonergic drugs are currently the first line of treatment of OCDs in humans. Clomipramine has been the drug of choice for treatment of animal repetitive disorders for many years, and some studies have found it to be more effective than desipramine or amitriptyline.[40,50] One study, however, used clomipramine for the treatment of psychogenic alopecia in cats and found no significant improvement.[68] In a study in which clomipramine was used to treat tail chasing in terriers, 75% of the patients demonstrated a 75% reduction in tail chasing behavior within 1 to 12 weeks.[39] Hewson and colleagues[69] found clomipramine treatment to be effective but not curative in a study of several different types of CDs in dogs. A study using clomipramine to treat anxiety-related disorders and CDs in 10 cats also documented improvement as did another study using clomipramine to treat separation anxiety, noise phobias, and CDs in dogs.[42,70] However, that multiple different diagnosis may have been represented by the study populations in these 3 papers brings the usefulness of the data into question.

One case report of shadow chasing in a dog used single-photon emission computed tomographic imaging studies to document alterations in the dopaminergic neurotransmitter systems (dopamine transporter [DAT] striatal-to-brain ratios), similar to those in humans with OCD. Clinical improvement was documented in this case after 7 days of treatment with clomipramine, and follow-up scans revealed that the DAT ratios returned to near normal levels.[43]

- Selegiline blocks monoamine oxidase (MAO)-B from breaking down dopamine, presumably boosting dopaminergic transmission. At higher doses (in humans), it bocks both MAO-A and MAO-B from breaking down norepinephrine, serotonin, and dopamine, potentially increasing transmission of all these neurotransmitters. Although no controlled studies on the use of selegiline to treat repetitive behaviors has been performed, there have been some anecdotal reports of its efficacy in treating compulsive licking.[71] Based on the growing body of knowledge suggesting that dopaminergic transmission and serotonergic transmission may be involved to varying degrees in repetitive behaviors, more research into the efficacy of selegiline is warranted.
- Fluoxetine is another serotonergic drug that has been found effective in treating both stereotypies and CDs in animals.[30,72–74] However, most studies have examined the drug in laboratory animals.[75,76] One randomized, placebo-controlled study has been published using fluoxetine in the treatment of CDs. As in previous studies, a variety of different repetitive behaviors were included in the study patients. Although dogs in this study treated with fluoxetine had a significant decrease in owner-reported severity of their CD, evaluation of owner diaries revealed no significant differences in the number or duration of compulsive behaviors documented.[30]
- Newer evidence suggests that altered glutamatergic transmission may play a role in human OCD; drugs that block the glutamate-sensitive N-methyl-D-aspartate (NMDA) receptors have been tried and found effective in treating some cases of OCD in humans. Memantine is one NMDA receptor antagonist that has shown promise in the treatment of canine CDs, as a single agent and in combination with fluoxetine.[33]

Nonpharmacologic Strategies

Basic principles
Avoidance of stimuli/triggers Behavioral management of repetitive behaviors begins with the identification and cataloging of as many stimuli or triggers for the behavior as possible. Not all triggers are readily apparent, but clients should be encouraged to keep a journal and describe the environmental conditions immediately before the initiation of the repetitive behavior. With this information, the clinician can help the client identify stimuli with the immediate goal of avoidance. The primary goal is to decrease the percentage of the time the pet engages in the repetitive behavior because repetition increases the likelihood of the behavior continuing.

Videotaping is often an additional step necessary to aid in recognizing triggers. Events that occur while the owner is away from the home may be major precipitating stimuli such as the arrival of delivery personnel or certain sounds or other events. In addition, videotaping in the client's absence helps to verify that the behavior is occurring whether the owner is present or not (to rule out attention-seeking behavior) and document what percentage of the time the animal is performing the repetitive behavior. Videotaping can also serve as a gauge to the severity of the problem, as well as the efficacy of any recommended treatment protocols.

Avoiding all stimuli that trigger the behavior can be challenging, so the clinician and pet owner need to work together to find the most feasible ways to do this in each individual case. In some cases, avoiding leaving the dog alone at home may be helpful and alternatives such as doggie day care, leaving the pet with a relative or friend, providing the pet with a temporary companion such as a friendly conspecific, or providing periodic interactions such as with a pet sitter or walker may be helpful. Every effort should be made to provide the pet with a place in the home where it feels most relaxed and comfortable. This place may be any preferred room or location where the pet is less likely to perform the repetitive behavior, such as a basement, car, or crate. Any and all options should be investigated and used to reduce the likelihood of the repetitive behavior occurring, and the additional methods described later are implemented to decrease overall stress in the environment and teach the pet appropriate alternative behaviors.

Physical prevention of behavior Another option or even necessity may be to physically prevent the repetitive behavior from occurring. Physical barriers that may be helpful include items such as baby gates, crates, and exercise pens (X-pens). In addition, in situations involving SIB, physical restraint may be necessary and would include items such as bandages, body covers, Elizabethan collars, soft neck wraps or braces, and buckets. Research in people indicates that the physical restriction of repetitive behaviors can potentially lead to collateral effects such as an increase in other undesired behaviors or a rebound effect when the restraint is removed.[77] The rebound effect has been documented in animals as well.[78] In humans, physically restraining the patient to prevent performance of a repetitive behavior has been shown to be extremely distressing,[79] so physical restriction should only be used to prevent physical harm while a comprehensive treatment protocol is initiated.

Use of head collar and dragline and/or tether Another way to decrease the percentage of time a pet performs repetitive behaviors is to keep the pet under direct observation and to interrupt the behavior sequence that leads to that repetitive behavior. The use of a head collar or harness along with a dragline allows easy access to the pet and rapid interruption of the behavior sequence and redirection of the pet to a more appropriate activity such as attention directed toward toys or food puzzles. The animal should be redirected immediately before the repetitive pattern begins (this is another reason why it is important for the pet owner to be aware of the stimuli likely to lead to the behavior); otherwise, the owner may inadvertently reinforce the behavior by providing attention to the pet. Tethering the pet to the owner or in immediate proximity to the owner also allows for close supervision of the pet and immediate intervention on an as-needed basis. Head collars may have the additional benefit of inhibiting behavior in some dogs.

Stop all punishment Punishment is not an effective behavior modification tool for most clients, and the use of punishment can be associated with increased aggression and injury.[80] In addition, as research continues to examine the repetitive behaviors, studies indicate that these behaviors frequently have a genetic and/or biologic basis to them.[7,31] Because they often occur as a result of conflict or frustration, they are a behavior and welfare concern, not a training issue. Up to 40% of SIBs in humans have an anxiety component associated with them.[81] Punishment increases anxiety and fear, potentially increasing the likelihood of a repetitive behavior being performed. Positive reinforcement or reward-based training should be used to decrease arousal, anxiety, and fear and to increase the likelihood of acceptable alternative behaviors occurring.

Environmental modification
Exercise Although there are no data indicating that exercise per se decreases repetitive behaviors, in general, most companion animals lead inactive lifestyles. The effect of regular exercise on the behavior and attitudes in humans is well documented.[82] Adoption of the 30 minutes of exercise for a minimum of 5 days a week guidelines established by the Center for Disease Control and Prevention for the maintenance of basic health should be a common sense starting point.[83] Walks provide the added benefit of enrichment by changing the animal's environment. Allowing a dog time to sniff and explore within the range of the leash can be enriching, as it allows the dog to exercise its exceptional sense of smell. This type of mental activity is a form of exercise that may be equally as beneficial as physical exercise. Just about any method of increasing activity should be acceptable as long as the activity does not increase the incidence of repetitive behaviors and the pet engages in the activity willingly.

Occupational training behaviorally appropriate activities Some researchers hypothesize that repetitive behavior originates from frustrated inherent behaviors.[16] Based on that theory, providing occupationally appropriate activities may decrease the incidence of stereotypies.[33] Examples would include terrier trials or digging pits for terriers, lure coursing or chasing fishing pole toys for sight hounds, herding opportunities including Treibball for herding breeds, tracking test or K9 Nose Work for scent hounds, and so on.

Environmental enrichment Environmental enrichment is covered elsewhere in this issue by Heath and Wilson. Enrichment can be provided at multiple levels and should engage all the senses. Being visually oriented, humans focus on visual stimuli, but scent and sound are likely to be much more important to companion animals. The use of pheromones, lavender, and catnip, as well as the use of classical music and natural sounds, can contribute positively to the quality of the animal's environment.[84]

Behavior modification
Predictable routines and interactions Stress is thought to play a significant role in the exacerbation of repetitive behaviors.[85] A predictable environment decreases stress, so the establishment of a routine is helpful. In addition, predictable, consistent interactions, referred to as a command (or cue) -response-reward interactions, help to further improve the pet-client bond. If the pet wants anything from the owner, the pet needs to do something to earn what the pet wants. If the pet responds to a cue, the pet is given access to what it wants, as well as verbal praise, and depending on the situations, food rewards. If the pet does not perform, it is ignored or redirected to another acceptable activity; this makes interactions predictable and structured. There are no penalties for failing to respond, but the pet is rewarded for responding appropriately. Command-response-reward interactions enhance the relationship, provide structure, and improve communication between the pet and the owner. Clear communication results in less anxiety associated with pet-owner interactions and gives the pet a reason to be more attentive to the owners' requests.

Teach relaxation If anxiety is contributing to the behavior, teaching the pet to relax is extremely helpful. There are several published protocols for teaching a pet to relax on cue.[46]

Ignore attention seeking, reward/reinforce relaxed behavior Ignoring attention seeking and rewarding and reinforcing relaxed behavior also contributes to decreasing overall anxiety. Attention-seeking behavior can include nudging, pawing, following, whining, crawling up on the owner, and possibly even the repetitive behavior itself. This behavior often occurs as a result of anxiety and the pet being unable to settle down and relax on its own. The animal needs to learn better coping skills and to not be so reliant on the owner for constant feedback. All attention-seeking behaviors should be ignored except repetitive behaviors that need to be interrupted as early in the cycle as possible. If the pet is persistent, the owner may have to move or redirect the pet, but they should not acknowledge the pet with eye contact or verbal instruction. Punishment, including saying things such as "No" or "Stop," should never be used for the reasons previously discussed; for some dogs, punishment is actually attention. Quiet praise should always be provided whenever the pet shows any inclination to be by itself or entertain itself. Food toys should be offered as mental exercise, possible distractions, and to encourage quiet independence.

Countercondition the pet to respond to the stimuli by performing an alternative behavior that is incompatible (response substitution) There are several behaviors that can be trained that may serve as an alternative to the repetitive behavior. Targeting, looking at the owner, and sitting are probably the most commonly used alternatives or "interrupters." As the pet is exposed to the provocative stimuli and begins to initiate the repetitive behavior, the owner requests that the pet "touch, "watch me," or "sit," in order to interrupt the behavioral sequence and prevent the repetitive behavior from occurring. Timing is crucial. Once the pet is fully engaged in the repetitive behavior, it may be difficult to interrupt. A head halter or harness with dragline or tether can be extremely helpful in implementing this behavior modification. Drug therapy also plays a key role in raising the arousal threshold and providing the client with additional time to be able to interrupt and prevent the behavioral sequence. The goal would be to have the pet begin to associate the stimulus that previously triggered the repetitive behavior with the new incompatible behavior and through operant conditioning learn a new, acceptable response to the stimuli.

Desensitization to stimuli and classic counterconditioning (reward calm behavior) If the triggers can be identified, isolated, and controlled, it may be possible to change the pet's internal response to the stimuli by pairing the stimuli with something desirable such as food. If, for example, the repetitive behavior is triggered by the sound of the doorbell, it may be possible to record the doorbell. Then while playing it at a volume so low that it does not trigger the repetitive behavior, begin pairing that sound with high-value food treats while cueing the pet to relax (see teaching relaxation discussed earlier). It may be possible to change the pet's emotional response to stimuli through food to one of rewarded relaxation.

EVALUATION, ADJUSTMENT, AND RECURRENCE

Most documented attempts to treat repetitive behaviors do not stop the behavior completely, and if it does, effects are often short term. Clients should be informed that there is much to learn about the actual causes and neurobiology underlying these behaviors, so treatment strategies are empiric at best.

- If the animal is responding to aspects of its environment that cause anxiety or stress, the repetitive behaviors may reoccur throughout its life any time that these conditions arise again.
- Animals that fail completely to respond to the recommended treatment program within 4 to 8 weeks should be carefully reevaluated for underlying disease processes and the presence of pain or neuropathy.

- Although many pet owners do not see repetitive behaviors as a problem, the practitioner, as an advocate for the pet should be prepared to educate owners about the possibility that it is reflective of poor animal welfare.
- The overriding goal of treatment should be aimed at eliminating or at least minimizing any chronic anxiety that the animal may be experiencing.

SUMMARY

Although much has been learned about the repetitive behavior in both humans and animals during the past 50 years, the neurophysiology underlying these problems remains unclear. Repetitive behaviors represent such a diverse array of behaviors in a large variety of species that it is possible that most do not even share the same underlying pathologic condition. Until more is known about what causes the different repetitive behaviors in animals, it may be best to avoid assigning them a particular label such as CD or stereotypy. The evidence is growing that stereotypies and compulsive/impulsive disorders have different neurophysiologic underpinnings, so the 2 terms should not be used interchangeably. To further complicate matters, it is becoming increasingly likely that many of the repetitive behaviors in dogs and cats may occur secondary to underlying disease processes not related to the neurologic system. Diseases or disorders causing pain or discomfort should never be overlooked too quickly simply because diagnostic tests initially fail to reveal a cause. Because these patients cannot speak, it behooves the practitioner to err on the side of caution and rule out pain or discomfort via empiric treatment if suspected, before assuming the condition is a mental health one. If signs of conflict, frustration, fear, or anxiety are apparent in the animal's environment, appropriate management for that problem is also necessary to treat the patient successfully.

REFERENCES

1. Low M. Stereotypies and behavioural medicine; confusions in current thinking. Aust Vet J 2003;81:192–8.
2. Powell SB, Newman HA, Pendergast JF, et al. A rodent model of spontaneous stereotypy: initial characterization of developmental, environmental, and neurobiological factors. Physiol Behav 1999;66:355–63.
3. Schwaibold U, Pillay N. Stereotypic behaviour is genetically transmitted in the African striped mouse, Rhabdomys pumilio. Appl Anim Behav Sci 2001;74: 273–80.
4. Houpt K. Ingestive behavior problems of dogs and cats. Vet Clin North Am Small Anim Pract 1982;12:683–92.
5. Blackshaw JK. Tail chasing or circling behavior in dogs. Canine Pract 1994; 19(3):7–11.
6. Moon-Fanelli AA, Dodman NH, Cottam N. Blanket and flank sucking in Doberman Pinschers. J Am Vet Med Assoc 2007;231(6):907–12.
7. Dodman NH, Karlsson EK, Moon-Fanelli A, et al. A canine chromosome 7 locus confers compulsive disorder susceptibility. Mol Psychiatry 2010;15:8–10.
8. Bhattacharyya S, Khanna S, Chakrabarty K, et al. Anti-brain autoantibodies and altered excitatory neurotransmitters in obsessive–compulsive disorder. Neuropsychopharmacology 2009;34(12):2489–96.
9. Maina G, Albert U, Bogetto F, et al. Anti-brain antibodies in adult patients with obsessive–compulsive disorder. J Affect Disord 2009;116:192–200.

10. Burns CC. A vicious cycle: a cross-sectional study of canine tail-chasing and human responses to it, using a Free Video-Sharing Website. PLoS One 2011; 6(11):e26553.
11. Bécuwe-Bonnet V, Bélanger M, Frank D, et al. Gastrointestinal disorders in dogs with excessive licking of surfaces. J Vet Behav 2012;7:194–204.
12. Frank D, Bélanger MC, Bécuwe-Bonnet V, et al. Prospective medical evaluation of seven dogs presented with fly-biting. Can Vet J 2012;53:1279–84.
13. Mills DS, Luescher AU. Veterinary and pharmacological approaches to abnormal repetitive behaviour. In: Mason G, Rushen J, editors. Stereotypic animal behaviour: fundamentals and applications to welfare. 2nd edition. Wallingford (WA): CABI; 2006. p. 294–5.
14. American Psychiatric Association. Diagnostic and statistical manual of mental disorders. 5th edition. Washington, DC: American Psychiatric Association; 2013.
15. Mason GJ. Stereotypies: a critical review. Anim Behav 1991;41:1015–37.
16. Rushen J, Mason G. A decade-or-more's progress in understanding stereotypic behavior. In: Mason G, Rushen J, editors. Stereotypic animal behaviour: fundamentals and applications to welfare. 2nd edition. Wallingford (WA): CABI; 2006. p. 1–18.
17. Garner JP. Perseveration and stereotypy – systems-level insights from clinical psychology. In: Mason G, Rushen J, editors. Stereotypic animal behaviour: fundamentals and applications to welfare. 2nd edition. Wallingford (WA): CABI; 2006. p. 121–52.
18. Mason GJ, Mendl M. Do the stereotypes of pigs, chickens and mink reflect adaptive species differences in the control of foraging? Appl Anim Behav Sci 1997;53:45–58.
19. Nicol CJ. Understanding equine stereotypies. Equine Vet J Suppl 1999;28:20–5.
20. Lyon M, Robbins TW. The action of central nervous system stimulant drugs: a general theory concerning amphetamine effects. Curr Dev Psychopharmacol 1975;2:79–163.
21. Longoni R, Spina L, Mulas A, et al. (D-Ala2) deltrophin II: D1-dependent stereotypies and stimulation of dopamine release in the nucleus accumbens. J Neurosci 1991;11:1565–76.
22. Weissman MM, Bland RC, Canino GJ, et al. The cross national epidemiology of obsessive compulsive disorder. The Cross National Collaborative Group. J Clin Psychiatry 1994;55(Suppl):5–10.
23. Fontanelle LF, Mendlowicz MV, Marques C, et al. Early- and late-onset obsessive–compulsive disorder in adult patients: an exploratory clinical and therapeutic study. Jpn Psychol Res 2003;37:127–33.
24. Graybiel AM, Rauch SL. Toward a neurobiology of obsessive compulsive disorder. Neuron 2000;28:343–7.
25. Mataix-Cols D, van den Heuvel OA. Common and distinct neural correlates of obsessive-compulsive and related disorders. Psychiatr Clin North Am 2006; 26:391–410.
26. Lewis MH, Presti MF, Lewis JB, et al. The neurobiology of stereotypy I: environmental complexity. In: Mason G, Rushen J, editors. Stereotypic animal behaviour: fundamentals and applications to welfare. 2nd edition. Wallingford (WA): CABI; 2006. p. 190–226.
27. Feusner JD, Bystritsky A. Managing treatment resistant OCD. Psychiatr Times 2005;22(8). Available at: www.lexisnexis.com/hottopics/lnacademic. Accessed 5 February, 2014.

28. Bourne SK, Eckhardt CA, Sheth SA, et al. Mechanisms of deep bran stimulation for obsessive compulsive disorder: effects upon cells and circuits. Front Integr Neurosci 2012;6(29):1–14.
29. Hewson C, Luescher U, Ball R. Measuring change in the behavioural severity of canine compulsive disorder: the construct validity of categories of change derived from two rating scales. Appl Anim Behav Sci 1998;60(1):55–68.
30. Irimajiri M, Luescher AU, Douglass G, et al. Randomized, controlled clinical trial of the efficacy of fluoxetine for treatment of compulsive disorders in dogs. J Am Vet Med Assoc 2009;235(6):705–9.
31. Ogata N, Gillis TE, Liu X, et al. Brain structural abnormalities in Doberman Pinschers with canine compulsive disorder. Prog Neuropsychopharmacol Biol Psychiatry 2013;45:1–6.
32. Reisner IR. The pathophysiologic basis of behavior problems. Vet Clin North Am Small Anim Pract 1991;21:207–24.
33. Schneider BM, Dodman NH, Maranda L. Use of memantine in treatment of canine compulsive disorders. J Vet Behav 2009;4(3):118–26.
34. Brown S. Naloxone responsive compulsive tail chasing in a dog. J Am Vet Med Assoc 1987;190(7):884–6.
35. Dodman NH, Shuster L. Animal models of obsessive compulsive behavior: a neurobiological and ethological perspective. In: Abramowitz JS, Houts AC, editors. Concepts and controversies in obsessive-compulsive disorder. New York: Springer; 2005. p. 53–71.
36. Hartigan PJ. Compulsive tail chasing in the dog: a mini-review. Ir Vet J 2000; 53(5):261–4.
37. Irimajiri M, Jay EE, Glickman LT, et al. Mild polycythemia associated with compulsive disorder in dogs. J Vet Behav 2006;1(1):23–8.
38. Moon-Fanelli AA, Dodman NH, Famula TR, et al. Characteristics of compulsive tail chasing and associated risk factors in Bull Terriers. J Am Vet Med Assoc 2011;238(7):883–9.
39. Moon-Fanelli AA, Dodman NH. Description and development of compulsive tail chasing in terriers and response to clomipramine treatment. J Am Vet Med Assoc 1998;212(8):1252–7.
40. Overall KL, Dunham AE. Clinical features and outcome in dogs and cats with obsessive-compulsive disorder: 126 cases (1989–2000). J Am Vet Med Assoc 2002;221(10):1445–52.
41. Leuscher AU. Diagnosis and management of compulsive disorders in dogs and cats. Clin Tech Small Anim Pract 2004;19(4):233–9.
42. Seksel K, Lindeman MJ. Use of clomipramine in treatment of obsessive-compulsive disorder, separation anxiety and noise phobia in dogs: a preliminary clinical study. Aust Vet J 2001;79(4):252–6.
43. Vermeire S, Audenaert K, Dobbeleir A, et al. A Cavalier King Charles dog with shadow chasing: clinical recovery and normalization of the dopamine trans-porter binding after clomipramine treatment. J Vet Behav 2010;5(6):345–9.
44. Landsberg G, Hunthausen W, Ackerman L. Stereotypic and compulsive disor-ders. In: Landsberg G, Hunthausen W, Ackerman L, editors. Handbook of behavior problems of the dog and cat. London: Elsevier; 2003. p. 195–225.
45. Hewson CJ, Luescher UA. Compulsive disorder in dogs. In: Voith VL, Borchelt PL, editors. Readings in companion animal behavior. New Jersey: Vet-erinary Learning Systems; 1996. p. 153–8.
46. Overall KL. Clinical behavioral medicine for small animals. St. Louis, Missouri: Mosby-Year Book, Inc; 1997.

47. Escriou C, Renier S, Tiira K, et al. Phenotypic and genetic characterization of "spinning" or "tail-chasing" in Bull Terriers. J Vet Behav 2012;7:e4–5.
48. Dodman NH, Knowles KE, Shuster L, et al. Behavioral changes associated with suspected complex partial seizures in Bull Terriers. J Am Vet Med Assoc 1996; 208:688–91.
49. Zulch HE, Mills DE, Lambert R, et al. The use of tramadol in a Labrador Retriever presented with self-mutilation of the tail. J Vet Behav 2012;7:252–8.
50. Goldberger E, Rapoport J. Canine acral lick dermatitis: response to the antiobsessional drug clomipramine. J Am Anim Hosp Assoc 1991;27:179–82.
51. Rappoport JL, Rylan DH, Kriete M. Drug treatment of canine acral lick. Arch Gen Psychiatry 1992;49:517–21.
52. Denerolle P, White SD, Taylor TS, et al. Organic diseases mimicking acral lick dermatitis in six dogs. J Am Anim Hosp Assoc 2007;43:215–20.
53. Shumaker AK, Angust JC, Coyner KS, et al. Microbiological and histopathological features of canine acral lick dermatitis. Vet Dermatol 2008;19:288–98.
54. White SD. Naltrexone for treatment of acral lick dermatitis in dogs. J Am Vet Med Assoc 1990;196:1073–6.
55. Wynchank D, Berk M. Fluoxetine treatment of acral lick dermatitis in dogs: a placebo-controlled randomized double blind trial. Depress Anxiety 1998;8:21–3.
56. Dellinger-Ness LA, Handler L. Self-injurious behavior in human and non-human primates. Clin Psychol Rev 2006;26:503–14.
57. Minert A, Gabay E, Dominguez C, et al. Spontaneous pain following spinal nerve injury in mice. Exp Neurol 2007;206.220–30.
58. Malais A. Compulsive targeted self-injurious behavior in humans with neuropathic pain: a counterpart of animal autotomy? Four case reports and literature review. Pain 1996;64:569–78.
59. Wiepkema PR. Developmental aspects of motivated behavior in domestic animals. J Anim Sci 1987;65:1220–77.
60. Bradshaw JW, Neville PF, Sawyer D. Factors affecting pica in the domestic cat. Appl Anim Behav Sci 1997;52:373–9.
61. Borchelt PL, Voith VL. Classification of animal behavior problems. Vet Clin North Am Small Anim Pract 1982;12:571–85.
62. Bamberger M, Houpt KA. Signalment factors, comorbidity, and trends in behavior diagnoses in cats: 736 cases (1991–2001). J Am Vet Med Assoc 2006;229:1602–6.
63. Marioni-Henry K, Vite CH, Newton AL, et al. Prevalence of diseases of the spinal cord in cats. J Vet Intern Med 2004;18:851–8.
64. Korman RM, Hetzel N, Knowles TG, et al. A retrospective study of 180 anaemic cats: features, aetiologies and survival data. J Feline Med Surg 2012;15:81–90.
65. Kohn B, Fumi C. Clinical course of pyruvate kinase deficiency in Abyssinian and Somali cats. J Feline Med Surg 2008;10:145–53.
66. Danford E, Darla H, Agnes M. Eating dysfunctions in an institutionalized mentally retarded population. Appetite 1981;2(4):281–92.
67. Willemse T, Mudde M, Josephy M, et al. The effect of haloperidol and naloxone on excessive grooming behaviour of cats. Eur Neuropsychopharmacol 1994;4: 39–45.
68. Mertens PA, Toress S, Jessen C. The effects of clomipramine hydrochloride in cats with psychogenic alopecia: a prospective study. J Am Anim Hosp Assoc 2006;42:336–43.
69. Hewson CJ, Luescher AU, Parent JM, et al. Efficacy of clomipramine in the treatment of canine compulsive disorder. J Am Vet Med Assoc 1998;213:1760–6.

70. Seksel K, Lindeman MJ. Use of clomipramine in the treatment of anxiety related and obsessive compulsive disorders in cats. Aust Vet J 1998;76:317–21.
71. Mills DS. Differential treatments for different repetitive behavior problems. In Proceedings Southern European Veterinary Conference. Barcelona, Spain; 2012.
72. Korff S, Stein DJ, Harvey BH. Stereotypic behaviour in the deer mouse: pharmacological validation and relevance for obsessive compulsive disorder. Prog Neuropsychopharmacol Biol Psychiatry 2008;32:348–55.
73. Poulson EM, Honeyman V, Valentine PA, et al. Use of fluoxetine for the treatment of stereotypical pacing in a captive polar bear. J Am Vet Med Assoc 1996;209: 1470–4.
74. Yalcin E, Aytug N. Use of fluoxetine to treat stereotypical pacing behavior in a brown bear (Ursus arctos). J Vet Behav 2007;2:73–6.
75. Arora T, Bhowmik M, Khanam R, et al. Oxcarbazepine and fluoxetine protect against mouse models of obsessive compulsive disorder through modulation cortical serotonin and CREB pathway. Behav Brain Res 2013;247:146–52.
76. Fontenot MB, Padgett EE, Dupuy AM, et al. The effects of fluoxetine and buspirone on self-injurious and stereotypic behavior in adult male Rhesus macaques. Comp Med 2005;55:67–74.
77. Rapp JT. Toward an empirical method for identifying matched stimulation for automatically reinforced behavior: a preliminary study. J Appl Behav Anal 2006;39:137–40.
78. McGreevy P, Nicol C. Physiological and behavioral consequences associated with short-term prevention of crib-biting in horses. Physiol Behav 1998;65: 15–23.
79. Barry S, Baird G, Lascelles K, et al. Neurodevelopmental movement disorders: an update on childhood motor stereotypies. Dev Med Child Neurol 2011;53: 979–85.
80. Herron ME, Frances S, Reisner IR. Survey of the use and outcome of confrontational and non-confrontational training methods in client-owned dogs showing undesired behaviors. Appl Anim Behav Sci 2009;117:47–54.
81. Iwata BA, Dorsey MF, Slifer KJ, et al. Toward a functional analysis of self-injury. J Appl Behav Anal 1994;27:197–209.
82. Salmon P. Effects of physical exercise on anxiety, depression, and sensitivity to stress: a unifying theory. Clin Psychol Rev 2001;21:33–61.
83. Centers for Disease Control and Prevention. Physical activity. Available at: http://www.cdc.gov/physicalactivity/everyone/guidelines/adults.html. Accessed October 31, 2013.
84. Wells DL. A review of environmental enrichment for kenneled dogs (Canis familiaris). Appl Anim Behav Sci 2004;85:307–17.
85. Cabib S. The neurobiology of stereotypy II: the role of stress. In: Mason G, Rushen J, editors. Stereotypic animal behaviour: fundamentals and applications to welfare. 2nd edition. Wallingford (WA): CABI; 2006. p. 227–55.

Intercat Aggression: Restoring Harmony in the Home:
A Guide for Practitioners

Christopher L. Pachel, DVM

KEYWORDS

- Feline aggression • Intercat aggression • Feline social behavior • Body language
- Environmental enrichment

KEY POINTS

- Understanding normal feline social behavior is extremely important to prevention and treatment of intercat aggression.
- Increasing the availability of resources, such as food and water, elevated resting locations, and litter boxes, can decrease motivations for territorial behavior and Intercat aggression.
- Treatment that consists of proactive management and desensitization/countercondi-tioning can be helpful for a variety of motivations that may contribute to intercat aggression, whereas additional strategies can be used when a more specific motivation is identified.
- Body language and interaction patterns provide confirmation of the intercat aggression diagnosis, and are also used to set the threshold for exposure sessions during treatment.
- A variety of medication and pharmaceutical options are available for augmentation of intercat aggression treatment plans, although there are no Food and Drug Administration–approved behavioral medications for cats.

INTRODUCTION

Aggressive behaviors between cats can be a source of stress for pet owners and a welfare concern for the individual cats involved. Recent pet ownership statistics show that roughly 36 million households in the United States are home to more than 74 million cats, with an average of 2.1 felines per cat-owning home.[1] Given the large number of cats sharing their homes with other cats, chances are high that social conflict is likely to occur, and relationships may be adversely affected.

Intercat aggression as been reported to occur at least once per month in 44.5% of multicat homes,[2] and aggression defined as biting and/or scratching occurred in 50% of homes after the adoption and introduction of a new cat to a household.[3]

Animal Behavior Clinic, 809 Southeast Powell Boulevard, Portland, OR 97202, USA
E-mail address: drpachel@animalbehaviorclinic.net

Vet Clin Small Anim 44 (2014) 565–579
http://dx.doi.org/10.1016/j.cvsm.2014.01.007 **vetsmall.theclinics.com**

A total of 185 of 736 cats presented to the Animal Behavior Clinic at Cornell University between 1991 and 2001,[4] and 101 of 336 cats presented to the Animal Behavior Clinic at the Barcelona School of Veterinary Medicine between 1998 and 2006[5] were diagnosed with this condition. Intercat aggression is also listed as a common reason for relinquishment or return to a shelter.[6]

Given these details along with the knowledge that even short-term exposure to stressors is correlated with an increase in sickness behaviors, such as vomiting, diarrhea, anorexia, and lethargy,[7] having an understanding of how to identify, treat, and prevent this condition is an essential aspect of providing veterinary care for domestic cats.

SOCIAL STRUCTURE OF FREE-LIVING CATS

The social structure of the free-living domestic cat is matrilineal, meaning that the social group is composed primarily of queens and their offspring. In addition, several queens may live together and share the responsibility of caring for offspring from another queen. Colonies consisting of multiple cats living within the same area are formed when there are sufficient food resources to support living within a group rather than as solitary individuals.[8] Domestic cats are somewhat unique in this regard in that their social structure is largely affected by such factors as population density and resource availability.

Colony members recognize other group members and frequently engage in a variety of friendly or affiliative social behaviors including rubbing of their head or body against another cat, referred to as allorubbing, and grooming of the head or neck area of another cat, a behavior known as allogrooming. Other affiliative interactions may include approaching with an elevated tail (**Fig. 1**); nose touching; sharing resources, such as food and water; and resting in close physical proximity to one another.

Although these colony groups are not definitively closed to new or unfamiliar individuals, the groups are somewhat insular and aggression is commonly displayed by resident colony members toward newcomers.[9] The process of joining an existing colony occurs gradually with the newcomer first on the physical and social periphery of the group and becoming more integrated over time, with this process often taking several weeks to occur.[10]

Cats rely on a variety of body language signals, vocalizations, and visual or olfactory marks to communicate with one another. Body language cues and vocalizations can

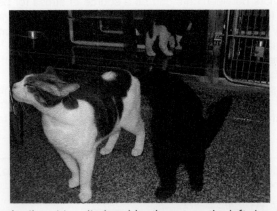

Fig. 1. The elevated tail position displayed by the cat on the left signals a willingness to engage in social interaction with the other cat shown in the photograph.

typically be categorized as neutral, affiliative (social, friendly), or agonistic (defensive or aggressive) based on the intent or the outcome of the interaction. These communication methods allow cats to establish relationships and also reduce the need for overt aggression during routine encounters.

The flexibility of the feline social structure and their tendency toward dispersal rather than reconciliation reduces the need for cats to resolve their differences for the purpose of survival or group living. This means that even minor conflicts have the potential to have significant consequences for the stability of individual relationships within the colony or group.

MULTICAT HOUSEHOLDS

The social and physical interactions displayed by free-living cats are also commonly observed between familiar cats living together within a home. One important difference between free and within-home living is that the movement patterns of indoor cats are restricted by their physical environment, and individual cats may not have the option of avoiding each other or maintaining adequate distance as they might otherwise do in an outdoor or unrestricted environment. As such, when cats live together in a home at higher densities than what might be observed in a free-living colony, "time-sharing" of specific locations may be observed in addition to space sharing or resting in close proximity to other household members.[11]

Another important difference for household cats is that resources, such as food and water, resting places, or elimination locations are provided by caregivers rather than being found naturally within the environment. Actual or perceived availability of those resources can have a significant impact on the level of competition between household cats and, by extension, the stability or strength of their relationships with each other.

IDENTIFICATION AND DIAGNOSIS OF INTERCAT AGGRESSION

The diagnostic term "intercat aggression" is broad and encompasses many different motivations for aggression including fear or defense, play or predation, territoriality, or redirection. Treatment recommendations listed in this article focus primarily on interventions that may be helpful for a wide variety of motivations, along with mention of additional strategies that can be used when more specific motivations for aggression are identified.

Early warning signs for intercat aggression within established multicat households may be as subtle as a lack of direct interaction between the cats, which may go unnoticed by many owners. In more obvious cases, the owners may describe spatial segregation with the cats avoiding each other or spending more time in parts of the home away from each other. The owners may also see active displacement of one cat by the other from favorite resting locations (**Fig. 2**), or they may see one of the cats resting in such a way as to block the other cat's access to food, water, or litter box locations (**Fig. 3**). As the severity of fighting increases and is more likely to include vocalizations, chasing, or physical contact between the cats, owners may be more likely to report the problem spontaneously or when questioned during a routine appointment.

Owners often interpret a lack of overt fighting as evidence that the cats are interacting comfortably, although that may not be true; careful questioning and observation may reveal findings consistent with intercat aggression. For example, such behaviors as self-grooming, oral behavior, scratching, and shaking of the head may be significantly elevated above baseline in the minute after a conflict with another household

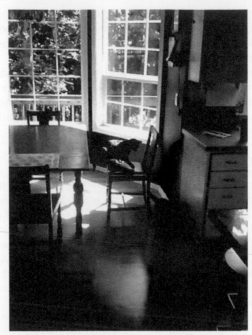

Fig. 2. Active displacement from resting places may include chasing and overtly offensive postures by the aggressor. The cat on the right shows body language associated with active avoidance and escape behavior in response to the other cat's advances.

cat[12] and these behaviors may be noted by observant owners and reported as part of the clinical history.

Owners may also describe periods of tension after situations, such as one returning from a veterinary appointment or after seeing an outdoor cat through one of the home windows. It may be necessary to ask specifically about these issues in multicat households during routine examinations rather than waiting for clients to self-report problems.

Play behavior in cats typically includes mutual interaction and can be very active with intense physical contact. However, if all of the physical interactions are

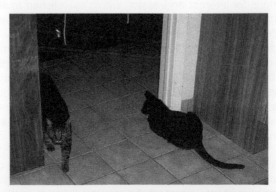

Fig. 3. Strategic position is most likely to occur at narrowed spaces, such as doorways. Note the avoidance of eye contact by the cat on the left and the direct, forward stare shown by the cat on the right.

characterized by one cat chasing or stalking the other or if the "target" of the perceived play behavior shows frequent hissing, swatting, or avoidance behaviors, diagnosis and intervention may be indicated.

Intercat aggression is most typically displayed in a unidirectional manner, with one cat consistently aggressing toward another; an aggressor and a victim were identifiable in 43 out of 50 cases of intercat aggression in one study.[13] This information can be helpful in guiding specific recommendations for each cat, because aggressors and victims frequently need to be treated somewhat differently.

The onset of aggressive behavior can occur in a variety of patterns. Tension may be evident from the first social interaction as is common in cases involving fear or territoriality as the primary motivation for aggression. The onset can also occur more gradually in response to the onset of social maturity between 2 and 5 years of age or perhaps in response to persistent play attempts from a younger cat to an older or more sedentary individual. An acute onset of aggression is commonly associated with redirected aggression; physical or physiologic illness; or perhaps in response to an acute change in the social or physical environment, such as a move or the addition of another person or pet to the household.

Cats affected by intercat aggression within the home may be presented to the veterinarian for assessment of other, seemingly unrelated problems, such as traumatic injuries, chronic weight loss, anxiety issues, or lack of consistent litter box usage. In addition to treatment of the primary concern, the assessment should also include questions about relationships between cats in the home to determine whether treatment of intercat aggression may also be indicated.

TREATMENT OF INTERCAT AGGRESSION

When intercat aggression is suspected or observed, clinicians should recommend early intervention rather than taking a more passive approach of waiting to see whether the problem intensifies or resolves itself. It is assumed for the purposes of this article that a comprehensive physical examination is performed on all involved cats in combination with appropriate diagnostic testing to rule out underlying medical conditions before initiating behavioral treatments of intercat aggression.

One of the most common questions asked by clients during the initial assessment is whether the cats should be separated from one another as part of treatment. It may be helpful to consider this recommendation in terms of the following categories (bullet point indicates recent clinical history):

"Green": Treatment not indicated at this time
- Sharing of resting places, allorubbing, and/or allogrooming
- Minimal incidence of overt conflicts and cats routinely show affiliative body language during interactions with each other

"Yellow": Treatment indicated, cats may not require separation
- Infrequent, or lack of affiliative interactions, such as allogrooming, allorubbing, or sharing of resting places
- Casual avoidance of one another and/or displacement from resting places without signs of overt anxiety or distress
- Infrequent negative interactions, such as blocked access to resources, or conflicts that include hissing, swatting, or offensive/defensive posturing
- No evidence of significant injury or chronic emotional distress for involved cats

"Red": Treatment indicated, cats would likely benefit from separation
- Overt conflict and/or aggressive interactions; may occur intermittently or may be consistent from one interaction to the next

- Intolerance of the presence of the other cat without signs of arousal, fear, anxiety, or aggression
- Physical contact and/or injury are common during interactions

Clients are often reluctant to separate cats because of the inconvenience of doing so, or because of the mindset that separation prevents cats from establishing a relationship with each other. Although it is true that interaction may be required for the cats to form a stable relationship, it should be stressed to the client that allowing uncontrolled, emotionally aversive interactions does more to damage the relationship than repair it. Separation may be indicated until an appropriate reintroduction plan can be created and implemented.

Separation can be accomplished in a variety of ways depending on the physical layout of the home, the availability of confinement locations, and each cat's tolerance of being confined. Confinement locations should provide convenient access to food, water, resting places, a litter box or access to an appropriate elimination location, and the opportunity for social interaction with people or other pets (provided that those interactions are safe and enjoyable for all involved parties).

When introducing a new cat to a household, allowing the resident cats full access to the core living area and gradually introducing the newcomer to that space fits most closely with the natural integration pattern of free-living cats. In cases in which one cat is offensively aggressive because of territoriality, confining the aggressor cat to a space on the periphery of the core area may allow the newcomer to establish residence more easily.

If any signs of aggression, threats, or intimidation occur at the boundary between confinement spaces, it may be necessary to create a "neutral zone" using an additional gate or closed door between the spaces to avoid rehearsal of aggressive behavior patterns.

WHEN SEPARATION IS NOT NECESSARY

Clients should be educated on the body language cues and vocalizations associated with offensive threat behavior, with defensive aggression, and with fear and anxiety so that they can accurately interpret the interactions they observe. This is helpful in determining the clinical response to interventions, and also enables owners to know when and if intervention is necessary during a particular interaction.

Plentiful Resources

Resource availability can have a tremendous impact on relationships, both in terms of limiting the need for competition and reducing territoriality, and on allowing cats to avoid each other within the home environment rather than clustering around limited resources.

Food should be distributed to multiple feeding stations throughout the home, provided none of the cats have dietary restrictions that make this impractical or unsafe. The cats do not need to be provided with more food, but rather have access to more locations from which food may be available. Water stations can be provided along with feed even though competition over water is less commonly reported than over food and the availability of water may have less impact on behavior.

A sufficient number of litter boxes should be made available throughout the home such that each cat has a box that is accessible at all times. Adequate spacing of litter boxes should ensure that each cat has the ability to access and use a box without a forced or close association with another cat. This is especially important for cases in which one or more cats are not using the litter box reliably. The "n + 1" rule is commonly given for how many litter boxes to provide, with "n" equaling the number of cats in the household. Distribution of boxes throughout the environment is perhaps as important, if not more important, than the actual number of boxes provided.

Cats should be provided with access to elevated perches and climbing areas and hiding boxes at or near floor level; this helps cats to maintain a social distance of 1 to 3 m from each other when needed.[14] Perches and boxes can be a variety of heights or sizes depending on what is preferred by the individual cat. These locations are especially important as a way of providing a retreat for the cat that is the target of the aggressive behavior. Creative placement of elevated perches or climbing trees is a great way to increase three-dimensional space in locations within the home in which the floor footprint is otherwise tight or limited.[11]

Physical and Mental Enrichment

In cases involving excessive play behavior or misdirected predatory/chase behavior, cats should be provided with opportunities for physical exercise and mental stimulation. Such options as using food-dispensing toys for meals, scheduling short play sessions throughout the day, or providing outdoor access (when it is determined to be a safe option) can provide appropriate outlets for these behaviors.

Interruption Strategies

Cat owners may instinctively react to a fight by attempting to restrain the aggressor or to protect the victim. This can be extremely unsafe because the owner may be bitten, scratched, or otherwise injured in the process. When conflicts are mild, creating an interruptive stimulus by leaving the area or walking through the room, making an unpleasant noise, or perhaps knocking at the front door or ringing the doorbell can be an effective way to shift the aggressor's focus and allow the victim time to leave the area. In more severe situations, it may be necessary to physically intervene by splashing the cats with water, tossing a blanket over the aggressor, pushing a couch cushion or other physical object between the cats, or by trapping one of the cats under an overturned laundry basket.

Clients should be made aware of the potential for redirected aggression during fights and also of the long latency period that may be required for cats to return to a normal resting level of arousal. It may be necessary to sequester one or more cats to individual confinement areas until they fully recover after an aggressive incident to ensure the safety of all individuals within the home.

Physical Adjuncts to Treatment

When one of the cats can clearly be identified as an offensive aggressor, securing a bell to that cat's collar may provide other cats with a means of identifying the aggressor's position and thereby improve their ability to avoid a conflict. Breakaway collars should be used for safety, and it may be necessary to introduce the collar gradually or through a desensitization protocol to ensure that it can be worn safely and comfortably.

Physical devices, such as a CatBib (Cat Goods, Inc, Portland, OR), a neoprene product designed to interfere with predatory behavior that is secured to a cat's collar, and the Thundershirt (ThunderWorks), a wrap that provides compressive pressure to the chest and thorax, have been anecdotally reported to help in reducing the frequency and intensity of aggressive displays when worn during social interactions. A desensitization or habituation period may be needed before devices such as these can be used successfully.

WHEN SEPARATION IS INDICATED

Separation is most likely to be needed when the frequency or intensity of aggression creates a safety or welfare concern for other cats in the home, or when therapeutic interventions applied to a group living situation have been unsuccessful. The first step is to establish a location for low-stress confinement, which includes providing the confined cat with adequate space for normal behaviors, reliable access to food and water sources, locations for perching or hiding, and convenient access to an appropriate litter box. After that has been accomplished, the next step is to create a treatment plan that focuses on reintroduction using desensitization and counterconditioning techniques.

It is difficult to make a specific recommendation as to the number of sessions required to accomplish a successful reintroduction. This depends on the severity and duration of the problem, the frequency with which the owner can perform the sessions, and the response of the individual cats involved. Rather than making a specific recommendation, clients should be instructed to proceed step-wise through the reintroduction process, and to check in with the veterinarian if they have any questions about when or how to proceed. It is important that clients not rush the steps or set a specific time limit for how long the reintroduction process should take, although they should be able to identify improvements in the social behavior or tolerance level of each cat throughout the treatment process.

Scent Transfer

This is done to collect scent and facial pheromones that would normally be deposited during bunting or facial marking on solid surfaces, or during allorubbing on another cat. Using a soft cloth, gently rub the cheek and perioral areas of one cat. The cloth is then taken to the second, who is given an opportunity to sniff and investigate the cloth. Assuming that the presence of the scented cloth is tolerated without any observable stress response, the cloth is then rubbed on the cheek and perioral area of the second cat before repeating the process again with the first cat. It can also be useful to countercondition by providing food rewards during the scent exchange. If the presence of the scented cloth or the act of rubbing the cloth on either cat causes stress or avoidance behavior, it may be necessary to approach this step more gradually.

This exercise should be performed several times before starting controlled introductions to establish a baseline of behavior, and to confirm that each cat is ready for the next step. Scent transfer can also be accomplished by giving each cat the opportunity to explore the main living area while the other is confined elsewhere, or by rotating each of the cats through a common confinement area, or by exchanging bedding or other cloth items between the confinement areas of each of the involved cats.

Gradual Introduction

This should initially be done using the principles of desensitization and classical conditioning. More specifically, the cats should be introduced to one another in a controlled environment, at a distance or intensity level at which each cat is aware of the other's presence but is nonreactive, nonfearful, and nonaggressive, and then the presence of the other cat is paired with an enjoyable experience, such as food or active play.

When using a physical barrier

Sessions can be performed with both cats on opposite sides of a barrier, such as a glass door (allows for visual contact) or screen door (allows for visual contact and acoustic and olfactory exposure). When such a barrier is not available, the same process can be performed using stacked baby gates across a doorway, or by using a combination of a cord/latch and a wood block (the cord/latch prevents the door from swinging open too wide and the block keeps it from closing).

When using a restraint device

The space between the cats can be controlled using a harness and leash for each cat, or by confining each cat to a carrier, condo, or tent. It may be necessary to introduce the restraint device or the confinement option before an actual introduction to ensure that the restraint itself does not add stress to the session.

Each cat should be managed in such a way that stress is low or nonexistent, and their preferred reward is used for reinforcement during sessions. This may require creative planning when multiple cats are involved, or when cats are not particularly food or toy motivated.

Although there is no an exact formula for the number or duration of sessions, general guidelines indicate that they should be short (perhaps no more than a few minutes at first) and frequent (as often as is convenient). To accomplish this efficiently, a single session can be broken up into several shorter ones. For example, the cats can be put into a carrier and placed at opposite ends of a room or hallway. Each cat is provided with a small amount of canned food or enjoyable treat, and then the carriers/cats are moved apart as soon as the food is finished by either cat. This can be repeated multiple times in succession to provide the greatest number of opportunities for associative conditioning to occur.

As each cat's comfort and tolerance improves over the course of several sessions, the cats can gradually be moved closer toward each other. When the cats are capable of remaining in close proximity to each other on a consistent basis, the owner can allow a greater level of contact by confining one cat while allowing the other to move about more freely, or by allowing the cats to have physical contact with each other for short periods of time before separating them once again.

One of the most common mistakes made by owners when working through these sessions is to progress at a rate that is faster than what an individual cat can tolerate, thereby increasing the risk of negative experiences rather than positive ones. Recommend that clients increase the intensity of sessions in small increments, or perhaps repeat sessions at a given intensity at least three times before making additional adjustments.

Additional Behavior Modification Options

Clicker training can be used in a variety of ways, either to mark and reward the specific moment in which one cat becomes aware of the other (classical conditioning) or to reward one of the cats for engaging in affiliative behaviors, such as bunting, rubbing, or moving forward with a relaxed, elevated tail.

For a cat that is likely to lunge, chase, or engage in offensively aggressive behaviors, using a combination of leash restraint and a clicker to reinforce behaviors, such as sitting, lying down, or disengaging focus from the other cat, can be useful. This takes more skill on the owner's part to use this technique successfully, but it can be extremely successful when implemented correctly.

Teaching a "go to" command (movement to a specific room or perch on cue) to one or both cats is a great way to allow more direct interactions between the cats during sessions by providing the owner with a way to intervene if any tension or hostility occurs.

RECOMMENDATIONS FOR USE OF PUNISHMENT DURING SOCIAL INTERACTIONS

Techniques aimed at punishing undesired behaviors should be used sparingly and extremely carefully, if at all. Although aversives, such as squirting a cat with water, can be an effective way to suppress or interrupt a particular behavior at the moment the aversive stimulus occurs, there are several limitations of this technique that clients should know before considering their use. Punishments must be (1) applied with reliable timing (ideally within 1 to 2 seconds of onset of the undesired behavior); (2) performed consistently (each time the undesired behavior occurs, not just when the pet is "caught in the act" by the owner); and (3) appropriate for the situation such that the likelihood of the undesired behavior decreases in the future, but without causing fear, anxiety, or unnecessary pain or discomfort in the process.

When punishments are used without proper technique, the cat is unlikely to understand the reason for the unpleasant experience, and their behavior is unlikely to change in the future even if the aversive stimulus stops the behavior in the moment. In addition, the use of aversives can be associated with an increase in fear, anxiety, or aggressive behaviors, which may intensify the intercat aggression problem.

Although it may be possible to use an aversive stimulus properly during a structured training session in which the criteria can be met, this still has the disadvantage of not providing the cat with feedback about which behaviors are desired within that interaction, which makes it difficult for behavioral improvement to occur reliably. As such, methods intended to punish specific behavior should generally be avoided as first-line therapy recommendations.

USE OF MEDICATION TO SUPPORT THE TREATMENT OF INTERCAT AGGRESSION

Many different medications and pharmaceuticals have been used to treat intercat aggression, although there is limited research on the topic to establish efficacy of treatment and there are no Food and Drug Administration–approved behavioral medications for use in cats.

When considering whether or not to include pharmacologic interventions in treatment recommendations, clinical experience suggests that cats with significant fear, anxiety, or impaired impulse control patterns may be more likely to respond to these interventions.

Treatment options can generally be categorized as situational/event or maintenance interventions. Situational options are used "as needed" and can be used during controlled sessions, or perhaps during initial introductions to reduce the likelihood of problems. If a behavior problem is nonresponsive to situational treatments, if treatment is required multiple times per day for the desired effect, or if the events leading to aggressive behavior are somewhat unpredictable, then choosing a maintenance therapy option is generally more suitable. In some cases, it may be desired to use situational and maintenance options for a combined therapeutic effect, or perhaps to achieve more immediate effects from the situational intervention while waiting for the maintenance medication to take effect.

Doses are discussed elsewhere in this issue. Also consult a veterinary formulary or behavior text for more comprehensive information regarding treatment indications, side effects, or possible contraindications of each medication listed below prior to use.

Situational/Event Intervention Options

Feliway (Ceva Animal Health, Inc, St. Louis, MO), a synthetic analogue of the F3 feline facial pheromone, has been studied for use in cats as treatment of urine marking, feline idiopathic cystitis, and for stress during hospitalization and medical procedures.

This product is available as a nonaerosol spray, as an electric room diffuser, and as a single-use disposal wipe. The spray and wipe formulations are best used situationally, whereas the diffuser is better suited to maintenance use. A synthetic analogue of the F4 feline facial pheromone shared in allomarking and bunting, Felifriend (Ceva Sante Animale), is distributed in some European countries for direct application to the cat (or to humans) to help facilitate social interactions.

Benzodiazepine medications, such as alprazolam (0.125–0.25 mg/cat every 8–24 hours) and lorazepam (0.125–0.25 mg/cat every 12–24 hours), target γ-aminobutyric acid receptors and can be effective anxiolytic medications for cats in addition to appetite-stimulating properties, which can be helpful for anorexic cats affected by anxiety or stress and for counterconditioning with food. This group of medications has been associated with behavior disinhibition, which can exacerbate pre-existing aggression issues for some cats, but may also have the effect of increasing confidence in a more fearful victim cat. Oral diazepam (0.2–0.5 mg/kg every 8–12 hours) should be used cautiously or not at all, because it has been associated with idiopathic hepatic necrosis in cats.[15,16]

Other options that may anecdotally provide benefit in the temporary management of intercat aggression include melatonin (1–3 mg every 12–24 hours), hydroxyzine (1–2.2 mg/kg every 8–12 hours), and Rescue Remedy (used according to package instructions).

Maintenance Intervention Options

Anxitane (Virbac Animal Health, Fort Worth, TX) contains an amino acid, L-theanine, which is found in green tea and has shown promise in treating anxiety disorders in cats.[17]

Selective serotonin reuptake inhibitors, such as fluoxetine (0.5–1.5 mg/kg every 24 hours), paroxetine (0.5–1.0 mg/kg every 24 hours), and sertraline (0.5–1.5 mg/kg every 24 hours), have anxiolytic and antiaggressive effects but may take 3 to 4 weeks or longer to be clinically effective as adjunctive treatment of intercat aggression.

Tricyclic antidepressants, such as clomipramine (0.25–1.0 mg/kg every 24 hours), exert a dual effect on serotonin and norepinephrine. Others, such as amitriptyline (0.5–1.0 mg/kg every 24 hours), are more selective for norepinephrine effects.

Buspirone (0.5–1.0 mg/kg every 12–24 hours) exerts an effect on serotonin, but through a different mechanism than selective serotonin reuptake inhibitor medications. It is nonsedating and may take effect within 1 to 3 weeks. This medication has been anecdotally associated with an increase in "affectionate" behaviors toward owners, which can be a desirable effect. It has also been associated with an increase in confidence and assertive behaviors, which can be beneficial or harmful depending on an individual cat's temperament or pre-existing behavior patterns. The use of buspirone as a treatment of intercat aggression has been associated with a significant decrease in likelihood of cure[13] but it can be useful in isolated cases.

Gabapentin (3–10 mg/kg every 8–12 hours) has pain-modulating properties and mild anticonvulsant and moderate antianxiety effects. This can be a helpful adjunct in cases with comorbid diagnoses related to pain or neurologic problems.

The Royal Canin Veterinary Diet CALM is a nutritionally balanced diet that contains three calming ingredients: (1) α-casozepine,[18] (2) L-tryptophan, and (3) nicotinamide (vitamin B_3). It can be used situationally in advance of stressful situations, or as part of adjunctive maintenance therapy in the treatment of anxiety conditions. A supplement (Zylkene) with α-casozepine alone is also available in some countries.

Although transdermal administration of medications can be highly convenient and potentially less stressful to administer, pharmacologic studies of transdermal preparations of fluoxetine,[19] amitriptyline, and buspirone[20] have not demonstrated serum levels comparable with oral administration in cats and should therefore not be recommended as first-line treatment options.

CASE EXAMPLE

The owner of a two-cat household presented both cats for evaluation of aggressive behavior. The owner first owned "Gilbert," a 6-year-old m/n Siamese cat. Gilbert was acquired as a kitten and lived as an only cat in the household until the addition of "Buttons," a 2-year m/n domestic shorthair cat, approximately 1 year ago. The owner reports a progressive frequency and intensity of conflicts between the cats with Gilbert as the aggressor. Buttons has shown progressively more fearful and avoidant body language and has been hiding in spaces throughout the home rather than interacting with other household members. Conflicts increased to a daily occurrence and include chasing, swatting, and hissing. No injuries were sustained, but there were several instances of Buttons expressing his bladder and bowels during conflicts. Physical examination and laboratory assessment of both cats including complete blood count, serum chemistry profile, urinalysis, and thyroid (T4) assessment were within normal limits.

Initial treatment consisted of increasing resource availability within the home, implementing the use of a belled collar for Gilbert, separating the cats to different areas of the home, and starting the process of reintroduction using desensitization and counterconditioning strategies as previously outlined. After a lack of clinical improvement within the initial 6 to 8 weeks of treatment, medical treatment was initiated for Gilbert with fluoxetine (0.5 mg/kg by mouth every day) and the use of Anxitane for Buttons.

Both cats were treated for approximately 4 months while reintegration was attempted and accomplished. Buttons was taken off Anxitane at that time without recurrence of conflicts or aggressive behavior. Fluoxetine was continued for an additional 3 months for Gilbert. He showed a recurrence of aggressive behavior when medication was tapered after 7 months of treatment; the decision was made to continue treatment for additional 1 to 3 years with the option of reattempting medication taper at that time.

PROGNOSIS

As with many behavioral problems, the prognosis for improvement or resolution of intercat aggression can vary widely from one case to the next. Factors affecting prognosis may include the following:

- Number of cats involved in conflicts and number of cats within the home (even if not involved)
- Ability of owner to comprehend, implement, and follow through with treatment recommendations
- Severity and duration of aggression at time of assessment and diagnosis
- Relative availability of resources and practicality of increasing availability of resources to meet the needs of the involved cats
- Accessibility of physical space for confinement (when required)
- Ability to administer medications to individual cats involved

In one study, 30 out of 48 cases of intercat aggression were rated as "cured" after treatment, and the likelihood of treatment success was not based on the gender of cats involved.[15] Clinical experience suggests that successful treatment of severe cases of intercat aggression may take upward of 3 to 6 months, or perhaps longer for complicated or refractory cases.

The prognosis is favorable for more rapid improvement in mild cases, or those in which the factors listed previously do not significantly impact the clinical presentation. Clients should be made aware that complete resolution of the problem may not be possible for all cases, and there is a possibility of relapse even after significant clinical improvement especially in cases presenting with a history of redirected aggression or severe emotional disturbances for one or more of the cats involved.

PREVENTION

The length of the primary socialization period for cats is generally considered to last from approximately 3 to an upward limit of 7 to 9 weeks. Having an opportunity to interact with other kittens and adult cats during this time provides for the development of social skills,[21] which may decrease the risk of developing fear-based intercat aggression later in life. Cats with a history of socialization have been shown to respond more favorably to stressors, such as the approach of an unfamiliar person, or the approach of a person with a cat or dog, compared with feral, nonsocialized cats[22]; this emphasizes the need for early social exposure as a preventative measure for avoiding social problems in adulthood. However, genetics also plays a role, with the paternal genes perhaps having a greater effect on social behavior.[23]

Choosing a New Addition

When deciding whether to add a kitten or an adult cat to a home, kittens may be better tolerated by resident adult cats and may have an easier time adapting to the new home environment. However, active and playful kittens can create social problems simply because of their exuberance and energy level, especially when combined with sedentary older cats or adult cats with socialization deficits.

Affiliative behavior is more common between littermates than nonlittermates, and between related than nonrelated cats, which supports the recommendation of acquiring littermates or perhaps a queen and her offspring.[23,24] Acquiring littermate kittens may not completely eliminate the possibility of intercat aggression, but does allow the kittens to acclimate to each other at a young age and may be more successful than introducing adult cats to one another.

Scientific information varies as to which gender combination is least likely to show intercat aggression. Two studies of multicat households showed no observed differences in affiliative or aggressive behaviors based on gender.[3,14] However, one of those studies evaluated same gender pairings and stated that females were never observed to allorub other females and male/male pairs spent more time in close proximity to one another,[14] which suggests that gender variation in behavior is possible.

In contrasting results, aggression between housemate cats was more likely to be initiated by male than female cats, although the aggression was equally likely toward other males or toward females,[13] whereas an additional study concluded that males were more likely to show aggression directed toward female than male cats within the household.[25]

In a study of households in which a new cat was introduced to a resident cat, the likelihood of current fighting at the time of study was positively associated with such factors as scratching and biting during initial introduction, provision of outdoor access, and the owner's perception of the first meeting as unfriendly or aggressive.[3]

Collectively, this information makes it difficult to make a definitive recommendation about which age or gender of cat to add to an existing cat household, or when acquiring multiple cats at the same time.

Introduction Recommendations

Unfamiliar cats should be introduced to one another gradually using the aforementioned methods, such as segregation, scent transfer, allowing cats to interact through a screen door, or introducing the cats with the help of confinement tools, such as carriers or harness/leash combinations. Remember that in free-living environments, new social group members are slowly accepted to the group after a period of time on the social and physical periphery. Arranging the physical environment and household routines to accommodate this pattern may be helpful during the introduction period.

Clients may find it tedious to plan gradual introductions for each new feline addition to the household. However, this process often goes more quickly when done preventatively, compared with the time required to work through the process after a problem has already developed, which should provide incentive for clients to adhere to recommendations. The actual timeline required to complete this process is affected by the response of each cat to the introduction, by how quickly the cats habituate to one another, and by the presence of prosocial behaviors that allow for interactions to occur comfortably for each cat.

Clients should be informed of the steps involved in the introduction process and the body language cues associated with threat or avoidance to watch for throughout the sessions. Reassessment before increasing the intensity of interactions allows a client to halt the process and spend more time at a particular integration step rather than pushing forward or putting the cats together prematurely.

REFERENCES

1. US pet ownership & demographics sourcebook. American Veterinary Medical Association; 2012.
2. Borchelt P, Voith V. Readings in companion animal behavior. Trenton (NJ): Veterinary Learning System; 1996.
3. Levine E, Perry P, Scarlett J, et al. Intercat aggression in households following the introduction of a new cat. Appl Anim Behav Sci 2005;90:325–36.
4. Bamberger M, Houpt KA. Signalment factors, cornorbidity, and trends in behavior diagnoses in cats: 736 cases (1991-2001). J Am Vet Med Assoc 2006;229:1602–6.
5. Amat M, Ruiz de la Torre JL, Fatjo J, et al. Potential risk factors associated with feline behaviour problems. Appl Anim Behav Sci 2009;121:134–9.
6. Casey RA, Vandenbussche S, Bradshaw JW, et al. Reasons for relinquishment and return of domestic cats (Felis Silvestris Catus) to rescue shelters in the UK. Anthrozoos 2009;22:347–58.
7. Stella J, Croney C, Buffington T. Effects of stressors on the behavior and physiology of domestic cats. Appl Anim Behav Sci 2013;143:157–63.
8. Crowell-Davis SL, Curtis TM, Knowles RJ. Social organization in the cat: a modern understanding. J Feline Med Surg 2004;6:19–28.
9. Liberg O, Sandell M. Spatial organization and reproductive tactics in the domestic cat and other felids. In: Turner DC, Bateson P, editors. The domestic cat: the biology of its behaviour. Cambridge (United Kingdom): Cambridge University Press; 1988. p. 67–81.

10. McDonald DW, Yamaguchi N, Kerby G. Group-living in the domestic cat: its sociobiology and epidemiology. In: Turner DC, Bateson P, editors. The domestic cat: the biology of its behaviour. Cambridge (United Kingdom): Cambridge University Press; 2000. p. 95–118.

11. Bernstein PL, Strack M. A game of cat and house: spatial patterns and behavior of 14 domestic cats (Felis catus) in the home. Anthrozoos 1996;9:25–39.

12. van den Bos R. Post-conflict stress-response in confined group-living cats (Felis silvestris catus). Appl Anim Behav Sci 1998;59:323–30.

13. Lindell EM, Erb HN, Houpt KA. Intercat aggression: a retrospective study examining types of aggression, sexes of fighting pairs, and effectiveness of treatment. Appl Anim Behav Sci 1997;55:153–62.

14. Barry KJ, Crowell-Davis SL. Gender differences in the social behavior of the neutered indoor-only domestic cat. Appl Anim Behav Sci 1999;64:193–211.

15. Center SA, Elston TH, Rowland PH, et al. Fulminant hepatic failure associated with oral administration of diazepam in 11 cats. J Am Vet Med Assoc 1996; 209:618–25.

16. Hughes D, Moreau R, Overall K, et al. Acute hepatic necrosis and liver failure associated with benzodiazepine therapy in six cats. J Vet Emerg Crit Care 1996;6(1):13–20.

17. Dramard V, Kern L, Hofmans J, et al. Clinical efficacy of l-theanine tablets to reduce anxiety-related emotional disorders in cats: a pilot open-label clinical trial. J Vet Behav 2007;5:85–6.

18. Beata C, Beaumont-Graff E, Coll V, et al. Effect of alpha-casozepine (Zylkene) on anxiety in cats. J Vet Behav 2007;2:40–6.

19. Ciribassi J, Luescher A, Pasloske KS, et al. Comparative bioavailability of fluoxetine after transdermal and oral administration to healthy cats. Am J Vet Res 2003;64:994–8.

20. Mealey KL, Peck KE, Bennett BS, et al. Systemic absorption of amitriptyline and buspirone after oral and transdermal administration to healthy cats. J Vet Intern Med 2004;18:43–6.

21. McCune S. The impact of paternity and early socialization on the development of cats behavior to people and novel objects. Appl Anim Behav Sci 1995;45: 109–24.

22. Yeon SC, Kim YK, Park SJ, et al. Differences between vocalization evoked by social stimuli in feral cats and house cats. Behav Processes 2011;87:183–9.

23. Bradshaw JW, Hall SL. Affiliative behaviour of related and unrelated pairs of cats in catteries: a preliminary report. Appl Anim Behav Sci 1999;63:251–5.

24. Curtis TM, Knowles RJ, Crowell-Davis SL. Influence of familiarity and relatedness on proximity and allogrooming in domestic cats (Felis catus). Am J Vet Res 2003; 64:1151–4.

25. Hart BL, Cooper L. Factors relating to urine spraying and fighting in prepubertally gonadectomized cats. J Am Vet Med Assoc 1984;184:1255–8.

Feline Aggression Toward Family Members: A Guide for Practitioners

Melissa Bain, DVM, MS*, Elizabeth Stelow, DVM

KEYWORDS

• Feline • Aggression • Behavior • Human-animal bond

KEY POINTS

- It is important to identify the underlying motivation for the aggression to provide the most effective treatment plan.
- Fear is a common reason for aggression toward people.
- Household management, including enrichment and avoidance of the triggers, is an important part of the overall treatment plan.
- A complete history, gathered using open-ended questions, helps determine the underlying motivation, owner attachment, and relationship between the owner and the cat.

RELEVANCE

Feline aggression toward people is a common, potentially dangerous problem that cat owners may face. It can lead to relinquishment or euthanasia of otherwise healthy cats. Despite the frequency with which it is reported, this aggression often presents a challenge to veterinarians to diagnose and prescribe a treatment plan. Complicating diagnosis and treatment is the fact that some cat owners believe that nothing can be done to help their cat,[1] or they seek help from someone other than their veterinarian.[2]

One study showed that almost 14% of cats presenting to the Animal Behavior Clinic at Cornell University were diagnosed with aggression directed toward people, with most of them showing aggression toward their owners. This finding represents an upward trend in this diagnosis, with an almost equal downward trend in cats diagnosed with urine marking, over a 10-year period.[3] In addition, approximately 50% of owners reported aggression between cats when introducing a new feline member to the household.[4] The most sobering statistic is from 1 study that reported that 15% and 12% of cats relinquished to shelters for behavioral reasons were relinquished because of aggression toward people and other cats, respectively.[5]

Clinical Animal Behavior Service, University of California School of Veterinary Medicine, 1 Shields Avenue, Davis, CA 95616, USA
* Corresponding author.
E-mail address: mjbain@ucdavis.edu

Vet Clin Small Anim 44 (2014) 581–597
http://dx.doi.org/10.1016/j.cvsm.2014.01.001
0195-5616/14/$ – see front matter © 2014 Elsevier Inc. All rights reserved.

NORMAL BEHAVIOR RELATED TO AGGRESSION
Role of Domestication

Contrary to common misconception, domestic cats are a social species. Many studies have shown that domesticated cats develop a bond with other cats, as well as with people.[6,7] Domestication is the process by which selective breeding changes the behavioral and morphologic characteristics of an animal.[8] By domesticating cats, their social structure has been changed from that of the ancestral species (Felis silvestris libyca), an asocial species, to a social, domesticated species. It is through domestication that cats have generally adapted to living in a social community with one another and with people. However, there is individual variation in behavioral and morphologic traits, which can be influenced by prenatal environment, early socialization, and life experiences.

Role of Genetics and Early Socialization

There is mounting evidence about the relationship between genetics and the behavior of cats.[9,10] Some of this evidence seems to be related to coat color. In 1 study, female cats with the color patterns of tortoiseshell, calico, or torbie (a tortoiseshell with a tabby pattern) were more frequently reported to be aggressive toward people. Male black and white cats were also reported to be more aggressive toward people, as well as toward other cats.[11] In this same study, it was shown that female cats were more likely to show aggression at the veterinarian's office.

Early socialization with people, which involves handling kittens during their first few weeks, leads to cats that are friendlier and less fearful toward people.[6,9] In addition, there is some evidence that hand-reared cats show more aggression.[11–14]

Communication Related to Aggression

Aggression is part of normal social communication, which includes visual, auditory, tactile, and olfactory components; this holds true whether the aggression is caused by fear, territorial, or hierarchal reasons. Communication occurs when 1 animal (or human) responds to the signals sent by another animal. Although it is expected that a cat recognizes and understands what another cat is communicating, humans do not intuitively speak cat, so they often miss (and misinterpret), what a cat is conveying. One of the most important reasons that animals show aggressive behaviors is to increase distance between themselves and another. If the respondent does not react in an appropriate manner to the earlier signals, a cat may present its repertoire in an increasingly more forceful manner until its goal is accomplished. Owners, understandably, generally do not wish to see these aggressive behaviors in their pets.

To fully understand cat aggression toward people, it is important to appreciate the aspects of communication that are used to express it. It is easier for owners to understand aggression when they can differentiate distance-increasing (aggressive) from distance-reducing (friendly) signals. One must take the entire cat into consideration when evaluating a cat's emotional state; even though a cat is rubbing up against a person, it does not preclude the cat biting them.

Domestication has helped change the communication signals that one cat delivers to another. Although not wild, feral cats show a different signaling repertoire compared with housecats.[15] Cats, like most domesticated species, have neotenized physical and behavioral characteristics.[8] In cats, these characteristics include their manners of vocal communication, including purrs, as well as their physical appearance.

Visual

Cats are adept at visual communication, via the posture of their body, ears, and tail, as well as a variety of facial expressions. Humans should learn to become adept at understanding this level of communication.

When a cat shows distance-increasing signals, one visual aspect it can alter is its apparent size. In a fearful, or fearfully aggressive, body posture, a cat stands sideways to the threat, often arching its back, raising its tail, and piloerecting. The result is the typical Halloween cat. A cat that wishes to withdraw from the encounter usually chooses to crouch low to the ground, pulling its head and tail closer to its body. An example of a fearfully aroused cat can be seen in **Fig. 1.**

A confidently aggressive cat also attempts to make its body appear larger; but instead of offering a side view to the threat or trigger, it leans forward and approaches head on, with its tail tip pointed down but with its tail head raised. It stares directly toward the object of its aggression. In this way, it appears not only larger but also more in command.

A cat's tail lashing side to side is often recognized by owners as an early sign of impending aggression, indicating general irritation, and is often seen with dilated pupils. A vertically held tail, often seen in combination with other affiliative behaviors such as rubbing up against a person or another cat, is associated with a distance-decreasing motivation.[16]

The cat's facial expressions give even more insight as to its internal emotional state. The position of its ears is easy for owners to identify, whether being pinned close to its head in fear or outwardly directed when more confidently aggressive. Dilated pupils are a nonspecific sign of arousal but should be identified when evaluating the entire animal. Some resources for cat body language can be found at the end of this article.

Auditory

Cat vocalizations are sometimes misinterpreted by owners, and for purposes of this article are divided into distance-increasing and distance-decreasing vocalizations.

Most people can identify sounds such as the purr and the chirrup, which are sounds usually made in greeting and with contact with another individual. Although the purr is usually interpreted as a sound made when comfortable and relaxed, some have reported that a cat's purr can help in the healing process.[17] Another

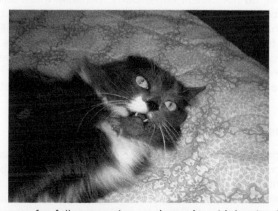

Fig. 1. Cat that is more fearfully aggressive, as shown by withdrawing its body from the person taking the picture. In addition, her ears are back and mouth is open.

distance-decreasing sound, the meiow, is distinctive, but owners can sometimes misinterpret a yowl as a meiow.[16]

Most aggressive vocalizations from cats are classified as strained intensity calls.[18] These sounds mostly include the yowl, growl, hiss, and spit. Research into feline communication shows that people can understand the meanings of different feline vocalizations.[19] A hiss, a growl, or a spit are shown during an aggressive encounter, whether based in fear or confidence. A cat can yowl when distressed, stemming from an aggressive encounter, or sometimes, when appearing to be lost or confused, such as when it cannot see or hear in its environment.

TACTILE

Cats can show distance-reducing behaviors such as allorubbing and allogrooming of people and other cats. These and other affiliative behaviors are often shown between preferred associates (where 2 cats choose to be in frequent, close contact) and are generally cooperative and sometimes reciprocated.[20,21] Humans may not appreciate allogrooming because of the roughness of the cat's tongue. Allorubbing is performed to develop a group scent, so that members of a colony or household can be recognized.[16]

Obvious distance-increasing behaviors include biting, scratching, and jumping onto another cat. Although some of these behaviors can be performed in play, it must be assumed that they are behaviors of aggression, or at least behaviors that can injure a person or another animal. Cats that are showing misdirected play usually do not vocalize, and appear to pounce on a person as if a toy. Often they crouch down, lash their tail, and chase.

FELINE SOCIAL HIERARCHIES

Despite behaviorists wanting to do away with the word dominance, because of its association with aversive methods of training, hierarchies occur among most animals, especially those in social species.[22] Humans are not included in the hierarchies of our domestic pets, because we have thumbs and open up the cans of food. Cats are no exception to this.

As with other animals, feline hierarchies are maintained by clear and consistent signaling that typically does not escalate to full-blown fights. Physical altercations resulting in injuries do not benefit either party, because these animals are at risk for developing abscesses, contracting an infectious disease, or other problematic outcomes. Alternatively, appropriate escalations in social signaling, as outlined earlier, are used to maintain the hierarchies. In normal animals, the subordinate cat avoids the more dominant cat, at least in specific situations, and the more dominant cat does not seek out the subordinate animal for a confrontation.[23] When fights do occur, it may be more likely that those animals involved are abnormal in their reactions.

GATHERING INFORMATION ON THE AGGRESSIVE FELINE PATIENT

It is important to gather all relevant information regarding the individual cat in question, other pets, and human family members, in addition to questions about the environment, the incident(s) in question, and the owner's relationship with the cat. **Table 1** summarizes some of the key points. One difference between behavioral and physiologic information gathering is the heavier reliance on owner-provided history and behavioral observations. To help make things more efficient for you and your staff,

Table 1 Gathering a behavioral history	
Basic information	Signalment Household members (people and animals) Medical history Acquisition
Environmental information	Daily activities Feeding routine Litterbox and hygiene information Household enrichment
Incident information	Frequency, intensity, and severity Antecedent to behavior Behavior of the cat during the incident Response of person or other cat Outcomes of treatments that owner has tried
Owner information	Level of bond with the cat Goals Willingness and ability of owner to implement treatment Risk assessment

you can use a history form that the owner can fill out and submit before the appointment, giving you time to review the information beforehand.

Another tool that can be used is video recording of the cat in its environment (safely). Even if an owner does not think that casual video of the cat is important, often there are subtle behavioral signs that show underlying motivations. A recording of the cat in its resting areas shows whether or not the cat is comfortable when approached while resting. Sometimes a video of the cat shows the subtle signs, such as dilated pupils or slightly crouched body posture. Other times it may show an owner interacting with the cat in an inappropriate manner, such as forcing the cat to remain on their lap. The recording can also provide important information on the layout of the home, including where litterboxes are placed, whether the home is environmentally enriched, and where alterations might be made to most effectively manage the problem. The owner should be counseled to not put themselves or the cat in any danger of being injured in order to collect video.

For the general practice veterinarian, asking behavior questions at each appointment leads owners to believe that you care about and understand behavior, which leads them to think of you when a problem behavior occurs. Most veterinarians do not ask the questions.[24–26] In a study on urine marking in cats, owners reported that veterinarians did not give advice on that problem behavior. However, those who were able to gather a complete history of the problem, and properly diagnose urine marking, reported a higher success rate than those veterinarians who did not.[2]

You may decide to see behavior cases either as a house call or an in-clinic visit. You may be able to gather more information from a house call, and this can lead to a more directed treatment plan. Owners may want you to see the cat in action, which is not advisable from a safety standpoint; a behavior plan should focus on preventing any further recurrence of the problem. You may also not even see cats that generally run from visitors. Another downside to a house call is the decreased ability to examine and draw blood, if necessary. An in-clinic visit gives you more control over the logistics of the visit. However, the cat may be stressed by a visit to the veterinary clinic. A case-by-case decision should be made on the best way to consult with the owner.

BASIC INFORMATION

As with all veterinary patients, it is important to gather detailed information about the cat's physical health, diet, current and past medical conditions, current and past medications, travel history, and human and animal household members. It is also important to complete your data gathering by performing a complete physical examination and any ancillary tests that are indicated based on your history.

ENVIRONMENTAL INFORMATION

Causes of aggression are often multifactorial, making underlying stressors important to elucidate. Stress has been shown to reduce impulse control, which can lead to aggression. Environmental information includes type and size of house; resting, feeding, and watering locations; time spent inside and outside; and litter and litterbox type, location, and hygiene schedule. A drawing of the layout of the house, a video tour of the house, or photographs of relevant areas are convenient ways for the owner to present this information when a house call is not possible.

HOUSEHOLD PET INFORMATION

Even if it may not seem relevant to the primary complaint, it is imperative to gather information on other pets in the household, their interactions with the problem cat, and the owner's relationships with each of them. This way, you identify factors that influence the amount of stress that the cat is under, such as the cat fighting with another household cat or having negative interactions with a household dog. These stressful interactions can lower the cat's threshold for tolerating any potentially stressful situations with people.

HUMAN FAMILY MEMBERS AND VISITORS

Before gathering information about the problem behaviors, it is necessary to know about the people with whom the cat interacts. The ages, genders, and relationships of people living in the household are important. It is also imperative to ascertain each person's individual relationship with the cat, to measure their bond and their willingness and ability to implement the treatment recommendations, as well as to be able to give the most appropriate safety recommendations. Even if the primary complaint is aggression toward human family members, it is important to collect information on any other behavior problems as well as how the cat interacts with visitors, veterinary staff, and other people it meets.

INCIDENT INFORMATION

Once the background information is collected, you need to collect information on specific aggressive incidents. To help owners through this process, it can be helpful to think of the ABCs of behavior: the antecedent (what happened before the incident), the behavior (what happened during), and the consequence (what did the person and cat do after). Owners often do not recognize early signs of anxiety, fear, and aggression; therefore, giving them an opportunity to view pictures or videos from which to identify what their cat looked like during an incident (as well as at other times) may be helpful.

ROLE OF OWNER

It is imperative to fully evaluate the relationship that the owner has with their cat, because behavioral counseling does not occur in a vacuum, and you do not treat just the cat. By the time an owner seeks help from a veterinarian, the behavior is often at crisis level, leading to a weakened or broken human-animal bond.[27,28]

It is perceived as risky to ask owners outright what their goals are, in case the veterinarian cannot meet their goals. It is also seems risky to ask owners outright if anyone has talked with them about (or if they have personally considered) euthanizing or rehoming a problem cat. But it is risky to not ask these questions, because they get to the heart of whether the owners are considering these options and can further guide a treatment plan and aid with the prognosis.

Another way to assess the owners' bond with the cat is their ability and willingness to implement the treatment plan that you outline. It is frustrating when owners expect a magic pill to cure the problem. However, it takes much discussion and negotiation to come to an acceptable compromise that achieves the best outcome for the cat, which is also acceptable and practical for the owners. This strategy often involves a multimodal approach to delivering the information, because owners often have a different recollection of what the treatment plan looks like after they leave the examination room.[2] Veterinarians have access to handouts, Web sites, and other resources to which they can refer their clients for further information,[29,30] and veterinarians need to be aware of their clients' communication styles.[31,32]

Veterinarians must also take into consideration the amount of risk that owners are able and willing to take, especially when it comes to an aggressive animal. This situation is where direct counseling of the owners about the different options for the cat should take place. Do small children live in the house? Is the owner someone who is potentially immunocompromised? Are the other pets in the house in danger? What are these pets' quality of life with the patient cat in the household? What is the patient's quality of life if it remains in the household? These and other concerns all need to be considered when delivering the prognosis and treatment plan.

CAUSES OF AGGRESSION
Overview

Cats show aggression toward people in many different situations, some of which overlap in their motivations. It is important to determine the motivation to deliver the best treatment plan and prognosis for the situation.

Human-Directed Aggression

In 1 study 35% of kittens adopted from a humane society showed aggression toward people at 1 year of age.[33] Feline aggression can be of great concern to owners, especially those who are most at risk for being physically injured or contracting a zoonotic disease, such as children or the elderly. There are many different reasons for aggression, including fear, inappropriate or misdirected play, petting-induced, and that based in confidence.

Fear-related aggression

Fear is a primary reason for cats to show aggression toward people. Behaviors that indicate fear, outlined earlier, make it simple to diagnose this problem, especially early in the development of the aggression. Over time, cats can learn to show more offensive or confident aggressive behaviors and fewer fearful behaviors, especially when people do not recognize the signs of fear and they keep doing what they are doing that the cat perceives as threatening. By the time owners seek help, the cat may no longer be showing any identifiable signs of fear. When asked, the owners are often able to identify specific triggers, which can include direct punishment (yelling, swatting) and visits to the veterinary office.

Inappropriate or misdirected play

This problem is more likely to be diagnosed in young cats, because younger animals are more likely than older ones to engage in play. Even although this behavior is based in play, it does not diminish the potential risk of physical injury to a person, especially when one considers that play is a component of, or prelude to, predation. Some owners encourage this problem by engaging kittens in play with their fingers, toes, or hair. As the cat ages and becomes larger, these play behaviors may become increasingly more injurious.

A subset of this problem can be categorized as inappropriate or misdirected predatory behavior. Although no domestic cat has been known to mistake a human as its prey, the behavior sequences look similar to those shown in play.

Petting-induced or handling-induced

Petting-induced or handling-induced aggression is a common problem reported by owners. There are no data elucidating the reason why cats show this behavior, especially if they actively seek out attention before biting the owners. One theory is that the cat becomes overstimulated, and early signals given by the cat are not recognized by the person. Another theory is that the cat is trying to control the situation and decides when the petting should end. A third potential reason is that petting is similar to feline allogrooming, but people perform it often using long strokes, rather than the short strokes typical of another cat's tongue; perhaps this difference is why cats tire of human petting. What is often a constant is that these cats become aggressive to anyone petting them in this manner, suggesting that it is the petting that they do not tolerate. In most cases, early signs of impending aggression include a lashing tail, ears moved back, and dilated pupils. Handling-related aggression is similar, but specific to just being handled. One sees this at the veterinarian's office, coupled with fear-related aggression. Owners also describe aggressive incidents surrounding being held, bathed, brushed, or trimming nails. In **Fig. 2**, you can see how this cat is pushing away from his owner, who is holding him tightly.

Confidence-based aggression

Although there is no evidence that cats consider humans to be part of their social structure, it cannot be denied that, rarely, cats show aggression toward people in a confident manner. It is imperative to rule out fear-related aggression, in which the cat has learned to be more offensive in its body posture. This behavior may also be classified under territorial aggression toward visitors to the house. Cats can also

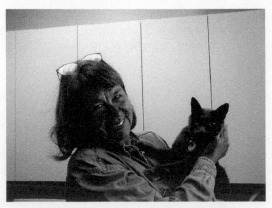

Fig. 2. Cat pushing away from his owner as she holds onto him.

show this behavior toward their owners, suggesting that cats may protect certain territories within their house from even familiar people.

Redirected aggression

To diagnose redirected aggression, you need to identify a primary trigger causing the redirected behavior.[34] In 1 study of feline aggression, a reaction to a loud noise or an interaction with another cat was determined to be the trigger in 95% of redirected aggression incidents. This same study showed that approximately 65% of these cats redirected toward people, most often their owner.[35] A common trigger identified by owners is the presence of an outdoor or stray cat, which triggers aggression in the indoor cat. The indoor cat, unable to aggress directly toward the other cat, redirects onto its owner or another inside cat. Redirected aggression can also be directed toward the owner after a fight with a household cat, especially if the owner tries to break up a fight.

TREATMENT
Overview

When developing a treatment plan, veterinarians should consider the owner's ability and willingness to follow their instructions. When discussing treatment options with owners, the veterinarian should continually check in with them to make sure that they understand the plan. One way to determine their level of understanding is by having them repeat what they have heard. They can even come up with their own options of how to implement the recommended treatment program, giving them a larger buy-in to the overall plan.

It may be beneficial to separate the steps into major categories, summarizing at the end of each section (chunk and check). An example is: management; medications and other related therapies; and desensitization (DS) and counterconditioning (CC) (**Table 2**). There is obvious overlap in these categories, and there are some instances in which you do not invoke all parts of the plan.

Table 2 Overview of treatment of human-directed aggression	
Physical health	Rule out and treat underlying medical problems Castrate or spay intact animals
Management	Provide household enrichment via hiding places, vertical resting space, multiple feeding locations and litterboxes, toys Provide social enrichment via safe, appropriate play Provide appropriate play objects for self-directed play Avoid identifiable triggers Confine as necessary Train cat to move to another room, off furniture, and so forth
DS/CC	Approach the cat from a distance it tolerates without fear or aggression Gradually decrease this distance or increase the stimulus in other ways (speed, intent of movement) If petting or handling-related aggression, gradually increase the length of time and relative intensity at which cat is handled or touched Give cat special treats or other food during above-mentioned steps
Additional treatments	Selective serotonin reuptake inhibitors or tricyclic antidepressants Pheromones Avoid buspirone, because it can increase aggression

Surgery, Medications, and Other Related Therapies

There have not been any studies reporting a positive effect from castrating or spaying a cat in decreasing human-directed aggression. However, castration has been shown to be effective in decreasing cat-directed aggression, spraying, and roaming, regardless of age at castration.[36,37] If a cat is very fearful or aggressive, owners should be counseled to not breed that individual, as well as counseled to look at the lineage of such cats when making decisions on which to breed.

Management

Tools and household enrichment

Indoor cats, which evolved to live an outdoor lifestyle, can show increased stress from the pressures of overcrowding, insufficient mental stimulation, and lack of physical activity. Studies have shown that increasing the activity levels and providing environmental enrichment for indoor cats can decrease their stress.[38] There are various simple ways to enrich a cat's indoor environment. Toys are an obvious method, both self-play toys (those that the cat can play with, without owner involvement) and interactive toys (those that are usually handled, at least in part, by people). Any positive interaction with a cat is a form of enrichment; exceptions are teasing a cat or playing with inappropriate toys or objects, such as hands or toes.

Many self-play toys dispense food, which motivates the cat to play with the toy, and perhaps take their focus away from another cat in the house or other stressor. The basic principle is that a person fills up the toy with dry kibble or treats, and the cat learns to manipulate the toy to release the food out of a hole. Self-play toys that do not dispense food are not nearly as exciting for the average cat. Some examples of simple food-dispensing toys are: toilet paper tube filled with kibble and ends folded over; dried water bottle filled with kibble; or a cleaned and dried plastic yogurt container with a hole cut in the lid, and filled with food (**Fig. 3**). Commercial food-dispensing toys are also available.

Interactive toys help strengthen the bond between owners and their cats. Both can have a great time playing with wand-type toys with strings, feathers, and fabric attached (**Fig. 4**). These wand-type toys provide an opportunity for the cat to engage in activities such as chase, pounce, and bite in a manner that is safe for people to use, because they keep the cat's claws and teeth away from the owner. Some cats enjoy playing with laser pointers, chasing the point of light around the house. Low-cost (or no-cost) toys are often the cat's preferred toys. Some suggestions are wadded-up paper or foil balls and plastic rings from milk jugs. Not every toy is right for every cat; for

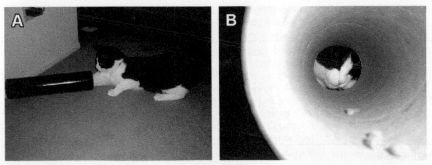

Fig. 3. (*A, B*) An example of a simple homemade food toy, where food is placed inside a cardboard tube.

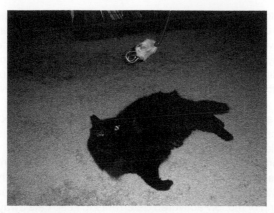

Fig. 4. An example of a wand-type toy with a feather on the end, enticing to many cats.

instance, plastic can lead to intestinal blockage and string can easily become a linear foreign body. So care must be taken to ensure that the toys are safe and serve their purpose of enriching the cat's life.

Instead of focusing on stopping a cat after it performs an unwanted behavior, it is more effective to focus on rewarding a cat for what you want it to do. One way an owner can achieve this goal is by trick-training their cat. Although some may snicker at this idea, cats can learn many commands. Three simple commands are come, sit, and target or touch. Realistically, all cats have the come command; just ask anyone who has opened up a can of cat food. Food or treats are often the most desirable reward, and using a clicker for training is 1 way to get the desired results. There are a lot of re-sources on the Internet that can help owners through this process.[39] By target training a cat, you can, for example, guide it away from scratching a piece of furniture to a different location in the house, or redirect it if it is ready to pounce on a person in play.

Indoor, elevated perches allow cats to virtually spend time outside and have a safe place to go to avoid conflicts with other cats or other fear-evoking stimuli, such as vis-itors. Something as easy as clearing off the back of a couch by the window can expand the amount of vertical space for the cat. However, owners need to be aware of roaming cats in the yard, because the sight of those other cats can trigger stress, and possibly urine marking and redirected aggression in the indoor cat. For more de-tails on stress management and environmental enrichment see the articles by Mills and colleagues and Heath and colleagues elsewhere in this issue.

Safety and avoidance
It is imperative that owners avoid the situations in which their cat has shown aggres-sion. An aggressive cat may even need to be housed separately from people or other cats. The reasons for this need are 3-fold: it provides a measure of safety for the aggressive cat, so that it does not become even more stressed; it provides safety for the potential victim; and it ensures that the cat does not continually practice an inappropriate behavior, causing the behavior to become more ingrained over time. Owners are sometimes reluctant to embrace avoidance; however, without curtailing the aggression in the first place, the cat is not in the right emotional state to be able to learn appropriate new behaviors. Often, this is a temporary solution while other treatment options are prepared.

Although usually not required, owners should be counseled that their cat may need to be confined in a separate room or part of the house, either away from people or other cats, for a longer than anticipated period. If this is the only option that keeps everyone safe, the welfare of the cat may be compromised, and this should be discussed with the owner. Another option is to make the cat an outside cat, at least partly. However, this may not be a feasible alternative, because of the potential safety issues for the cat or wildlife. In addition, a cat may engage in aggressive encounters with stray cats, increasing its stress levels and, subsequently, aggression toward people and household cats.

In addition to avoiding the triggers, owners must be counseled to avoid using confrontational methods, such as yelling, swatting, or other aversives, because these actions can escalate the aggression.

If a cat is responding aggressively toward an outside cat, treatment options include blocking the cat's access to the windows, blocking the view out the windows, and decreasing the attractiveness of the yard to other cats. It may be necessary to install cat-specific fencing or motion-activated deterrents to keep cats away. This strategy is also important if a cat is redirecting toward another cat or person after seeing or smelling an outdoor cat.

Medications and Other Related Therapies

Medications can be an important part of treating cats with aggression that stems from fear, stress, and anxiety. They do not provide long-lasting effects without concurrent behavior modification.[40] However, they can provide the owner with a means by which behavior modification can proceed more smoothly. Selective serotonin reuptake inhibitors, such as fluoxetine at 0.5 to 1 mg/kg once daily, or tricyclic antidepressants such as clomipramine at 0.25 to 0.5 mg/kg once daily are options that are often recommended.[29] Buspirone should be avoided, because it might lead to an increase in aggression in some cats, potentially caused by disinhibition.[41]

Treatment with commercially available pheromones is another option and may be more efficacious in treating intercat aggression compared with human-directed aggression.[42] It may also be effective in decreasing stress in hospitalized cats.[43] However, there is some question as to whether the clinical trials for urine marking provide sufficient evidence for efficacy.[44,45]

DS and CC

DS and CC are the hallmark of most behavior modification plans. DS is the gradual exposure of a trigger stimulus below the level of an animal's reactivity, and CC is pairing that stimulus with something that is rewarding for that animal, thus causing the formerly fear-inducing stimulus to now induce a positive emotional response.[29] DS/CC can be used to treat several feline problem behaviors, including human-directed aggression.

Cats that are aggressive toward people, whether based in fear or confidence, usually respond to this process. We start by allowing the cat the ability to leave and, hence, avoid the situation during each session; this serves to decrease the cat's fear and aggression. This strategy is especially effective if the cat has a safe haven where it has learned to go for relaxation and security. Educating owners to move slowly in the DS/CC process and set reasonable goals is important. Offering food at the cat's comfortable distance from the person is 1 way to implement DS/CC. Playing with the cat using toys that are tossed toward the cat (ie, wadded-up paper balls or food-filled toys), and wand-type toys, offers the owner a way to positively interact with the cat while building a positive association (CC).

Cats with petting-induced aggression are particularly challenging, because owners typically have cats with the express desire to be able to pet and hold them. Educating owners on the early signs of arousal (ears back, tail twitching) is imperative. They should be counseled to stop their interaction at the first sign of intolerance, or ideally, before the behavior begins and to not push the cat away. Instead, they should either simply stop their petting and wait for the cat to leave, or they can stand up and allow the cat to jump to the ground without having the owner touch it. Owners can attempt to begin DS and CC by petting for a short time, and gradually increasing those sessions, while feeding the cat some special treats.

For cats that are aggressive at veterinary clinics because of fear, there are many available resources for practitioners to use during the appointment. Ideally, slow, gentle interactions combined with high-value rewards are most appropriate.[46,47] Because of the sometimes painful treatments required, sedation or full anesthesia may be a more appropriate tool for some cats. Veterinarians and their staff can be proactive in conditioning their calmer feline patients to accept treats at the veterinary clinic, much as we do with dogs.

Misdirected play, which usually dissipates as the cat ages, can still pose a problem. Although DS and CC can be undertaken, the general recommendation is to manage the problem by offering appropriate outlets for the play. Wand-type toys and toys that can be tossed away from the person are safe (and fun) ways to engage the cat in its play session. To best implement this play, the owners should be prepared with these toys at the ready, so that they can interrupt the behavior at the initiation of the sequence. Although it should not be necessary to state this necessity, owners should be discouraged from playing with their cat with their hands or feet. Allowing the cat outdoor time on a leash and harness or in a cat-proof enclosure or obtaining a second compatible cat may be effective at providing acceptable alternative outlets for play aggression. However, the risk of compatibility issues when introducing a new cat must be weighed against the potential benefits. See the article by Pachel, elsewhere in this issue for more information about preventing and treating intercat aggression.

PREVENTION

Most of the treatment of aggression also falls under the category of prevention. We have all heard "an ounce of prevention is worth a pound of cure". It equally applies to problem behaviors. Proper socialization to potential stimuli that a cat encounters in its adult life is the gold standard. However, the primary socialization period is in the cat's early weeks of life, and a cat's future behavior is dependent not only on socialization but also on its genetic predisposition.[6,9,10,48] There are many different types of situations that a cat can be exposed to for socialization, including but not limited to different types of people, cats, sounds, and situations.

Some veterinarians are offering Kitten Kindergarten to clients and their kittens.[49] Although sessions are usually held after the end of a kitten's primary socialization period and likely do not have a great influence on the cat's future behavior, they offer owners a chance to interact with other cat owners and to be educated outside the usual veterinary office call. Although little has been directly studied about these sessions, puppies that attend puppy classes are more likely to remain in the home a year later.[50] It could also serve to bond clients to the veterinary practice offering these classes.

Appropriate handling of young kittens is important, including having owners play only with toys and not with fingers, and so forth. Some limited research has shown that, contrary to popular belief, hand-reared (orphaned) cats may be friendlier and not as aggressive as believed if raised in an environment with sufficient play-type toys and the presence of other cats.[12] However, other people claim that hand-reared cats are more aggressive.[51] Owners who find themselves with a hand-reared cat should be counseled to avoid playing with human appendages.

Also, although not proved, there is anecdotal evidence that, if a hand-reared cat is raised with at least 1 other kitten, it will be less likely to develop unwanted behaviors.

Owners should be instructed to interact with their cat in a positive manner. They should not use direct punishment, such as yelling, scruffing, flicking the nose, or smacking/hitting in response to an unwanted behavior. Although not studied specifically in cats, research in dogs has shown that owners who use aversive training methods are significantly more likely to be bitten.[52]

In addition to alleviating underlying stress, household enrichment also helps to prevent problem behaviors. If a cat has appropriate outlets to show species-typical behaviors, such as scratching, running, playing, resting, and eating, it is less likely to develop unwanted behaviors later. See the article elsewhere in this issue by Heath and colleagues for more information on how to effectively enrich a cat's environment to help prevent problems.

SUMMARY

As cats continue to be members of our families, it is important to be able to house them in an appropriate manner. Not only do we have to take the cat into consideration, we also have to consider the safety of the people who interact with the cat. By understanding why cats act like they do, and taking appropriate steps to ameliorate their stress, anxiety, and aggression, veterinary staff can affect the care and well-being of their patients.

Cat Behavior Resources

The Catalyst Council, http://www.catalystcouncil.org/

The Ohio State University Indoor Pet Initiative, http://indoorpet.osu.edu/cats

University of California-Davis Clinical Animal Behavior Service, http://behavior.vetmed.ucdavis.edu

ASPCA Cat Behavior, http://www.aspca.org/pet-care/virtual-pet-behaviorist/cat-behavior

Cat Channel.com How to Read Cat Body Language, http://www.youtube.com/watch?v=rihLUk9Xr1E

REFERENCES

1. Notari L, Gallicchio B. Owners' perceptions of behavior problems and behavior therapists in Italy: a preliminary study. J Vet Behav 2008;3(2):52–8.
2. Bergman L, Hart BL, Bain MJ, et al. Evaluation of urine marking by cats as a model for understanding veterinary diagnostic and treatment approaches and client attitudes. J Am Vet Med Assoc 2002;221(9):1282–6.
3. Bamberger M, Houpt KA. Signalment factors, comorbidity, and trends in behavior diagnoses in cats: 736 cases (1991–2001). J Am Vet Med Assoc 2006;229(10):1602–6.
4. Levine E, Perry P, Scarlett J, et al. Intercat aggression in households following the introduction of a new cat. Appl Anim Behav Sci 2005;90(3–4):325–36.
5. Salman MD, Hutchison J, Ruch-Gallie R, et al. Behavioral reasons for relinquishment of dogs and cats to 12 shelters. J Appl Anim Welf Sci 2000;3(2):93–106.
6. Collard RR. Fear of strangers and play behavior in kittens with varied social experience. Child Dev 1967;38(3):877–91.
7. Turner D. The human-cat relationship. In: Turner DC, Bateson P, editors. The domestic cat: the biology of its behaviour. Cambridge (MA): Cambridge University Press; 2000. p. 193–206.

8. Price EO. Behavioral development in animals undergoing domestication. Appl Anim Behav Sci 1999;65(3):245–71.

9. McCune S. The impact of paternity and early socialisation on the development of cats' behaviour to people and novel objects. Appl Anim Behav Sci 1995; 45(1–2):109–24.

10. Reisner IR, Houpt KA, Erb HN, et al. Friendliness to humans and defensive aggression in cats: the influence of handling and paternity. Physiol Behav 1994;55(6):1119–24.

11. Stelow E. The relationship between coat color and behaviors in the domestic cat. In: Proceedings from the Veterinary Behavior Symposium. Chicago, July 19, 2013. p. 38.

12. Chon E. The effects of queen (Felis sylvestris)-rearing versus hand-rearing on feline aggression and other problematic behaviors. In 5th International Veterinary Behavior Meeting. Minneapolis (MN): Purdue University Press; 2005. p. 201–2.

13. Seitz PF. Infantile experience and adult behavior in animal subjects: II. Age of separation from the mother and adult behavior in the cat. Psychosom Med 1959;21(5):353–78.

14. Mellen JD. Effects of early rearing experience on subsequent adult sexual behavior using domestic cats (Felis catus) as a model for exotic small felids. Z Biol 1992;11(1):17–32.

15. Yeon SC, Kim YK, Park SJ, et al. Differences between vocalization evoked by social stimuli in feral cats and house cats. Behav Processes 2011;87(2):183–9.

16. Bradshaw J, Cameron-Beaumont C. The signalling repertoire of the domestic cat and its undomesticated relatives. In: Turner DC, Bateson P, editors. The domestic cat: the biology of its behaviour. Cambridge (MA): Cambridge University Press; 2000. p. 67–94.

17. Rubin C, Pope M, Chris Fritton J, et al. Transmissibility of 15-Hertz to 35-Hertz vibrations to the human hip and lumbar spine: determining the physiologic feasibility of delivering low-level anabolic mechanical stimuli to skeletal regions at greatest risk of fracture because of osteoporosis. Spine 2003;28(23):2621–7.

18. Moelk M. Vocalizing in the house-cat; a phonetic and functional study. Am J Psychol 1944;57(2):184–205.

19. Nicastro N, Owren MJ. Classification of domestic cat (Felis catus) vocalizations by naive and experienced human listeners. J Comp Psychol 2003;117(1):44–52.

20. Barry KJ, Crowell Davis SL. Gender differences in the social behavior of the neutered indoor-only domestic cat. Appl Anim Behav Sci 1999;64(3):193–211.

21. Curtis TM, Knowles RJ, Crowell-Davis SL. Influence of familiarity and relatedness on proximity and allogrooming in domestic cats (Felis catus). Am J Vet Res 2003;64(9):1151–4.

22. Shizuka D, McDonald DB. A social network perspective on measurements of dominance hierarchies. Anim Behav 2012;83(4):925–34.

23. Knowles RJ, Curtis TM, Crowell-Davis SL. Correlation of dominance as determined by agonistic interactions with feeding order in cats. Am J Vet Res 2004;65(11):1548–56.

24. Patronek GJ, Dodman NH. Attitudes, procedures, and delivery of behavior services by veterinarians in small animal practice. J Am Vet Med Assoc 1999; 215(11):1606–11.

25. Roshier AL, McBride EA. Canine behaviour problems: discussions between veterinarians and dog owners during annual booster consultations. Vet Rec 2013; 172(9):235.

26. Roshier AL, McBride EA. Veterinarians' perceptions of behaviour support in small-animal practice. Vet Rec 2013;172(10):267.

27. Houpt KA, Honig SU, Reisner IR. Breaking the human-companion animal bond. J Am Vet Med Assoc 1996;208(10):1653–9.

28. Serpell JA. Evidence for an association between pet behavior and owner attachment levels. Appl Anim Behav Sci 1996;47(1–2):49–60.

29. Landsberg G, Hunthausen W, Ackerman L. Handbook of behavior problems of the dog and cat. 2nd edition. New York: Saunders; 2003.

30. Lifelearn client education. 2013. Available at: http://www.lifelearn.com/veterinary-practice-success/client-education/. Accessed February 4, 2014.

31. Dysart LM, Coe JB, Adams CL. Analysis of solicitation of client concerns in companion animal practice. J Am Vet Med Assoc 2011;238(12):1609–15.

32. Shaw JR. Four core communication skills of highly effective practitioners. Vet Clin North Am Small Anim Pract 2006;36(2):385–96.

33. Wright JC, Amoss RT. Prevalence of house soiling and aggression in kittens during the first year after adoption from a humane society. J Am Vet Med Assoc 2004;224(11):1790–5.

34. Chapman BL, Voith VL. Cat aggression redirected to people: 14 cases (1981–1987). J Am Vet Med Assoc 1990;196(6):947–50.

35. Amat M, Manteca X, Brech SL, et al. Evaluation of inciting causes, alternative targets, and risk factors associated with redirected aggression in cats. J Am Vet Med Assoc 2008;233(4):586–9.

36. Hart BL, Barrett RE. Effects of castration on fighting, roaming, and urine spraying in adult male cats. J Am Vet Med Assoc 1973;163(3):290–2.

37. Hart BL, Cooper L. Factors relating to urine spraying and fighting in prepubertally gonadectomized cats. J Am Vet Med Assoc 1984;184(10):1255–8.

38. Buffington CA, Chew DJ, Kendall MS, et al. Clinical evaluation of multimodal environmental modification (MEMO) in the management of cats with idiopathic cystitis. J Feline Med Surg 2006;8(4):261–8.

39. Clinical Animal Behavior Service. University of California-School of Veterinary Medicine. Available at: http://behavior.vetmed.ucdavis.edu. Accessed October 1, 2013.

40. Pryor PA, Hart BL, Bain MJ, et al. Effects of a selective serotonin reuptake inhibitor on urine spraying behavior in cats. J Am Vet Med Assoc 2001;219(11):1557–61.

41. Lindell EM, Erb HN, Houpt KA. Intercat aggression: a retrospective study examining types of aggression, sexes of fighting pairs, and effectiveness of treatment. Appl Anim Behav Sci 1997;55(1–2):153–62.

42. Ogata N, Takeuchi Y. Clinical trial of a feline pheromone analogue for feline urine marking. J Vet Med Sci 2001;63(2):157–61.

43. Griffith CA, Steigerwald ES, Buffington CA. Effects of a synthetic facial pheromone on behavior of cats. J Am Vet Med Assoc 2000;217(8):1154–6.

44. Mills DS, Redgate SE, Landsberg GM. A meta-analysis of studies of treatments for feline urine spraying. PLoS One 2011;6(4):e18448.

45. Frank D, Beauchamp G, Palestrini C. Systematic review of the use of pheromones for treatment of undesirable behavior in cats and dogs. J Am Vet Med Assoc 2010;236(12):1308–16.

46. The Catalyst Council. Available at: http://www.catalystcouncil.org/. Accessed October 1, 2013.

47. Yin S. Low stress handling, restraint and behavior modification of dogs and cats: techniques for developing patients who love their visits. Davis (CA): CattleDog Publishing; 2009.

48. Wilson M, Warren JM, Abbott L. Infantile stimulation, activity, and learning by cats. Child Dev 1965;36(4):843–53.
49. Seksel K. Training your cat. Flemington (Australia): Hyland House Press; 2001.
50. Duxbury MM, Jackson JA, Line SW, et al. Evaluation of association between retention in the home and attendance at puppy socialization classes. J Am Vet Med Assoc 2003;223(1):61–6.
51. Khuly P. Bottle-fed kittens: nightmares in the making? 2008. Available at: http://www.petmd.com/blogs/fullyvetted/2008/july/bottle-fed-kittens-nightmares-making. Accessed October 1, 2013.
52. Herron ME, Shofer FS, Reisner IR. Survey of the use and outcome of confrontational and non-confrontational training methods in client-owned dogs showing undesired behaviors. Appl Anim Behav Sci 2009;117(1–2):47–54.

Canine Aggression Toward People: A Guide for Practitioners

Karen Lynn C. Sueda, DVM[a],*, Rachel Malamed, DVM[b]

KEYWORDS

- Aggression • Body language • Dominance • Fear • Territorial aggression
- Behavior history • Canine

KEY POINTS

- Aggression is not a diagnosis; dogs may exhibit human-directed aggression because of fear, conflict, possessive behavior, territorial behavior, redirected aggression, play, predatory behavior, and pathophysiologic reasons.
- Once physical causes have been ruled out, the clinician can differentiate between the various behavioral causes of human-directed aggression based on a complete history and client and first-hand observations of the dog's body language and behavior.
- The clinician must counsel clients regarding risk assessment, management options, and reasonable treatment goals, as well as manage client expectations of the prognosis.
- Treatment of human-directed aggression includes client education, avoidance of confrontational training techniques and other situations that trigger aggressive behavior, positive-reinforcement training, behavior modification techniques, and occasionally the use of psychopharmaceuticals.
- Clinicians play a key role in preventing human-directed aggression by educating clients regarding signs of anxiety and aggression, modeling positive-reinforcement training, and advocating early socialization and appropriate behavioral intervention.

INTRODUCTION

With roughly 4.5 million people who report being bitten by a dog each year[1] and an unknown number of bites going unreported, human-directed aggression has not only a substantial impact on public safety but also damages the critical relationship between our clients and their dogs. Clients may feel angry, betrayed, or even frightened of their own pets. Many clients cannot accept the liability of owning an aggressive animal and contemplate rehoming or euthanasia; bites and aggressive behavior

Disclosures: None.
[a] Behavior Service, VCA West Los Angeles Animal Hospital, 1900 South Sepulveda Boulevard, Los Angeles, CA 90025, USA; [b] Dr. Rachel Malamed Behavior Consulting, 7119 West Sunset Boulevard, Los Angeles, California 90035, USA
* Corresponding author.
E-mail address: Karen.Sueda@VCAHospitals.com

Vet Clin Small Anim 44 (2014) 599–628
http://dx.doi.org/10.1016/j.cvsm.2014.01.008
0195-5616/14/$ – see front matter © 2014 Elsevier Inc. All rights reserved.

toward people are the most commonly cited behavioral reasons for owner relinquishment to shelters.[2] If a client elects to keep their dog and attempts to curb aggressive behavior though physical punishment or confinement, they may severely negatively impact the dog's welfare and can further increase the risk of owner-directed aggression.[3]

When presented with patients exhibiting human-directed aggression, the ultimate goal is to provide the best quality of life for both the clients and their dogs. The first step toward that goal is to determine the cause of the aggressive behavior, be it physical or behavioral. Once a diagnosis has been made, owners can be counseled regarding risk assessment and treatment options to minimize future aggression. Because prevention is more effective than treatment, veterinarians should educate clients on the early signs of aggression and how they might avoid injury before it occurs.

APPROACH TO DIAGNOSING AND TREATING HUMAN-DIRECTED AGGRESSION: AN OVERVIEW

Why Is a Diagnosis Important?

The term *aggression* is not a diagnosis. Aggression is simply a clinical sign that warrants formulation of a list of differential diagnoses, including both physical and behavioral causes. The veterinarian's role is to determine which of these differentials is most likely and to make appropriate recommendations. Without fully investigating the cause of aggressive behavior and the circumstances surrounding it, one cannot properly assess the risk and prognosis or formulate an accurate treatment plan. Misdiagnosis or the absence of a diagnosis may also present a liability issue for the veterinarian.

How Do I Make a Behavioral Diagnosis?

Distinguishing different categories of aggression requires knowledge of normal canine body language, common initiating factors, targets and triggers, and an understanding of how aggressive behavior is reinforced. Information pertinent to the specific patient is then gathered through history taking, observation of the pet, and diagnostic tests to rule out physical causes of aggression.

From the collected subjective (eg, client history) and objective data (eg, clinician observations, physical examination, laboratory data), a problem list can be created. The clinician then determines differential diagnoses for each behavioral problem, keeping in mind that comorbidity and multiple behavioral diagnoses are common[4] and that patients may possess multiple or mixed motivations for exhibiting the same behavior. For example, a dog that barks at visitors may exhibit fear aggression toward some (eg, male guests) and territorial aggression toward others (eg, postman). Additional information may be required before the clinician can arrive at a diagnosis or diagnoses.

How Do I Obtain Behavioral Information?

A large body of information is necessary for an accurate behavioral diagnosis (Table 1). A verbal history may be obtained from the client during the appointment but may not be comprehensive because of time constraints. Clients can be asked to complete a general history form before the appointment, allowing time for more detailed questioning during the consultation. Printable history forms are available in most veterinary behavior textbooks.

Historical information obtained from the client is subjective and may be colored by the client's perception and interpretation. Clients often need to be reminded to tell you exactly what happened and not what they think happened or what they believe the dog was thinking or feeling during a particular aggressive event. Witnessing the dog's body language and behavior first hand provides the clinician with more objective

Table 1 Obtaining behavioral information	
Preappointment	*History forms:* History forms are used to elicit information about acquisition, household/environment, socialization, aggression screen, description of primary behavior, body postures, specific incidents, progression, frequency, attempts to treat, owner interactions, the use of confrontation or positive punishment, perceived severity of problem, and owner goals. *Video:* Video is used to help elucidate triggers, body language, and handler responses and is obtained only if it can be done safely without risk to any person or animal. *Journal:* Owners are encouraged to keep a record of specific incidents, triggers, body language, frequency and intensity of response in order to obtain baseline information. *Attendance:* All household members/involved parties are encouraged to attend in order to obtain a complete and accurate history, determine the goals of all family members, and improve compliance and understanding of treatment plan. *Other preappointment considerations:* Liability forms may be needed.
During appointment	*Clinician observations:* These observations are made to gain information about general temperament; personality; reaction to specific triggers (eg, movement, noise, other animals, people); motivations (eg, food, toy, attention); responsiveness to commands; and the presence of a confident, conflicted, or fearful demeanor. • Interaction between pet and handler • Body language (handout/picture) • Behavior assessment (temperament testing) • Observations both inside and outside the clinic (eg, on a walk) *History taking:* History taking is used to clarify and gather additional information through the use of open-ended questions. Questioning should be nonjudgmental because clients may feel embarrassed, guilty, or sensitive regarding their pet's behavior. *Physical examination, diagnostic tests:* Whenever possible, a physical exam, complete chemistry panel, total thyroid level, and urinalysis should be completed to rule out medical causes of aggression. Reviewing medical records may alert the veterinarian to conditions that may contribute to or exacerbate aggressive behavior. *Medical record:* Description of behaviors should be as objective as possible in order to provide an accurate record of the dog's baseline behavior and as a means to compare behaviors and assess progress on subsequent appointments. Awareness of subtle signs of fear and reactivity can better enable the clinician to interact with the pet safely.

data. In addition to observing client-pet and clinician-pet interactions, the clinician may also choose to replicate common situations in order to observe the dog's response. For example, a dog's reaction to a technician entering the examination room may approximate how he might act toward a visitor entering the house. Alternatively, the clinician may choose to see the appointment at the client's home (**Table 2**), or clients can provide video of the behavior in the context in which it occurs but only if it can be obtained safely without endangering people or the pet. The clinician should always use good judgment so as not to put any person or animal at risk.

What Tests Should Be Performed to Rule Out Physical Causes for Aggression?

The development of aggression may be the result of an underlying physical illness, a behavior problem, or a combination of the two. The index of suspicion for a primary

Table 2
House call appointments: pros versus cons

Pros	Cons
• Potential for pet and client to be more relaxed in their home environment and exhibit more typical behavior; avoidance of travel-related stress	• Increased cost to client
	• Significantly greater time allotment because of travel
• Improved attendance of household members and the ability to observe interactions with household members and other pets	• Potential difficulty in performing physical examination and diagnostic testing
• Potential to observe the problematic behavior and perform behavior modification exercises in the context in which the behavior normally occurs (eg, territorial aggression)	• Inability to use hospital support/technical staff (unless accompanying consultant to visit)
	• Potential for pet's behavior to be altered by the clinician's (stranger's) presence in their home
• Identification of triggers specific to the home environment that would not be noticeable in a clinical setting	• Increased potential for the client and pet to be distracted or the appointment interrupted in their home

Depending on the circumstances, appointments may be conducted at the clinic or as a house call. If feasible, a house call may be more informative; however, each setting has its own advantages and disadvantages.

medical cause is higher if the aggression is of sudden onset or lacks a distinct pattern or identifiable external trigger, especially in an older animal.

A minimum database for all patients presenting with aggression should include

- Review of prior medical records
- Behavioral history
- Complete physical examination
- Complete blood count
- Serum chemistry panel
- Total thyroid level (**Box 1**)
- Urinalysis

Examples of physical conditions that may result in aggressive behavior include but are not limited to

- Any chronic or acute medical illness causing pain, discomfort, or irritability, which may lower a dog's tolerance and exacerbate preexisting aggression or result in the pet acting in an uncharacteristically aggressive manner
- Neurologic conditions, especially those affecting the limbic system
- Sensory deficits, such as impaired vision or auditory acuity, that could impact the dog's startle reaction

Even if the pet is currently healthy, negative associations with the client may have formed while the pet was previously ill and persisted beyond resolution of the disease. For example, a dog may have developed a classically conditioned fear response to having his or her head touched secondary to the treatment of otitis externa.

Ultimately, it may be necessary to pursue further diagnostics if the pet's behavior does not improve with behavioral therapy.

What Is the Pet's Prognosis?

The prognosis for human-directed aggression depends on a myriad of factors but is usually guarded. The clinician should manage client expectations early in the

> **Box 1**
> **Hypothyroidism and aggression: the facts**
>
> A common misconception is that there is a direct link between hypothyroidism and canine aggression. Currently, there is a lack of well-controlled clinical studies that support this hypothesis. In fact, most dogs with behavior problems are not hypothyroid; if alterations in total thyroid (TT4) concentrations are present, they are usually higher. Carter and colleagues[5] compared TT4 and thyroid-stimulating hormone (TSH) levels of dogs presenting for behavioral issues with healthy control dogs without behavioral issues. Higher TT4 concentrations were reported in dogs with behavioral issues, but no values were out of the reference range for either group. There was no significant difference in TSH level between the two groups. Radosta and colleagues[6] compared thyroid analytes in dogs aggressive to familiar people with those of nonaggressive dogs and found no significant difference. In a study by Dodman and colleagues,[7] dogs diagnosed with owner-directed aggression and borderline low thyroid hormone levels were treated with either thyroxine or a placebo. Thyroxine-treated dogs did not show significant improvement in aggression frequency when compared with dogs in the placebo group.
>
> Although a consistent relationship between aggression and hypothyroidism has not been demonstrated, it is still beneficial to evaluate thyroid function in dogs presenting for aggressive behavior. Any physical illness, including hypothyroidism, can cause discomfort and irritability resulting in aggressive behavior. A thyroid panel is indicated if hypothyroidism is suspected based on history or clinical signs in addition to aggression and/or if a routine screening TT4 is low. Baseline thyroid levels should also be obtained before initiating treatment with a behavior-modifying medication. Clomipramine, a tricyclic antidepressant, may cause a 35% to 38% decrease in serum TT4 and free T4 concentrations during administration; if baseline levels are not obtained, the dog may later be misdiagnosed with hypothyroidism because of an iatrogenic decrease in thyroid levels.[8]

counseling process. Clients must be advised to view human-directed aggression as a chronic but treatable condition that can be managed but not cured, similar to diabetes. Successful treatment reduces the severity and frequency of clinical signs like biting and provides an improved quality of life for both the dog and client.

What Are Our Client's Options?

In general, clients have 4 options when faced with a behavioral problem: management/avoidance, behavior modification and other treatment, relinquishment, and euthanasia (**Table 3**).

How Do We Treat a Dog with Human-Directed Aggression?

If the client elects to keep their dog and the cause for the aggression is determined to be of nonmedical origin, a customized treatment plan to manage and reduce their dog's aggression must be formulated. General elements of this plan may include (**Table 4**)

Client education
Understanding why their dog is aggressive and how the treatment plan works will improve client compliance.

Safety and management
Providing instruction on how to effectively avoid triggers and manage their dog safely is the most important part of the treatment plan (**Figs. 1–3**).

Communication and training
Positive-reinforcement training provides a way for clients and their dogs to communicate.

Table 3
Clients' options when faced with a behavioral problem (risk assessment)

Management/avoidance
  No changes occur other
    than avoiding triggers
	• Safety and avoidance of triggers should *always* be recommended.
	• However, if the trigger is difficult to avoid, aggression often worsens because the dog practices unwanted behavior.
	• Aggression rarely improves with time or age alone.
	• Consider if
	  ○ Aggression is very minor (eg, limited to barking).
	  ○ The trigger situation is rare or easily avoided (eg, only possessive of rawhides).
	  ○ The dog is easily managed (eg, small dog that can be picked up and held).

Behavior modification and
  other treatment
    Implement appropriate
      behavior modification
      treatment plan
	• It is the best chance at improving the dog's behavior and keeping him or her in the home.
	• There is an ongoing risk of aggression during treatment; safety measures must be taken.
	• It may be difficult for owners to implement treatment recommendations.
	• Owners must be counseled regarding risk assessment and short- and long-term prognosis.
	• Consider if
	  ○ Owners want to keep the dog and are willing to implement treatment recommendations.
	  ○ Owners are willing to accept ongoing risks.
	  ○ The dog does not pose a significant safety hazard to family or public; owners are able to mitigate danger by rigorous implementation of safety recommendations.

Relinquishment or
  rehoming
    Relinquishment to a
      shelter, rescue agency,
      or sanctuary; rehome
      with family, friends, or
      adopter
	• Aggressive behavior is likely to occur in the new home.
	• Consider if
	  ○ The situation that triggers aggressive behavior occurs less frequently or is more manageable in a different home (eg, dog that is aggressive toward children is rehomed in a household without children).
	  ○ Adoptive owners are better equipped to work with or train the dog.
	  ○ Shelter or rescue group is able to implement behavior modification and training to improve behavior before readoption.
	• Adoptive owners must be made aware of the dog's historic aggression, accept the risk, and be willing and able to continue behavior modification and training after adoption; legal (liability) issues may be present.
	• It may take months to years to find an appropriate adoptive home; often an adoptive home is never found.
	• Additional problems may arise in a shelter, rescue, or sanctuary environment.
	• Relinquishing owners should take into consideration their dog's quality of life in a shelter, rescue, or sanctuary.

(continued on next page)

Table 3 (continued)	

Euthanasia	• It may be the most humane option in some cases.
	• The quality of life of the dog and the other household members (human and animal) must be taken into consideration.
	• Consider if
	   ○ Aggression is severe or likely to cause injury to humans (especially children, elderly, or infirm).
	   ○ Triggers are frequent, difficult to avoid, or unpredictable.
	   ○ Owners are unable or unwilling to implement safety recommendations.
	   ○ There is continued or worsening aggression despite treatment.
	   ○ Owners are unable or unwilling to accept ongoing risk.
	   ○ There is actual or potential litigation.
	   ○ Owners are scared of the dog.
	• These dogs are often emotionally or mentally ill even if they are not physically ill; euthanasia may prevent long-term suffering and further decline.

Consistent, positive, predictable interactions

Unpredictable or unsolicited attention may cause anxiety and aggression. To prevent this, every person who interacts with the dog should follow the same command-response-reward (CRR) format.

Desensitization and counter-conditioning

Once a trigger is identified, it is presented in an attenuated form that does not elicit aggressive behavior; calm behavior is rewarded. Over multiple training sessions, the trigger intensity may be gradually increased but always kept below the dog's threshold for aggressive behavior. If aggression occurs, the dog is moved away or the trigger intensity decreased until the dog calms and can be rewarded for appropriate behavior. Refer to the article "Common Sense Behavior Modification" by Dr Debbie Horwitz and Dr Amy Pike to learn more about these techniques.

Response to aggressive behavior

Clients must avoid positive punishment, confrontational methods, or flooding when dealing with aggressive behavior. Hitting, kicking, forcing the dog to lie down, pinning the dog on his or her side (alpha roll), or staring at the dog may elicit aggressive behavior and do not teach the dog anything useful.[3]

Negative punishment by withdrawing attention and isolating the dog in a safe, quiet room for a short period of time (social isolation) is a more humane approach that avoids confrontation and further aggression.

Anxiolytics (pheromones, wraps, dietary, pharmaceutical)

Anxiolytics are products and therapies that may decrease anxiety and reactivity and, thus, aggressive behavior.

Pheromones Studies on dog-appeasing pheromone (Adaptil) have demonstrated that it may decrease barking at a friendly stranger,[9] but it failed to reduce aggressive behavior during physical examination by a veterinarian.[10]

Wraps Wraps that apply pressure around the dog's body use a swaddling effect that may calm the animal. Their effects on aggression have not been studied.

Dietary Dogs exhibiting dominance (conflict) or territorial aggression may benefit from a low-protein (18%) diet supplemented with the amino acid tryptophan, the precursor

Table 4
General treatment recommendation for human-directed canine aggression

Client education	Discuss diagnosis and treatment plan Address questions and misconceptions
Safety and management	*Avoidance:* Specific situations that trigger aggressive behavior are identified, and owners are counseled how to avoid them for safety reasons and to prevent the dog from becoming increasingly sensitized to the trigger. *Training aids* provide physical control, particularly when there is a size or strength disparity between the dog and client. • *Head halters:* By controlling the dog's head, the halter facilitates training and redirection during an aggressive encounter. • *Front-attachment body harness:* The leash attaches to a ring located over the dog's sternum. When the dog pulls, the harness encourages the dog to turn to the side and focus on the handler. • *Basket muzzle:* Muzzles may prevent a dog from biting but do not stop aggressive behavior. Basket muzzles are preferred because they allow food rewards without compromising safety and may be worn for an extended period of time with supervision. Gradually accustom the dog to wearing the muzzle in a positive manner.
Communication and training	*Positive reinforcement training:* Dog is taught commands, such as sit, down, stay, and so forth, through consistent, reward-based training. Training provides a way for owners to communicate with their dogs. *Response substitution:* The dog is instructed to perform a calm, acceptable behavior in a situation that would otherwise elicit aggressive behavior. Usually paired with desensitization. • For example, the dog is instructed to lie on his or her bed when a visitor arrives rather than lunge and bark. The client may practice this command when a family member (who does not trigger barking) returns home before working with visitors.
Consistent, positive, predictable interactions Also known as "Nothing in Life is Free,"[54] "Learn to Earn,"[55] "Leadership Exercises"[56]	*Command-response-reward (CRR):* All interactions with people follow a CRR format in which the dog earns attention, food, walks, or anything desirable by performing a command. • Rewards are contingent on performing the command. The dog is not reprimanded, but attention or the reward is withheld for failure to follow the command. • Attention-seeking behavior is discouraged and ignored. Benefits include • Aggression is less likely to occur because the dog is not forced to interact with the person or punished for disobeying a command but rather does not get rewarded (ie, negative punishment). • The dog is given a choice whether to interact or avoid the person without resorting to aggressive behavior. Hesitation to approach or reluctance to follow command can be interpreted as apprehension or fear. • The dog's anxiety is decreased when interactions with people follow a predictable routine. • Rewards, especially attention, become more motivating because they are no longer given when the dog begs without performing a command. • The dog becomes hungrier for attention and, thus, more tolerant of human interaction.

(continued on next page)

Table 4 (*continued*)	
Desensitization and counter-conditioning	*The trigger* is presented in an attenuated form that does not elicit aggressive behavior, and the dog is rewarded for remaining calm. Over multiple training sessions, the trigger intensity is gradually increased but always kept below the dog's threshold for aggressive behavior, and calm behavior is reinforced. *Gradient:* Commonly used gradients include distance between the person and dog, speed or abruptness of movement, degree of interaction with the dog, type of person, location of the interaction, and value of the coveted resource.
Response to aggressive behavior	*Avoid positive punishment, confrontational methods, and flooding* because these increase aggression and fear. *Negative punishment (social isolation):* The owner's attention is withdrawn by placing the dog in a separate room or having the owner leave the room. If aggressive behavior occurs on a walk, the owner and dog immediately return home and the dog placed in isolation on arrival if he or she is still aggressively aroused. A verbal cue (eg, time out!) may act as a bridging stimulus to pinpoint and associate the aggressive act with the consequence (eg, isolation or cessation of walk).
Anxiolytics (pheromone, physical, dietary, pharmaceutical)	*Pheromone:* Synthetic pheromones in the form of sprays, diffusers, or collars may reduce anxiety.[9,10,28–30] *Physical:* Wraps that apply pressure around the dog's body use a swaddling effect that may be calming.[31,32] *Dietary:* Low-protein (18%) diet and/or tryptophan supplementation may reduce some forms of aggression.[12] Nutraceutical supplements, such as L-theanine[14] or alpha-casozepine, or a commercial diet containing both alpha-casozepine and tryptophan,[14] S-Adenosyl methionine (SAM-e), or melatonin may reduce aggression. *Pharmaceutical:* Drugs that increase serotonin, norepinephrine, dopamine, and GABA may decrease anxiety and reactivity in some dogs. Medications should always be used in conjunction with behavior modification. Because medications are used in an extralabel fashion to treat aggression, owners must be informed of the risks and benefits involved.
Alternative therapy	Modalities such as *acupuncture, music therapy,*[33] *aromatherapy,*[34] *homeopathy,*[35,36] *and grooming*[37] may reduce anxiety. *Herbal* preparations may decrease anxiety but should be used with caution to avoid adverse effects, incorrect dosing, and drug interactions.[38] Query clients regarding any over-the-counter herbal preparations they may be administering.
Surgery	*Castration* may decrease some forms of human-directed aggression regardless of age.[18] *Ovariohysterectomy* prevents maternal aggression, but the role estrogen plays in modulating aggressive behavior is not fully understood.[21,22] *Heritability:* Because aggression may be a heritable trait, gonadectomy of aggressive dogs is recommended. *Dental disarming:* This term encompasses various dental procedures aimed to prevent a dog from inflicting injury from a bite. It may involve crown reduction to the gingival margin or extracting some or all of a dog's teeth. Although it may reduce bite-related injury, these procedures affect the dog's welfare and do not address the underlying cause of aggressive behavior. Dogs may still injure people through other means.[27]

(*continued on next page*)

Table 4 (continued)	
Documentation and aftercare	*Journal:* Owners are encouraged to maintain a log of aggressive events noting the frequency, intensity, duration, and triggers as well as their dog's response to behavior modification and training. *Video:* Videotaping allows observation of situations that may be impossible to replicate in the clinic environment (eg, trigger situations), are difficult to describe verbally or in writing (eg, training techniques), or are more easily understood when viewed in slow motion (eg, dog's body language). Owners must be cautioned not to purposefully trigger aggression for the sake of capturing it on camera. *Ongoing communication* via recheck appointments, phone calls, e-mails, videoconferencing, and so forth should occur in a timely manner based on the individual patient, client, and severity or complexity of the behavior problem.

to serotonin.[11,12] Owner- and stranger-directed aggression were reduced in dogs fed a commercial diet containing tryptophan and alpha-casozepine, a protein that has structural similarities to gamma-aminobutyric acid (GABA).[13] L-theanine, an amino acid that may increase GABA and other neurotransmitters, may also decrease anxiety in some dogs.[14]

Pharmaceutical Drugs that increase serotonin, norepinephrine, dopamine, and GABA may decrease aggression, anxiety, and reactivity in some dogs. Decreased serotonin levels have been implicated in canine aggression. Serum 5-hydroxytryptophan (5-HT) was significantly lower in human-directed aggressive dogs than nonaggressive

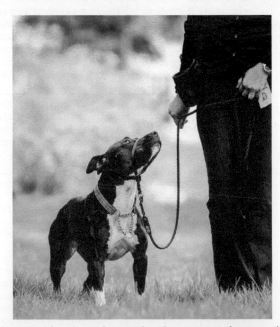

Fig. 1. A head halter provides physical control and encourages focus on the handler (Gentle Leader; PetSafe, Knoxville, TN). (*Courtesy of* MaoMau Images, Redondo Beach, CA; with permission.)

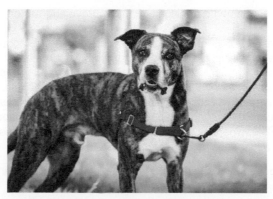

Fig. 2. When using a front-attachment body harness, the leash attaches to a ring located over the dog's sternum (Easy Walk harness; PetSafe, Knoxville, TN). (*Courtesy of* MaoMau Images, Redondo Beach, CA; with permission.)

controls, with the lowest 5-HT levels occurring in dogs with defensive aggression.[15] The cerebrospinal fluid (CSF) of dogs exhibiting dominance (conflict) aggression contained lower levels of 5-hydroxyindoleacetic acid (5-HIAA), a serotonin metabolite, compared with nonaggressive dogs. This level was especially low in dogs that bit without warning.[16] Lower CSF 5-HIAA have been reported in violent humans who have problems with impulse control.[17]

Medications should always be used in conjunction with behavior modification. Because these medications are used extralabel to treat aggressive behavior, owners must be informed of the potential risks involved.

Alternative (eg, homeopathy, herbalism, aromatherapy, acupuncture, massage)
There is a lack of controlled scientific studies to determine their safety and/or efficacy in treating human-directed aggression.

Surgery
Gonadectomy Research investigating the role of sex hormones in aggressive behavior has yielded variable results. Castration, regardless of age, reduced aggression by more than 50% in approximately 30% of dogs exhibiting aggression toward human

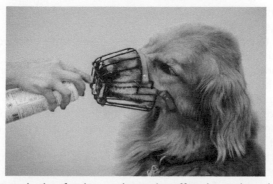

Fig. 3. Spray cheese and other food rewards may be offered to a dog while wearing a basket muzzle. (*Courtesy of* MaoMau Images, Redondo Beach, CA; with permission.)

family members; castration did not significantly improve aggression toward strangers or intruders.[18]

Except in rare cases,[19] ovariohysterectomy prevents maternal aggression. Estrogen and oxytocin have anxiolytic effects,[20] which possibly accounts for the findings that spaying may worsen aggressive behavior in dogs exhibiting aggression before surgery[21] and increase some dogs' reactivity toward unfamiliar people.[22]

Evidence that human-directed aggression is a heritable trait has been shown in several different breeds (golden retrievers,[23,24] English cocker spaniels,[25] English springer spaniels[26]). Owners of aggressive dogs should be counseled to neuter or spay their pets to avoid passing on genes related to aggression.

Tooth reduction or removal Clients may inquire about dental disarming to prevent bite-related injury. The American Veterinary Dental College states

When presented with an aggressive animal case where other corrective measures have failed (including but not limited to behavior modification) the veterinarian at his/her discretion may recommend full mouth extraction, crown reduction (to the gingival margin) or euthanasia. ...It must be understood that removal or reduction of teeth as a treatment for canine or feline aggression will not absolutely prevent injury to people or to other animals.[27]

These procedures affect the dog's physical and behavioral welfare and do not address the underlying cause of aggression. Subjecting a dog who has undergone a dental disarming procedure to the situation that provokes aggressive behavior will continue to stress and traumatize the dog and may still result in injury to the people involved.

Documentation and follow-up care
Ongoing and frequent communication is necessary to troubleshoot and support the client during the treatment process (**Table 5**). Gathering objective data by journaling or videotaping permits the clinician and client to gauge progress and identify areas that need further work.

BEHAVIORAL CAUSES OF HUMAN-DIRECTED AGGRESSION
Fear Aggression

Fear aggression is one of the most common forms of human-directed aggression seen by veterinary behaviorists (**Tables 6** and **7**). Dogs with fear aggression exhibit defensive aggression directed at familiar or unfamiliar people who the dog perceives to be a threat. Types of triggers that tend to elicit a fear response may include the following:

- Stature/height, sex, or age
  - Tall or large individuals
  - Men (tend to trigger a fear response more frequently than women)
  - Elderly individuals, children
- Physical characteristic or appearance not frequently encountered by the dog
  - Attire (eg, hoodie, hat, poncho, uniform)
  - Skin color, presence of facial hair
- Intrusive, sudden, unpredictable, or unusual interactions or movement
  - Direct approaches, staring, petting, reaching, bending over, hugging, sudden movement, and handling for procedures
  - Change in body position (eg, sitting to standing), entering a room, awkward or unusual movement or gait, large gesticulations
  - Carrying or using unfamiliar or frightening objects (eg, walking aids or wheelchairs, leaf blower, bags, stroller)

Table 5
Answers to common client questions regarding canine aggression

Is my dog trying to dominate me when he is aggressive?	Your dog's aggression is not motivated by a desire to be dominant over you. Dogs exhibit aggressive behavior for many different reasons, such as illness, pain, or fear. It is natural for dogs to guard resources, such as food, toys, or personal space, though this behavior is considered unacceptable in most households. Dogs exhibiting guarding behavior are not trying to be dominant but are simply acting in their own best interests.
Is it true that I need to alpha roll my dog to show him who is boss?	Pinning your dog on his or her side or back (alpha rolling) is not recommended. In fact, research has shown that that alpha rolling and yelling no *increases* the likelihood that your dog will be aggressive. Confrontational or painful techniques, such as alpha rolling, forcing your dog to lie down, hitting, kicking, or glaring at your dog, not only increases the risk that your dog will bite you but may make your dog afraid of you. More importantly, these techniques do not address the underlying cause for your dog's aggressive behavior.
Can my dog's aggression be cured? How long will it take?	Like many chronic conditions (eg, arthritis, diabetes), aggression cannot be cured but can be treated and managed to maximize your and your dog's quality of life. Treatment may reduce the intensity and frequency of aggressive behavior over time. How quickly your dog improves depends on many factors, including diagnosis (ie, why your dog is aggressive), how severe his or her aggression is, and your ability to carry out the treatment plan. In most cases, treatment will last months to years, but your dog may require some degree of management for the rest of his or her life.
Will medications decrease my dog's aggressive behavior?	Unfortunately, there are no magic pills to treat canine aggression. Medications can be used as adjunctive therapy for some types of aggression that are caused by fear or reactivity and impulsivity. Decreasing a pet's anxiety may allow him or her to learn faster and respond better to training. Once your dog has been examined and diagnosed, your veterinarian may recommend behavior medication in conjunction with a behavior modification plan. Always follow your veterinarian's instructions regarding dosage and safety precautions. Medication alone is unlikely to stop your dog's aggression.

- Children (especially boys between 5 and 9 years of age who have the highest incidence of being bitten[39])
- Environment/context
  - Unfamiliar, confining, or loud/bustling environments (may lower a dog's threshold for fear aggression)
  - Environments associated with negative experiences (eg, veterinary clinic) in a confined space or other location where the dog has had prior negative experience (eg, veterinary clinic)

Diagnosis of fear aggression is based on the pet's body language, acquisition of a thorough history, and ruling out medical causes. Fear-aggressive dogs may not exhibit fearful behavior before an attack. If the trigger is repeatedly encountered, the dog may become sensitized to the situation and rapidly escalate to using aggressive behavior as a defensive mechanism (**Fig. 4**). Over time, avoidance and fearful body language are skipped in favor of aggressive behavior once the dog learns that threats are most effective at making the person retreat.

Table 6
Differential diagnoses of human-directed aggression in dogs: common historical findings and behavioral observations

	History	Observations	Example
Fear	• Triggers may be related to sex, age, appearance, unfamiliarity, movement or interaction, environment • May have been inadequately socialized with a variety of people • Prior negative experiences and/or use of punishment or confrontational training techniques may have occurred • Possible comorbidity with other anxiety disorders	• Fearful and defensive body language • Assertive body postures may develop over time	• Dog barks, growls, bares teeth (horizontal lip retraction), retracts ears, cowers, and tucks tail when stranger approaches dog in the home; dog lunges as person gets closer.
Conflict	• Triggers: confrontation over resources or personal space; when thwarted, frustrated, or disciplined • Often fearful in other situations, anxious temperament • Historically labeled *dominance aggression*	• Mixture of fearful and assertive body language • May display appeasement or submissive behavior immediately following an attack	• Dog growls and bares his or her teeth with vertical lip retraction (assertive) while his or her ears are pinned back and body weight shifted away (fearful) when approached while chewing a bone.
Possessive	• Triggers: approached or challenged while in possession of a resource (food, toys, people/attention, or other animals) • May be a component of conflict aggression	• Primarily assertive body language, though elements of defensive body language may also be apparent	• When approached while eating, the dog stiffens, leans forward over the food bowl, growls and bares his or her teeth with vertical lip retraction.
Territorial	• Aggression only or primarily occurs at the edge of a defensible area (yard/fence line, entrance way) • Not aggressive toward strangers away from defended area	• Primarily assertive body language	• When visitor approaches fence or door, the dog barks, lunges, growls with ears erect/forward, and tail up and wagging stiffly.

Redirected	• Unable to get to focus of aggression and instead attacks a third party • Secondary to another type of aggression (eg, interdog aggression) • Target of attack nearby when first attack occurred; during subsequent attacks, initial target may be preferentially sought out	• High arousal	• A handler is bitten during attempts to separate a dogfight or when applying leash, corrections, or other attempts to thwart aggression directed toward another dog during leash walks.
Play	• Young, high-energy dog; mouthy • May have inadequate training or exercise, may exhibit poor impulse control or have difficulty calming down once aroused, may lack conspecific playmates • Trigger: excitement • May progress to fear or frustration-related aggression	• No signs of fear or agonistic behavior • Play-bow or a loose body and face may be evident even while dog barks or growls	• Young, outdoor dog barks, jumps on and mouths the owner's arms when he enters the yard; bites become harder and more persistent when the owner attempts to push the dog away.
Predatory	• Rare • Trigger: preylike humans, may be directed toward infants • Intent is to injure or kill, though not necessarily consume	• Silent; visual fixation on target • All or part of the predatory sequence: stare, head down, stalk, chase, catch, bit/attack, kill, consume	• Dog's body is tense as he or she silently stares at the infant; ears are forward and alert; quiet but extreme arousal.
Idiopathic, pathophysiologic	• Severe aggressive behavior without apparent trigger or motive • May be more prevalent in certain breeds (eg, springer spaniels; cocker spaniels)	• Sudden, explosive attack with little warning; poor impulse control	• Dog who was lying quietly suddenly runs across the room and attacks a seated person without apparent trigger or prior warning signs.

Table 7
Specific safety/avoidance and desensitization and counter-conditioning treatment recommendations for the various forms of human-directed aggression

	S/A	DS/CC
Fear	*Visitors:* Place pet in another room before arrival.	*Visitors:* While seated, ask visitor to ignore dog. Bring dog out on leash and maintain comfortable distance. If calm, gradually move dog closer to visitor. Visitor tosses treats to the dog at a distance. Progress to visitor instructing the dog to perform commands.
		Movement: The dog may be reinforced for lying down across the room from a seated stranger. Calm behavior is continually reinforced as the intensity of the stranger's movements gradually increases: sitting, shifting in his or her seat, standing, walking away, walking toward the dog, and so forth. Response substitution may be added by rewarding the dog for making eye contact with the owner vs staring at the stranger.
	Pedestrians: Increase distance by crossing to the opposite side of the street, walking in the opposite direction, turning down a side street, or walking up a driveway or alley; use a parked car or hedge as a visual barrier.	*Pedestrians:* Sit and focus on the owner while the person walks by at maximum distance (beyond threshold) and with low intensity (eg, type of movement, speed, direction of approach). High-value treats are administered until the person is no longer in sight. The dog is rewarded for a behavior that is incompatible with the unwanted behavior of (eg, sitting instead of lunging). The dog can then be moved closer to the passerby in small increments (eg, 1–2 ft).
Conflict	*Resources:* See "Possessive Aggression"	*Resources:* See "Possessive Aggression"
	Personal space: Block access to furniture; encourage the dog to rest on a dog bed in a low-traffic area.	*Personal space:* Stand at a distance from the resting dog, toss a treat to the dog, and leave. Gradually decrease distance from which you toss the treat as long as the dog remains calm.
	Limit petting and handling; use consistent owner interaction (CRR) for predictability. Use management tools (eg, head halter, long leash, basket muzzle) if necessary.	*Handling:* Pet or brush once, followed by a reward if the dog remains calm. Gradually increase duration and/or intensity of handling.
	Discipline: Avoid physical punishment; use social isolation.	*Frustration:* Implement sit- or down-stay exercises that reward the dog for remaining calm in a difficult or distracting situation for progressively longer periods of time.

(continued on next page)

Table 7 (*continued*)		
	S/A	**DS/CC**
Possessive	*Food/toys:* Feed the dog separately or only offer coveted items in locations where the dog will not be disturbed; trade object for a higher-value item.	*Food/Toys:* • *Distance:* Toss a treat to the dog from a distance while he or she has possession of a coveted item, and then walk away. Gradually decrease the distance from which you can toss the treat, staying below the dog's aggression threshold. • *Item value:* Teach the dog to drop a low-value item on command. Gradually increase the value of the item you instruct the dog to drop (eg, ball<food).
	People/animals: Call the dog away from the person or animal rather than approach.	*People/Animals:* Gradually decrease the distance from which you call the dog away from the person or animal; reward the dog for remaining calm during the approach and coming when called.
Territorial	*Pedestrians approaching the house:* Avoid leaving the dog in the yard; if outdoor access is unavoidable, solid, secure fencing is best. Use white noise or music to reduce auditory stimuli (eg, car engine, voices). Use window covering if access to windows is unavoidable. *Visitors:* Before visitor arrival, confine dog to a separate room/area. Provide food-dispensing toy as a distraction. Instruct visitors to call rather than knocking or ringing the doorbell.	*Pedestrians approaching the house:* Begin exercises outside (eg, in front of yard/fence or door) with dog on leash. Provide high-value item as pedestrian passes at varying distances, eventually approaching door. Reward desirable behavior. *Visitors:* • *Knocking/doorbell:* Sound may be recorded and played back at a lower volume, or a familiar person may knock lightly on the door. The dog alerts but does not respond aggressively to the lower volume noise; the dog is directed to lie on his or her bed and rewarded. The volume of the doorbell or knock is gradually increased. • *Entrance:* The dog is rewarded for staying on his or her bed while a familiar person, then eventually a stranger, enters the house. Initially the dog may down-stay further from the front door and is encouraged to stay while the owner walks to the front door and opens it without a person present.
Redirected	*High-arousal situations:* Avoid situations when possible. Avoid physical interaction during high-arousal situations. Use management tools if necessary (eg, head halter, long leash, basket muzzle, citronella spray to remotely disrupt behavior).	Address the primary diagnosis.

(*continued on next page*)

Table 7 (continued)	S/A	DS/CC
Play	*Excitable play, high-arousal situations:* Avoid these situations. Engage in structured play sessions that follow a CRR format (eg, sit before throwing the ball). Do not encourage dog to bite hands or feet.	*Excitable play, high-arousal situations:* Identify situations that cause the dog to become overly excited and reinforce calm behavior (eg, sit-stay) while gradually increasing the intensity of the trigger. For example, reward the dog for staying on his or her dog bed for progressively longer periods of time while children run and play in the yard.
Predatory	*Safety of the child is the priority:* Completely separate dog from the child; dog may need to be rehomed either temporarily (until the child is older) or permanently. Accustom the dog to wearing a basket muzzle or keep him or her leashed in the presence of child. *Chasing fast-moving objects:* The dog is likely motivated by fear or play.	*Chasing fast-moving objects:* DS/CC to movement may be implemented.
Idiopathic, pathophysiologic	*Triggers are unknown or minor:* Focus is on safety and management through the use of basket muzzle, head halter, or complete separation from people (confinement, tethering). Consider MRI and/or EEG to rule out neurologic conditions.	The prognosis is grave; euthanasia may be the safest option. Owners may attempt treatment with serotonergic medication.

Client education, positive-reinforcement training, and avoidance of confrontational techniques play a role in all forms of human-directed aggression and are discussed under general treatment recommendations.

Abbreviations: DS/CC, desensitization and counter-conditioning; EEG, electroencephalogram; MRI, magnetic resonance imaging; S/A, safety/avoidance.

In these cases, fear aggression is differentiated from assertive (offensive) aggression in 2 ways:

- History: Knowledge of the dog's early history including progression of the dog's behavior and body language may indicate that the dog initially showed signs of fear in the presence of people. Clients may describe their dog being shy or aloof around people long before the onset of aggression.
- Body language: Pinned ears, lip licking, yawning, rear weight distribution, avoidance, and horizontal lip retraction distinguish fear from assertive aggression (see **Fig. 4**).

Fear aggression should be addressed early on before it progresses and becomes more difficult to treat. The goal of treatment is to change the pet's negative emotional

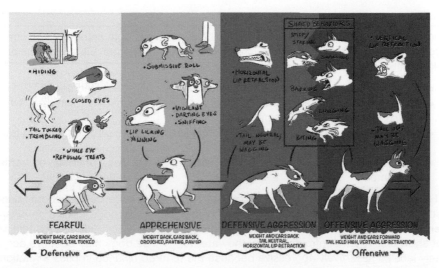

Fig. 4. Canine body language: how a dog responds to stressful or threatening situations. Categories are not mutually exclusive; dogs may exhibit a mixture of signals depending on the underlying motivation for their behavior. (Illustration by Valerie Fletcher, *Courtesy of* Dr Rachel Malamed and Dr Karen Sueda, all rights reserved.)

response to the trigger to a positive response. Fear-eliciting situations must be avoided during the treatment process to prevent sensitization to the trigger. If this is not possible, tools such as head halters and basket muzzles are used to manage the pet safely. The trigger (eg, visitor, pedestrian) is then gradually reintroduced through desensitization and counter-conditioning (DS/CC) exercises (see **Table 7**).

If accidental exposure to a fear-eliciting trigger occurs and the pet reacts, the dog can either be removed from the situation (social isolation) or redirected to perform a substitute response (eg, sit, watch) that can then be rewarded in order to change the dog's emotional state. Because most dogs will ignore treats when fearful, acceptance of a food reward may indicate a more relaxed state.

Care should be taken to withhold rewards when the dog is actively barking, lunging, or biting to prevent inadvertent reinforcement of aggressive behavior. Although a behavioral response can be reinforced, the emotional state cannot be rewarded. Therefore, if the dog can be redirected and reoriented away from the trigger with a treat or lure, it can be immediately rewarded with less concern for rewarding the behavior.

At home, a CRR program may help to create more consistent, positive, and predictable interactions with people. This protocol can be extended to include visitors once the dog is sufficiently comfortable to respond to commands and accept treats from strangers.

Pharmacologic intervention, such as the use of selective serotonin reuptake inhibitors (SSRIs) or tricyclic antidepressants (TCAs), may be indicated in cases refractory to behavior modification or if the pet's reactivity or fear is so pronounced that counter-conditioning cannot take place, even at the lowest trigger intensity. In these cases, anxiolytic medication may reduce arousal and anxiety levels enough to allow behavior modification to occur. Clients must be advised of off-label use and the potential for behavioral disinhibition. In dogs that are hyporesponsive to other pharmacologic treatment, as-needed use of clonidine, an alpha-2 agonist, may be useful for the treatment of fear-based behaviors, including fear aggression. Further studies are needed to evaluate the safety and efficacy of clonidine in dogs.[40]

Conflict Aggression

Dogs demonstrating conflict aggression exhibit a mixture of both defensive and offensive body language and behavior toward people when challenged. Situations that provoke conflict aggression may include

- Confrontations over resources (eg, food, toys, stolen or coveted items)
- Intrusion into the dog's personal space (eg, approached or disturbed while resting; grooming or handling)
- When thwarted or frustrated (eg, restricting movement, preventing the dog from performing a desired activity)
- When threatened or disciplined (eg, staring at the dog, physical or verbal punishment)

Historically, these dogs were diagnosed with dominance aggression without taking body language or motivation into account. In retrospect, most dogs labeled *dominant* were likely exhibiting conflict aggression. Although supremely confident dogs that do not show fear when confronted exist, they are rare. These dogs may be more accurately labeled *assertively aggressive* because the term *dominance* implies a relationship in which one individual consistently defers to another, which is not the case in human-canine interaction.

Conflict aggression lies along a spectrum ranging from fear aggression on one extreme to assertive aggression on the other. Dogs with fear aggression exhibit primarily defensive body language and may attempt to flee, whereas conflict aggression occurs when dogs are sufficiently motivated or confident enough to stand their ground but are uncomfortable with the confrontation or consequences. The conflict between these motivations produces the mixture of defensive and offensive body language and behavior. The proportion of defensive and offensive behavior may vary, but both are evident (**Fig. 5**).

An important aspect of treating conflict aggression is the recognition that fear plays a significant role. Clients who believe their dog is dominant may be tempted to use punishment-based training methods that will increase aggressive behavior. Instead, situations that elicit aggressive behavior should be avoided while clients gradually accustom their dog to being approached, handled, or restrained through DS/CC training (see **Table 7**).

Because dominant (conflict) aggressive dogs exhibited lower levels of serotonin metabolites compared with nonaggressive dogs,[16] treatment with medication, such as an

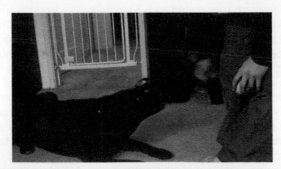

Fig. 5. Dog with conflict aggression growling as her owner removes her toy. Note that the dog's ears are back, her body weight is shifted back, and she exhibits a "whale eye" (defensive) while simultaneously exhibiting vertical lip retraction and a direct stare (offensive). (*Courtesy of* Dr Karen Sueda, Los Angeles, CA.)

SSRI, to increase serotonin levels may be beneficial. In a single-blinded, crossover study, fluoxetine decreased owner-directed dominance aggression after 3 weeks of treatment compared with placebo.[41] However, treatment of dominance aggression in dogs with clomipramine in a double-blinded placebo-controlled study in the absence of behavior modification failed to show a significant difference in reduction of aggression compared with placebo. Similarly, treatment of aggressive dogs with amitriptyline failed to show a significant difference compared with placebo.[42]

Possessive Aggression

Possessive aggression occurs when a dog uses aggressive behavior to prevent another individual from having access to a resource. Resources may include food, toys, people/attention, other animals, and so forth. Which items are worth defending depends on the individual preference of the dog. Possessive aggression is a normal and evolutionarily advantageous behavior that prevents competitors from stealing or monopolizing valuable resources. Although normal, this behavior is not necessarily acceptable in a domestic situation.

Aggression typically occurs once the dog possesses the resource and is in a position to defend it. For example, a dog may not guard a food bowl if the dog is only allowed a few mouthfuls of kibble before it is removed. However, possessive aggression may occur if the dog is permitted to eat from it for several seconds (enough time to establish ownership) before the bowl is taken. The faster ownership is established, the more objects are guarded, and the more difficult it is to avoid the triggers, the more severe the behavior and the poorer the prognosis.

Possessive aggression may be a component of conflict aggression or may occur alone. Offensive body language predominates, though some degree of defensive body language may be apparent.

Treatment of possessive aggression is similar to conflict aggression. If aggression is limited to a few objects, then management may be all that is necessary to prevent aggressive behavior. Clients may avoid feeding treats (eg, rawhides) that elicit aggressive behavior or only provide coveted toys outside where the dog is not likely to be disturbed. On rare occasions when the dog guards an item, clients may trade a higher-value reward (eg, treat, toy) for that item (**Box 2**). Trading should not occur frequently because some dogs will learn to steal items in expectation of a reward from the client.

If triggers are unavoidable, occur frequently, or elicit severely aggressive behavior, then CRR exercises and DS/CC to the client's approach are warranted. DS/CC exercises may use distance or object value as gradients, always staying below the dog's threshold for exhibiting aggressive behavior. A dog guarding food or toys may also be taught to leave it and drop it. Response substitution may also be used to encourage dogs to go to a specific area, such as their bed, when food is being prepared or when they begin to exhibit possessive behavior. Treatment with an SSRI or TCA may be beneficial as with conflict aggression.

Territorial Aggression

Territorial aggression is directed toward people that encroach on an area or space that dogs perceive to be their own. Because aggressive behavior is used in an assertive manner to keep the person out of the territory, offensive body postures predominate (see **Fig. 4**). Areas that may be defended include physical boundaries, such as a fence line or front door; enclosures, such as a room or car; and defined space, such as the area around the dog's bed.

Box 2
Retrieving stolen items

How to retrieve stolen items

- First, try trading the dog for a high-value reward, such as a turkey hot dog.
- Never trade directly in front of the dog and the object, many dogs will quickly eat the food item and quickly grab the stolen object, possibly resulting in a bite.
- Show the dog the delectable food, and then toss several of them across the room and encourage the dog to follow them.
- If the dog goes far enough away, it may be safe to pick up the item.
- Otherwise the dog should be lured with the food away from the stolen item and into a safe location.
- Lure the pet by holding onto the food and using a series of *come* and *sit* commands until the dog is at a safe distance.
- For additional safety, lure the dog into a secure room or crate and close the door before picking up the item.
- If another person is in the home, they can go and pick up the item and dispose of it properly.
- In some cases, changing the subject, such as ringing the doorbell and retrieving the stolen object after the dog drops it and while its focus remains on the door, may distract a dog.

Courtesy of Debbie Horwitz and Amy Pike, St Louis, MO.

It can be difficult to differentiate territorial aggression from fear aggression. A dog who barks at a visitor entering the house may be motivated by fear rather than defense of his or her home. The dog's body language and behavior in other circumstances are used to differentiate between the two diagnoses. Dogs with territorial aggression exhibit primarily offensive body language during the encounter and are friendly toward people outside the territory. In contrast, fearful dogs display defensive aggression at home and are fearful or fear aggressive toward strangers outside the territory.

Territoriality can be managed or treated, but the prognosis is poor when owners are unable or unwilling to avoid triggers and cannot manage the dog safely. Clients desiring guard dogs that discriminate between welcome and uninvited guests should be informed that this is an unrealistic expectation for most dogs.

In addition to denying access to locations where territorial behavior is practiced (eg, yard, front door, rooms with windows), the dog can be desensitized and counter-conditioned to people passing, approaching, or entering the home. As stated previously, lower-protein diets or supplementation with tryptophan may improve territorial aggression.[11,12] SSRIs and TCAs may also reduce reactivity leading to aggression.

Redirected Aggression

Redirected aggression occurs when a dog becomes aroused, is unable to access the intended target, and instead attacks a third party. Redirected aggression occurs secondary to another type of aggression and is defined as such (eg, redirected aggression toward the client secondary to interdog aggression). In most cases, the victim of the attack is the closest available target. A common scenario is a client being injured while holding the dog back from attacking another person.

Treatment of redirected aggression focuses on addressing the primary behavioral diagnosis. High-arousal situations or triggers for redirected aggression should be avoided whenever possible. If unavoidable, the use of safety tools (eg, basket muzzle, head halter, citronella spray [SprayShield, PetSafe, Knoxville, TN]) is advised. The prognosis is poor to guarded if the dog is easily aroused and the situation/trigger is difficult to avoid.

Play Aggression

The term *play aggression* is a misnomer. The playful dog is not trying to harm his or her playmate or drive him away. Injuries to humans that occur in the context of play may be caused by a dog that is highly aroused, mouthy, or has poor bite inhibition or impulse control. These dogs are often young, very energetic, and have a difficult time calming down once excited. They have not been taught proper play etiquette with humans and play with people as they would another dog, including jumping, chasing, pawing, mouthing, and biting. These dogs do not exhibit signs of fear or agonistic behavior before or during the attack. Instead they lack body tension and may play-bow even while growling and barking. Play aggression may occur more frequently if the dog does not have access to conspecific playmates. Play aggression may lead to fear or conflict aggression if punishment-based training is used or dogs are not given an acceptable outlet for their energy and become frustrated.

Dogs exhibiting play aggression benefit from training aimed at rewarding calm behaviors and teaching self-control. Basic commands, such as sit, down, stay, wait, and so forth, should be practiced and reinforced especially in the face of distractions. Discourage clients from roughhousing, wrestling, or other activities that promote high-arousal, physical play. Instead, encourage clients to engage in play that promotes interactions that follow a CRR format, such as instructing the dog to sit before a ball is thrown. If tooth-to-skin contact occurs, play immediately ends, and client is instructed to separate himself or herself from the dog until he or she calms down (negative punishment). Increasing mental and physical exercise and allowing supervised play with conspecifics may redirect the dog's energy and promote proper social interaction. Because play is a normal behavior, drug treatment is not typically recommended or needed.

Predatory Aggression

Predatory aggression is motivated by intent to hunt and possibly, though not necessarily kill and/or consume prey items. Since the dog's motivation is not to drive the prey item away, the term "predatory aggression" is also a misnomer.

Although rare, predatory aggression toward humans is extremely dangerous. Predatory aggression is most often directed toward infants who seem and act preylike to the dog. Dogs may exhibit all or part of the predatory sequence toward the baby: stare/visually fixate (giving eye), head down stalk, chase, catch, bite/attack, kill, consume. Attacks are usually silent and may occur with little warning. Given the severity of the consequences, complete separation from the infant is recommended for any dog exhibiting predatory behavior toward a child. The safest route is to rehome the dog either temporarily (until the child is older) or permanently. If rehoming is not an option, the dog must be kept in a separate part of the house, muzzled or on leash whenever the baby is present. The dog may stop exhibiting predatory aggression once the infant reaches a certain age or developmental state and no longer acts preylike. For example, aggression may desist once the child is mobile or bipedal.

In the authors' opinions, dogs that are aggressive toward fast-moving people, such as joggers, bicyclists, skateboarders, and so forth, are most commonly motivated by fear rather than predatory behavior. These dogs typically bark during attacks and exhibit fearful body language. Some dogs may chase fast-moving objects in a playful manner or because of an innate drive, as may be the case in herding breed dogs. Because these dogs were selected to stare, stalk, chase, and sometimes nip, herding breeds tend to exhibit elements of the predatory sequence regardless of the underlying behavioral motivation (eg, fear, play, territorial behavior). Predatory behavior exhibited by semiferal dog packs that attack joggers or hikers may be socially facilitated or involve an element of territorial behavior.

Impulsive Behavior: Idiopathic and Pathophysiologic Aggression

Clients often claim that their dog's aggression occurred out of the blue. Explanations for unpredictable aggression include

- Subtle signs of fear and aggression were present before the attack but were not recognized by the client (most common).
- History taking reveals that the dog previously exhibited warning signs but began bypassing milder forms of aggression in favor of biting, particularly if growling was punished.
- The dog rarely gave warning and has always rapidly escalated to biting. These dogs exhibit a lack of impulse control.

In human psychiatric medicine, patients with poor impulse control are unable to resist urges that may be harmful to themselves or others. Impulsive behaviors seem to occur with minimal forethought and may be inappropriate for or disproportionate to the situation.[17] Poor impulse control is not a diagnosis but a trait common to many different psychiatric conditions. Impulsivity is associated with low levels of serotonin and elevated dopaminergic activity.[43] Other neurochemicals that affect aggressive behavior, such as gamma-aminobutyric acid (GABA), noradrenaline, nitric oxide, Monoamine oxidase A (MAOA), and steroid hormones, may also be involved.[44]

Dogs that are quick to exhibit unpredictable aggressive behavior may be characterized as impulsive. Although impulsive behavior may occur with any type of human-directed aggression, it is most commonly associated with conflict aggression. A subset of these dogs manifest sudden, explosive aggression either without an apparent trigger or grossly disproportionate to the stressor. This form of canine aggression shares similar characteristics to intermittent explosive disorder in humans[17] and has been variously called "idiopathic aggression"[45]; "impulsive aggression"[46]; "impulse-control aggression"[47]; or, colloquially, "rage syndrome."[48]

The prognosis for dogs exhibiting this form of aggression is extremely guarded to grave. Because triggers are unpredictable or absent, it is difficult to avoid attacks that may seriously injure the victim. In many cases, euthanasia may be the safest and most humane option. Treatment, if attempted, should focus on safety and management, including muzzling the dog whenever it is around people, tethering, and/or separation from people through the use of gates, pens, or confinement in a crate or room. Thought should be given to the dog's welfare and quality of life if human contact is severely limited. Treatment with an SSRI or TCA may be attempted if clients are cautioned regarding the potential for increased aggression and behavioral disinhibition. If a serotonergic depletion exists as is hypothesized for impulse control disorders in humans, dogs may respond well to medications that enhance serotonin levels.

Some cases of aggression may be caused by an undiagnosed physiologic problem. Neurologic conditions ranging from congenital or acquired anatomic disorders, neoplasia, and seizures may result in aggressive behavior. For example, it is hypothesized that some cases may be caused by a seizure disorder based on abnormal electroencephalogram and response to anticonvulsant therapy.[49]

AFTER THE APPOINTMENT AND FOLLOW-UP
What Should I Do After the Appointment?

Written discharge instructions outlining the diagnosis and treatment plan should be sent to the client soon after the appointment. The client may use the summary as a reference throughout the treatment process as well as to update family members who were not present at the behavior appointment.

Discharge instructions may consist of a write-up by the clinician and/or preprinted handouts (available in reference books). Regardless of the form of the instructions, the clinician must tailor their recommendations to meet the individual needs of each patient and client. For example, a general handout may recommend confining a dog to another room when visitors arrive, but if a patient has separation anxiety in addition to fear aggression toward visitors, other approaches, such as tethering the dog within sight of the owner, need to be considered.

How Do I Monitor Treatment?

Frequent communication between the client and clinician is essential for successful management of human-directed aggression. Follow-up may be conducted through

- Recheck appointments (in-clinic or house call visits)
- Phone calls
- E-mail
- Written/faxed communication
- Video conference or exchange of video recordings

The appropriate frequency of follow-up communication varies with the severity of the problem, clinician preference, client and patient needs, and so forth. In general, the more frequent the contact the better the potential prognosis is for patients. The authors recommend contacting clients by phone or e-mail at least once during the first week following the appointment and then every 1 to 2 weeks thereafter. In-person recheck appointments are recommended approximately 8 weeks after the initial appointment, depending on the patients' rate of improvement and client need. In the authors' experience, 8 weeks provides enough time for clients to implement and evaluate the efficacy of the treatment plan provided at the initial appointment. If medication was prescribed, 8 weeks is usually sufficient time to determine its effectiveness.

When Do We End Treatment?

Clients may ask when their dog will be cured, but aggression is never cured because there is always some risk of future aggressive behavior. Clinicians should seek to answer the following questions: When will my dog's aggressive behavior be manageable? When will my dog's aggression be in remission? The answer to either of these questions depends on several factors, such as the initial severity of the aggression, the response to treatment, client goals, how easily the aggressive behavior is triggered, and how well clients can manage their pet's treatment.

The authors' rule of thumb for a successful course of treatment is for the dog's behavior to be manageable, or reaching a level that the clients can live with or find acceptable, for at least 2 months. At that point, the authors may consider altering the treatment protocol to reduce the frequency of training, behavior modification, and CRR interactions.

If the dog is receiving behavior medication, the medication may be gradually tapered to a lower dose, usually a 25% reduction every 1 to 2 weeks. How slowly the dose is reduced will depend on the type of medication as well as the duration of

Table 8 Clinician's role in preventing human-directed canine aggression	
In-clinic modeling of behavior	*Staff body language/approach:* Allow dog to approach first and adopt nonthreatening body postures. *Classical conditioning:* Offer high-value rewards, such as food items or long-lasting treats, during vaccinations, nail trims, or other procedures. *Advocate reward-based training:* Demonstrate how to reward the dog for performance of commands and desirable behaviors (eg, sitting calmly on the examination table). *Avoid confrontational techniques:* • Use low-stress handling techniques and minimal restraint when possible, especially for fearful dogs. • Avoid positive punishment (eg, verbal and physical reprimands) and flooding methods. • Discuss ways that owners can minimize stress when administering medications at home.
Advocate socialization	*Relay the importance of early socialization (<16 wk of age):* Animals who are not socialized during this period are at risk for developing fears and fear aggression later on in life. *Schedule fun visits:* The pet receives treats (no procedures) to create positive associations with veterinary clinic and staff. *Encourage puppy classes:* • Puppies can begin classes as early as 7–8 wk of age, 1 week after first set of vaccinations and deworming.[50] • Conduct puppy classes at the clinic. • There is supporting evidence that vaccinated puppies attending puppy classes during the primary socialization period are at no great risk of contracting canine parvovirus (CPV) infection than vaccinated puppies that do not attend these classes.[51]
Client education	*Body language:* Discuss and provide handouts/pictures/videos that help owners identify defensive/offensive canine body language and human interactions that may trigger a fear response. *Prevention:* Relay common causes of aggression and how to prevent them. Stress the importance of avoiding confrontational training techniques. *Resources:* Direct clients to appropriate handouts, Web sites, books, and videos.
Preemptive steps	*Pet selection:* • Assist selection of individual animal and breed compatible with the owner's lifestyle, personality, and expectations. • Discuss types of behaviors to watch for when making selection. • Discourage the acquisition of pets from sources/environments such as pet stores and commercial breeding facilities (puppy mills) that increase risk for the development of behavioral issues, such as social and nonsocial fears[52] and aggression toward people.[53] *Record behavioral information:* The behavior history should be noted in every pet's medical record along with behavior observations during visits. *Prepare environment:* Optimize clinical setting for animals identified as fearful or aggressive. *Anticipate behavior problems:* Identify critical times in which behavior problems may arise (eg, addition of new pet or family member, relocation or travel, arrival of a baby, age-related changes) and prepare owners/pets accordingly.

treatment and severity of aggression. Drugs with shorter half-lives should be tapered more slowly to avoid physiologic withdrawal. A slower tapering schedule that provides more opportunity to detect the resurfacing of aggressive behavior is recommended for dogs who initially exhibited severe aggression for a longer period of time before treatment.

Clinicians should prepare clients to manage their dog's behavioral health for the rest of their lives. At minimum, clients will need to avoid situations that have triggered aggressive behavior in the past or follow a strict routine when unfamiliar or less familiar persons interact with the dog (eg, instruct the dog to sit before petting him). Ongoing behavior modification and training may also be necessary depending on the severity of aggression. In general, most owners find these restrictions tolerable once they become a routine part of their life and find it preferable to relinquishment or euthanasia.

What If the Dog's Behavior Does Not Improve?

For severe cases or for those patients refractory to treatment, clinicians should strongly consider referral to a veterinary behaviorist.

THE CLINICIAN'S ROLE IN PREVENTING HUMAN-DIRECTED AGGRESSION

The primary care clinician should be the first to educate and advise clients regarding the prevention and treatment of behavioral problems, particularly aggression (**Table 8**). Unfortunately, clients more often turn to the Internet, television, or other media outlets for guidance, resulting in the propagation of harmful, unreliable, and scientifically inaccurate information and treatment techniques. Veterinarians can combat this misinformation by proactively engaging clients in discussion about their pet's behavior rather than waiting for clients to engage them once a problem occurs. The sooner a problem is identified, the better the treatment prognosis. Clinicians play a key role in preventing human-directed aggression by educating clients about canine body language, how to recognize early signs of fear, positive-reinforcement techniques, and the importance of early socialization.

SUMMARY

When addressing human-directed canine aggression, the clinician must first determine the underlying cause of the behavior be it fear or conflict related, possessive behavior, territorial behavior, redirected aggression, play, predatory behavior, or pathophysiologic in nature. Once medical causes of aggression have been ruled out, the clinician uses information gathered through client history and behavior observations to differentiate between behavioral diagnoses and customize a treatment plan for patients. Because human-directed aggression is a manageable chronic disease but not curable, frequent communication between the client and clinician throughout treatment is necessary for a successful outcome. Ultimately, the best way to address human-directed aggression is through prevention; clinicians can reduce the frequency of human-directed aggression among their patients by advocating positive-reinforcement training, early socialization, and appropriate behavioral intervention with all clients.

REFERENCES

1. Centers for Disease Control and Prevention. Dog bite prevention. In: Centers for Disease Control and Prevention Web site. Available at: http://www.cdc.gov/HomeandRecreationalSafety/Dog-Bites/biteprevention.html#howbig. Accessed July 2013.

2. Kogan L, New JC, Kass PH, et al. Behavioral reasons for relinquishment of dogs and cats to 12 shelters. J Appl Anim Welfare Sci 2000;3:93–106.

3. Herron ME, Shofer FS, Reisner IR. Survey of the use and outcome of confrontational and non-confrontational training methods in client-owned dogs showing undesired behaviors. Appl Anim Behav Sci 2009;117:47–54.

4. Bamberger M, Houpt KA. Signalment factors, comorbidity and trends in behavior diagnosis in dogs: 1,644 cases (1991-2001). J Am Vet Med Assoc 2006;229:1591–8.

5. Carter GR, Luescher AU, Moore G. Serum total thyroxine and thyroid stimulating hormone concentrations in dogs with behavior problems. J Vet Behav 2009;4(6):230–6.

6. Radosta LA, Shofer FS, Reisner IR. Comparison of thyroid analytes in dogs aggressive to familiar people and non-aggressive dogs. Vet J 2012;192(3):472–5.

7. Dodman NH, Aronson L, Cottam N, et al. The effect of thyroid replacement in dogs with suboptimal thyroid function on owner-directed aggression: a randomized, double-blind, placebo-controlled clinical trial. J Vet Behav 2013;8:225–30.

8. Gulikers KP, Panciera DL. Evaluation of the effects of clomipramine on canine thyroid function tests. J Vet Intern Med 2008;17(1):44–9.

9. Tod E, Brander D, Waran N. Efficacy of dog appeasing pheromone in reducing stress and fear related behaviour in shelter dogs. Appl Anim Behav Sci 2005;93:295–308.

10. Mills S, Ramos D, Gandia Estelles M, et al. A triple-blind placebo-controlled investigation into the assessment of the effect of dog appeasing pheromone (D.A.P.®) on anxiety related behavior of problem dogs in the veterinary clinic. Appl Anim Behav Sci 2006;98:114–26.

11. DeNapoli JS, Dodman NH, Shuster L, et al. Effect of dietary protein content and tryptophan supplementation on dominance aggression, territorial aggression, and hyperactivity in dogs. J Am Vet Med Assoc 2000;217:504–8.

12. Dodman NH, Reisner I, Shuster L, et al. Effect of dietary protein content on behavior in dogs. J Am Vet Med Assoc 1996;208:376–9.

13. Kato M, Miyaji K, Ohtani N, et al. Effect of prescription diet on dealing with stressful situations and performance of anxiety-related behaviors in privately owned anxious dogs. J Vet Behav 2012;7:21–6.

14. Araujo AA, de Rivera C, Ethier JL, et al. Anxitane® tablets reduce fear of human beings in a laboratory model of anxiety-related behavior. J Vet Behav 2010;5:268–75.

15. Rosado B, Garcia-Belenguer S, Leon M, et al. Blood concentrations of serotonin, cortisol and dehydroepiandrosterone in aggressive dogs. Appl Anim Behav Sci 2010;123:124–30.

16. Reisner IR, Mann JJ, Stanley M, et al. Comparison of cerebrospinal fluid monoamine metabolite levels in dominant-aggressive and non-aggressive dogs. Brain Res 1996;714:57–64.

17. Sadock BJ, Sadock VA. Impulse-control disorders not elsewhere classified. In: Grebb JA, Pataki CS, Sussman N, editors. Synopsis of psychiatry. 10th edition. Philadelphia: Lippincott Williams and Wilkins; 2007. p. 773–85.

18. Neilson JC, Eckstein RA, Hart BL. Effects of castration on problem behaviors in male dogs with reference to age and duration of behavior. J Am Vet Med Assoc 1997;211:180–2.

19. Misner TL, Houpt KA. Animal behavior case of the month. Aggression that began 4 days after ovariohysterectomy. J Am Vet Med Assoc 1998;213(9):1200–2.

20. McCarthy MM, McDonald EH, Brooks PJ, et al. An anxiolytic action of oxytocin is enhanced by estrogen in the mouse. Physiol Behav 1997;60:1209–15.
21. O'Farrell V, Peachey E. Behavioural effects of ovariohysterectomy on bitches. J Small Anim Pract 1990;31:595–8.
22. Kim HH, Yeon SC, Houpt KA, et al. Effects of ovariohysterectomy on reactivity in German shepherd dogs. Vet J 2006;172:154–9.
23. Liinamo A, van den Berg L, Leegwater P, et al. Genetic variation in aggression-related traits in golden retriever dogs. Appl Anim Behav Sci 2007;104:95–106.
24. van den Berg L, Schilder MB, de Vries H, et al. Phenotyping of aggressive behavior in golden retriever dogs with a questionnaire. Behav Genet 2006;36: 882–902.
25. Perez-Guisado J, Lopez-Rodrigue R, Munoz-Serrano A. Heritability of dominant-aggressive behavior in English cocker spaniels. Appl Anim Behav Sci 2006; 100(3-4):219–27.
26. Reisner IR, Houpt KA, Shofer FS. National survey of owner-directed aggression in English springer spaniels. J Am Vet Med Assoc 2005;227:1594–603.
27. American Veterinary Dental College. Aggressive dogs and cats – dental treatment: removal or reduction of teeth as a treatment for canine or feline aggression. 1988. Available at: http://www.avdc.org/aggressivetreatment.html. Accessed July 6, 2013.
28. Levine ED, Ramos D, Mills DS. A prospective study of two self-help CD based desensitization and counter-conditioning programmes with the use of dog appeasing pheromone (D.A.P.®) for the treatment of firework fears in dogs (Canis familiaris). Appl Anim Behav Sci 2007;105:311–29.
29. Gaultier E, Pageat P. Effects of a synthetic dog appeasing pheromone (D.A.P.®) on behaviour problems during transport. In: Proceedings of the 4th International Behaviour Meeting. Caloundra (Australia): 2003. p. 33–5.
30. Kim Y, Lee J, Abd el-aty AM, et al. Efficacy of dog-appeasing pheromone (DAP) for ameliorating separation-related behavioral signs in hospitalized dogs. Can Vet J 2010;51:380–4.
31. Cottam N, Dodman NH. Comparison of the effectiveness of a purported anti-static cape (the Storm Defender®) vs. a placebo cape in the treatment of canine thunderstorm phobia as assessed by owners' reports. Appl Anim Behav Sci 2009;119:78–84.
32. Cottam N, Dodman NH, Ha JC. The effectiveness of the Anxiety Wrap in the treatment of canine thunderstorm phobia: an open-label trial. J Vet Behav 2013;8:154–61.
33. Leeds J, Spector L, Wagner S. Bioacoustic research and development (BARD) canine research summary. 2007. Available at: http://throughadogsear.com/pdfs/BardExecutiveSummary.pdf. Accessed July 31, 2013.
34. Wells DL. Aromatherapy for travel-induced excitement in dogs. J Am Vet Med Assoc 2006;229:964–7.
35. DePorter TL, Landsberg GM, Araujo JA, et al. Harmonease chewable tablets reduces noise-induced fear and anxiety in a laboratory canine thunderstorm simulation: a blinded and placebo-controlled study. J Vet Behav 2012;7:225–32.
36. Cracknell NR, Mills DS. A double-blinded placebo-controlled study into the efficacy of a homeopathic remedy for fear of firework noises in the dog (Canis familiaris). Vet J 2008;177:80–8.
37. McGreevy PD, Righetti J, Thomson PC. The reinforcing value of physical contact and the effect on canine heart rate of grooming in different anatomical areas. Anthrozoos 2005;18(3):236–44.

38. Fugh-Berman A, Ernst E. Herb-drug interactions: review and assessment of report reliability. J Clin Pharmacol 2001;52:587–95.

39. Weiss HB, Friedman DI, Coben JH. Incidence of dog bite injuries treated in emergency departments. JAMA 1998;279(1):51–3.

40. Ogata N, Dodman NH. The use of clonidine in the treatment of fear-based behavior problems in dogs: an open trial. J Vet Behav 2011;6:130–7.

41. Dodman NH, Donnelly R, Shuster L, et al. Use of fluoxetine to treat dominance aggression in dogs. J Am Vet Med Assoc 1996;209(9):1585–7.

42. Virga V, Houpt KA, Scarlett JM. Efficacy of amitriptyline as a pharmacologic adjunct to behavioral modification in the management of aggressive behaviors in dogs. J Am Anim Hosp Assoc 2001;37:325–30.

43. Seo D, Patrick CJ, Kennealy PJ. Role of serotonin and dopamine system interactions in the neurobiology of impulsive aggression and its comorbidity with other clinical disorders. Aggress Violent Behav 2008;13(5):383–95.

44. Nelson RJ, Trainor BC. Neural mechanisms of aggression. Nat Rev Neurosci 2007;8:536–46.

45. Hart BL, Hart LA. Aggressive behavior in dogs. In: Canine and feline behavioral therapy. Philadelphia: Lea & Febiger; 1985. p. 282–301.

46. Amat M, Manteca X, Mariotti VM, et al. Aggressive behavior in the English cocker spaniel. J Vet Behav 2009;4(3):111–7.

47. Overall KL. Abnormal canine behaviors and behavioral pathologies involving aggression. In: Manual of clinical behavioral medicine for dogs and cats. St Louis (MO): Elsevier; 2013. p. 214–8.

48. Podberscek AL, Serpell JA. The English Cocker Spaniel: Preliminary findings on aggressive behavior. Appl Anim Behav Sci 1996;75–89.

49. Dodman NH, Niczek KA, Knowles K, et al. Phenobarbital-responsive episodic dyscontrol (rage) in dogs. J Am Vet Med Assoc 1992;210:1580–3.

50. American Veterinary Society of Animal Behavior. AVSAB position statement on puppy socialization. 2008. Available at: http://avsabonline.org/uploads/position_statements/puppy_socialization.pdf. Accessed July 31, 2013.

51. Stepita ME, Bain MF, Kass PH. Frequency of CPV infection in vaccinated puppies that attended puppy socialization class. J Am Anim Hosp Assoc 2013;48(2):95–100.

52. McMillan FD, Duffy DL, Serpell JA. Mental health of dogs formerly used as "breeding stock" in commercial breeding establishments. Appl Anim Behav Sci 2011;135(1–2):86–94.

53. Franklin DM, Serpell JA, Duffy DL. Differences in behavioral characteristics between dogs obtained from pet stores and those obtained from noncommercial breeders. J Am Vet Med Assoc 2013;242(10):1359–63.

54. Voith VL, Borchelt PL. Diagnosis and Treatment of Dominance Aggression in Dogs. Vet Clin North Am 1982;12:655–63.

55. Yin S, Sophia. Yin's Learn to Earn Program for Puppies. In: Perfect puppy in 7 days: How to start your puppy off right. Davis, CA: CattleDog Publishing; 2011. p. 67–126 p.

56. Landsberg G, Hunthausen W, Ackerman L. Figure 3.20 Establishing leadership and control. In: Handbook of behavior problems of the dog and cat. 2nd Edition. Edinburgh: Saunders; 2003. p. 48.

Appendix: Drug Dosage Chart

Caroline Perrin, BVSc, MACVSc[a], Kersti Seksel, MRCVS, FACVSc[a],*,
Gary M. Landsberg, BSc, DVM, MRCVS[b]

KEYWORDS

- Behavioral management • Pharmakokinetics • Behavior problems • Drug dosages
- Drug dose table

KEY POINTS

- For many medications, the pharmacokinetics and pharmacodynamics in pets have not yet been established and even where studies have been done, there is widespread species and individual variation.
- Practitioners should start with the lower end of the dose range and titrate up to maximum doses where there is insufficient therapeutic effect and no adverse effects or contraindications.
- A complete blood count and serum chemistry profile, as well as urinalysis, should be performed on an animal before initiating the use of any medication, but especially with the use of off-label medications.
- Pharmacologic intervention for the treatment of behavior problems should be considered just one aspect of a comprehensive behavioral management and treatment protocol.

With the rare exception (fluoxetine, clomipramine, selegiline), drugs used in veterinary behavioral medicine are human medications, used off-label, that have not been licensed for use in pets. In fact, for many of these drugs, the pharmacokinetics in pets have not yet been established, and even where studies have been done, there is widespread species and individual variation. Therefore, there is a wide range of published doses based on many variables, such as the intended application, the target outcome, individual variability in effects, and side effects.

This article is intended to provide a drug dose table (**Table 1**) that has been compiled by the authors and editors to serve as a reference. Veterinarians are advised to see the individual articles within the issue to find specific recommendations and applications and to view the references within the articles and at the end of this article for greater details on mechanism of action, indications, and contraindications. As a general rule of thumb, practitioners should start with the lower end of the dose range and titrate up to maximum doses, where there is insufficient therapeutic effect and no adverse effects or contraindications.

[a] Sydney Animal Behaviour Service, 55 Ethel Street, Seaforth, New South Wales 2092, Australia;
[b] North Toronto Veterinary Behaviour Specialty Clinic, 99 Henderson Avenue, Thornhill, ON L3T 2K9, Canada
* Corresponding author.
E-mail address: sabs@sabs.com.au

Vet Clin Small Anim 44 (2014) 629–632
http://dx.doi.org/10.1016/j.cvsm.2014.01.012
0195-5616/14/$ – see front matter © 2014 Elsevier Inc. All rights reserved.

Table 1
Drug Dosage Chart

Class	Drug Name	Dogs	Cats	Contraindications	Adverse Effects
Amphetamine	Dextroamphetamine	5–10 mg/dog PO q8h (narcolepsy) or 0.2–1.3 mg/kg (hyperkinesis)	N/A		
	Methylphenidate	0.5–2.0 mg/kg PO q12h	N/A	Seizures, cardiac disease, hypertension, aggression	
Anticonvulsant	Gabapentin	5–30 mg/kg PO q8–12h	3–10 mg/kg PO q8–24h	Severe renal dysfunction	Sedation
Antihistamine, Serotonin antagonist	Cyproheptadine	1.1 mg/kg PO q4–6h for serotonin syndrome	2–4 mg/cat PO q4–6h for serotonin syndrome		
Azapirones	Buspirone	0.5–2 mg/kg PO q8–24h	0.5–1 mg/kg PO q8–12–24h		
Benzodiazepine	Alprazolam	0.01–0.1 mg/kg PO PRN	0.125–0.25 mg/kg PO q8 h	Severe liver dysfunction	Paradoxic excitement
	Clonazepam	0.1–1 mg/kg PO q8–12h	0.05–0.2 mg/kg PO q12–24h	Reported to be safer for liver dysfunction	
	Clorazepate	0.5–2.2 mg/kg PO q4–6h	0.2–0.4 mg/kg PO q12–24h	Severe liver dysfunction, aggression	
	Diazepam	0.5–2.2 mg/kg PO q4–6h	0.2–0.5 mg/kg PO q12–24h	Severe liver dysfunction, aggression	Paradoxic excitement, rare liver hepatonecrosis reported in cats
	Lorazepam	0.02–0.1 mg/kg PO q8–12h	0.03–0.08 mg/kg PO q12–24h or 0.125 to 0.25 mg/cat	Reported to be safer for liver dysfunction	
	Oxazepam	0.2–1.0 mg/kg PO q12–24h	0.2–0.5 mg/kg PO q12–24h	Acute narrow-angle glaucoma, reported to be safer for liver dysfunction	
Dibenzazepine	Carbamazepine	4–8 mg/kg PO q12h	2–6 mg/kg q12h	MAOIs, bone marrow suppression	
Ergot alkaloid	Nicergoline	0.25–0.5 mg/kg PO q24h	0.25–0.5 mg/kg PO q24h		
Hormone	Melatonin	1.5–12 mg PO q8–24h	1.5–12 mg PO q12–24h	Severe liver dysfunction	

Class	Drug	Dose	Dose	Contraindication	Side effect
MAOI-B	Selegiline	0.5–1.0 mg/kg PO q24h	0.25–1.0 mg/kg PO q24h	SSRIs, TCAs, SNRIs	
NMDA antagonist	Memantine	0.3–1.0 mg/kg PO q12h	N/A		
Opiate	Hydrocodone	0.25 mg/kg PO q8–12h	0.25–1 mg/kg PO q8–24h	MAOIs	Sedation
Opiate antagonist	Naloxone	0.01 mg/kg SC		Cardiac disease	
	Naltrexone	1–2.2 mg/kg PO q12–24h	5–10mg/kg PO q24h	Hepatic dysfunction	
SARI	Trazodone	3–7 mg/kg PO q12h	1–2 mg/kg PO q12h	MAOIs	Sedation
SSRI	Citalopram	0.5–2.0 mg/kg PO q24h		MAOIs	
	Fluoxetine	1–3 mg/kg PO q24h	0.5–1.5 mg/kg PO q24h	MAOIs, seizures	Appetite suppression
	Fluvoxamine	1–2 mg/kg PO q12–24h	0.25–0.5 mg/kg PO q24h	MAOIs, cisapride	Appetite suppression
	Paroxetine	0.5–2 mg/kg PO q24h	0.5–1.0 mg/kg PO q24h	MAOIs	Constipaton cats
	Sertraline	1–3 mg/kg PO q24h	0.5–1.5 mg/kg PO q24h	MAOIs, cisapride	
TCA	Amitriptyline	1–2 mg/kg PO q12h	0.5–2.0 mg/kg PO q12–24h	MAOIs, cardiac arrhythmias, seizures	Urine retention
	Clomipramine	1–3 mg/kg PO q12h	0.25–1.0 mg/kg PO q24h	MAOIs, cardiac arrhythmias	Urine retention
	Doxepin	3–5 mg/kg PO q8–12h	0.5–1 mg/kg PO q12–24h	MAOIs	Urine retention
	Nortriptyline	1–2 mg/kg PO q12h	0.5–2.0 mg/kg PO q12–24h	MAOIs	
	Imipramine	2.2–4.4 mg/kg PO q12–24h	0.5–1.0 mg/kg PO q12–24h	MAOIs, seizures	Urine retention
TeCA	Mirtazapine	0.6 mg/kg PO q24h	1 mg PO q24h		
Xanthine derivative	Propentofylline	2.5–5 mg/kg PO q12h	12.5 mg/cat PO q24h		
α-2 agonist	Clonidine	0.01–0.05 mg/kg PO q12h	N/A	Advanced cardiovascular disease	
β-blocker	Pindolol	0.125–0.25 mg/kg PO q12h			
	Propranolol	0.2–1.0 mg/kg PO q8h	0.2–1.0 mg/kg PO q8h	Cardiac disease	Bradycardia

Specific drug recommendations are made within the individual articles. Medications should be selected on the basis that an accurate diagnosis has been made. It is generally recommended to start at the lower end of the dose range and titrate up, as needed. Sufficient time needs to be given to allow each medication to reach therapeutic levels before increasing the dose or adding another medication. Particular care should always be taken when using multiple medications concurrently. Be certain to review for any potential contraindications before combining medications.

Abbreviations: MAOI, monoamine oxidase inhibitor; NMDA, N-methyl-D-aspartate; PO, orally; PRN. as needed; q, every; SARI, serotonin antagonist and reuptake inhibitor; SC, subcutaneously; SNRI, serotonin-norepinephrine reuptake inhibitor; SSRI, selective serotonin reuptake inhibitor; TCA, tricyclic antidepressant; TeCA, tetracyclic antidepressant.

Whenever possible, a complete blood count and serum chemistry profile, as well as urinalysis, should be performed on an animal before initiating the use of any medication, but especially with the use of off-label drugs. Although there is no documentation suggesting that these drugs can lead to specific organ damage, most are metabolized by the liver and excreted by the kidney, so confirming that those organs are functioning normally is the prudent thing to do when possible. In some cases, restraint for sample collection may be too stressful for the pet or dangerous for the pet and handlers, so each case will need to be assessed on an individual basis with the clinician determining the likely risk-to-benefit ratio of sample collection on a case-by-case basis.

Pharmacologic intervention for the treatment of behavior problems should be considered just one aspect of a comprehensive behavioral management and treatment protocol. It is unlikely that any drug will provide a long-term solution to most behavior problems. Appropriate management and behavior modification are usually needed to change the animal's relationship to a particular stimulus. Medication has been demonstrated to improve the likelihood of success, as well as speed the rate of success with behavior modification in many cases.

If any particular case is not responding as well as expected, then it may be that the medication, the dose, the time given for the medication to take effect, or another aspect should be reevaluated. Referral to a veterinary behaviorist should always be an option.

SUGGESTED READINGS

Ogata N, Dodman NH. The use of clonidine in the treatment of fear-based behavior problems in dogs: an open trial. J Vet Behav 2011;6:130–7.

Hickman MA, Cox SR, Mahabir S, et al. Safety, pharmacokinetics and use of novel NK-1 receptor antagonist maropitant (Cerenia) for the prevention of emesis and motion sickness in cats. J Vet Pharmacol Ther 2008;31:220–9.

Gruen ME, Sherman BL. Use of trazodone as an adjunctive agent in the treatment of canine anxiety disorders: 56 cases (1995–2007). J Am Vet Med Assoc 2008;233: 1902–7.

Quimby JM, Gustafson DL, Samber BJ, et al. Studies on the pharmacokinetics of mirtazapine in healthy young cats. J Vet Pharmacol Ther 2011;34:388–96.

Beaver BV. Canine behavior: insights and answers. 2nd edition. Philadelphia: Saunders Elsevier; 2009.

Beaver BV. Feline behavior: a guide for veterinarians. 2nd edition. St Louis (MO): Saunders; 2003.

Crowell-Davis S. Veterinary psychopharmacology. Hoboken (NJ): Blackwell Publishing; 2005.

Crowell-Davis S, Landsberg GM. Pharmacology and pheromone therapy. In: Horwitz DF, Mills DS, editors. BSAVA manual of canine and feline behavioural medicine. 2nd edition. Gloucester (United Kingdom): BSAVA; 2009. p. 245–58.

Kuehn NF. North American companion animal formulary. 9th edition. Port Huron (MI): North American Compendiums; 2010.

Landsberg G, Hunthausen W, Ackerman L. Behavior problems of the dog and cat. 3rd edition. St Louis (MO): Saunders, Elsevier; 2013.

Overall K. Manual of clinical behavioral medicine for dogs and cats. St Louis (MO): Elsevier; 2013.

Plumb D. Plumb's veterinary drug handbook. 7th edition. Ames (IA): Wiley Blackwell; 2011.

Seksel K. Behavior modifying drugs. In: Madison JE, Page SW, Church B, editors. Small animal clinical pharmacology. 2nd edition. St Louis (MO): Saunders Elsevier; 2008. p. 126–47.

Index

Note: Page numbers of article titles are in **boldface** type.

Moving?

Make sure your subscription moves with you!

To notify us of your new address, find your **Clinics Account Number** (located on your mailing label above your name), and contact customer service at:

Email: journalscustomerservice-usa@elsevier.com

800-654-2452 (subscribers in the U.S. & Canada)
314-447-8871 (subscribers outside of the U.S. & Canada)

Fax number: 314-447-8029

Elsevier Health Sciences Division
Subscription Customer Service
3251 Riverport Lane
Maryland Heights, MO 63043

*To ensure uninterrupted delivery of your subscription, please notify us at least 4 weeks in advance of move.

Printed and bound by CPI Group (UK) Ltd, Croydon, CR0 4YY

03/10/2024

01040496-0010